AF544930

Atlas of
Pediatric Infectious Diseases

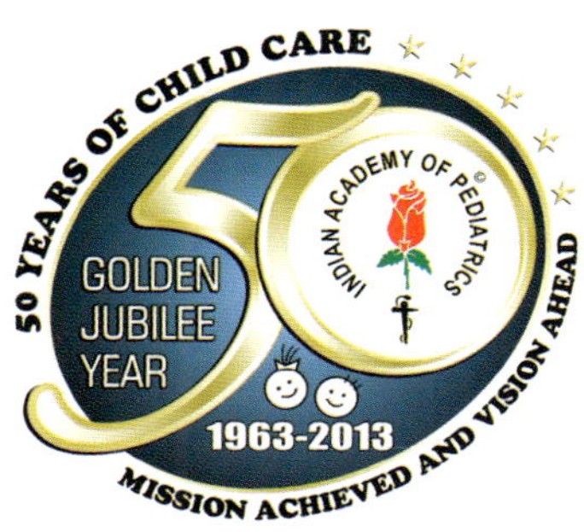

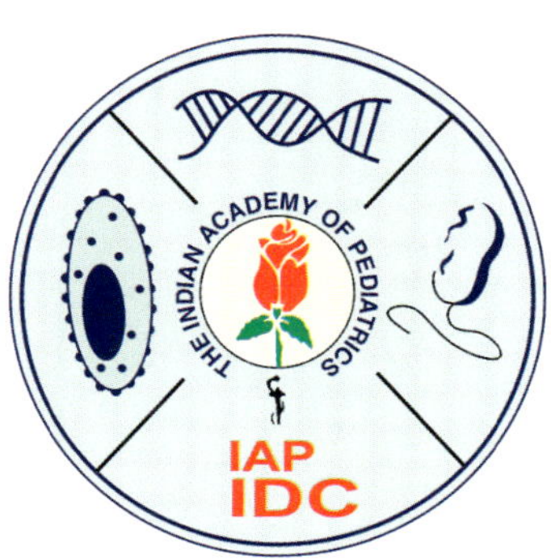

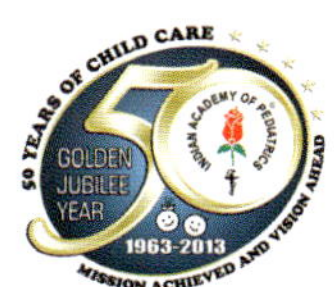

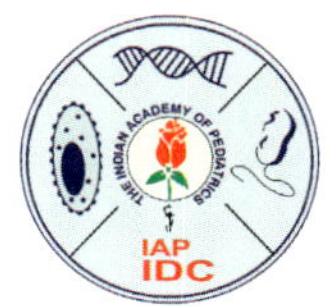

Atlas of Pediatric Infectious Diseases

Editor-in-Chief

A Parthasarathy
Distinguished Professor
The Tamil Nadu Dr MGR Medical University
Retd Senior Clinical Professor of Pediatrics
Madras Medical College
Deputy Superintendent
Institute of Child Health and Hospital for Children
Chennai, Tamil Nadu, India
apartha2020@gmail.com

Chief Academic Editors

Rohit C Agrawal
Director and Consultant Pediatrician
Chandrajyoti Children Hospital
Mumbai, Maharashtra, India
Visiting Consultant
Kohinoor Hospital
Mumbai, Maharashtra, India
drrohitag@gmail.com

Ritabrata Kundu
Professor of Pediatrics
Institute of Child Health
Kolkata, West Bengal, India
rkundu22@gmail.com

Chief Executive Editors

Vijay N Yewale
Director and Consultant Pediatrician
Dr Yewale's Multispeciality Hospital for Children
Navi Mumbai, Maharashtra, India
Honorary Pediatric Consultant
Mathadi Trust Hospital
Navi Mumbai, Maharashtra, India
vnyewale@gmail.com

Jaydeep Choudhury
Associate Professor
Institute of Child Health
Kolkata, West Bengal, India
drjaydeep_choudhury@yahoo.co.in

Academic Editors

Abhay K Shah
Senior Consultant Pediatrician
Children Hospital
Ahmedabad, Gujarat, India
drabhaykshah@yahoo.com

Digant D Shastri
CEO and Senior Pediatrician
Killol Children Hospital and NICU
Surat, Gujarat, India
drdigant@hotmail.com

Publication Editor

Dhanya Dharmapalan
Consultant Pediatrician
Dr Yewale's Multispeciality Hospital for Children
Navi Mumbai, Maharashtra, India
drdhanyaroshan@gmail.com

Forewords

Rohit C Agrawal
CP Bansal

IAP National Publication House, Gwalior

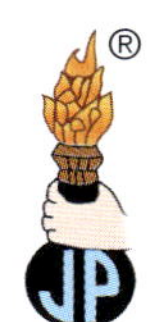

JAYPEE BROTHERS MEDICAL PUBLISHERS (P) LTD.

New Delhi • London • Philadelphia • Panama

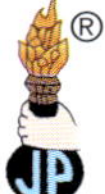

Jaypee Brothers Medical Publishers (P) Ltd.

Headquarters

Jaypee Brothers Medical Publishers (P) Ltd.
4838/24, Ansari Road, Daryaganj
New Delhi 110 002, India
Phone: +91-11-43574357
Fax: +91-11-43574314
Email: jaypee@jaypeebrothers.com

Overseas Offices

J.P. Medical Ltd.
83, Victoria Street, London
SW1H 0HW (UK)
Phone: +44-2031708910
Fax: +02-03-0086180
Email: info@jpmedpub.com

Jaypee-Highlights Medical Publishers Inc.
City of Knowledge, Bld. 237, Clayton
Panama City, Panama
Phone: 507-301-0496
Fax: +507-301-0499
Email: cservice@jphmedical.com

Jaypee Brothers Medical Publishers Ltd.
The Bourse
111, South Independence Mall East
Suite 835, Philadelphia, PA 19106, USA
Phone: + 267-519-9789
Email: joe.rusko@jaypeebrothers.com

Jaypee Brothers Medical Publishers (P) Ltd.
17/1-B, Babar Road, Block-B, Shaymali
Mohammadpur, Dhaka-1207
Bangladesh
Mobile: +08801912003485
Email: jaypeedhaka@gmail.com

Jaypee Brothers Medical Publishers (P) Ltd.
Shorakhute, Kathmandu
Nepal
Phone: +00977-9841528578
Email: jaypee.nepal@gmail.com

Website: www.jaypeebrothers.com
Website: www.jaypeedigital.com

Inquiries for bulk sales may be solicited at: jaypee@jaypeebrothers.com

Atlas of Pediatric Infectious Diseases

First Edition: **2013**

ISBN 978-93-5090-378-0

Printed at : Ajanta Offset & Packagings Ltd., New Delhi

Dedicated to

Those little ones who emerged victorious and also to those who lost the battle against the bad bugs, offering learning opportunities to generations of doctors.

Contributors

Editor-in-Chief

A Parthasarathy
Distinguished Professor
The Tamil Nadu Dr MGR Medical University
Retd Senior Clinical Professor of Pediatrics
Madras Medical College
Deputy Superintendent
Institute of Child Health and Hospital for Children
Chennai, Tamil Nadu, India
apartha2020@gmail.com

Chief Academic Editors

Rohit C Agrawal
Director and Consultant Pediatrician
Chandrajyoti Children Hospital
Mumbai, Maharashtra, India
Visiting Consultant
Kohinoor Hospital
Mumbai, Maharashtra, India
drrohitag@gmail.com

Ritabrata Kundu
Professor of Pediatrics
Institute of Child Health
Kolkata, West Bengal, India
rkundu22@gmail.com

Chief Executive Editors

Vijay N Yewale
Director and Consultant Pediatrician
Dr Yewale's Multispeciality Hospital for Children
Navi Mumbai, Maharashtra, India
Honorary Pediatric Consultant
Mathadi Trust Hospital
Navi Mumbai, Maharashtra, India
vnyewale@gmail.com

Jaydeep Choudhury
Associate Professor
Institute of Child Health
Kolkata, West Bengal, India
drjaydeep_choudhury@yahoo.co.in

Academic Editors

Abhay K Shah
Senior Consultant Pediatrician
Children Hospital
Maninagar, Ahmedabad, Gujarat, India
drabhaykshah@yahoo.com

Digant D Shastri
CEO and Senior Pediatrician
Killol Children Hospital and NICU
Surat, Gujarat, India
drdigant@hotmail.com

Publication Editor

Dhanya Dharmapalan
Consultant Pediatrician
Dr Yewale's Multispeciality Hospital for Children
Navi Mumbai, Maharashtra, India
drdhanyaroshan@gmail.com

SECTION 1: INFECTIONS IN NEONATES

Editors

Rhishikesh Thakre
Professor
Department of Pediatrics
Mahatma Gandhi Mission's Medical College and Hospital
Aurangabad, Maharashtra, India
rhishikesht@gmail.com

Sandeep Kadam
Pediatric Consultant and Neonatologist
Ravi Polyclinic
Pune, Maharashtra, India
drsandeepkadam@yahoo.com

Contributors

Snehal Thakre
Professor
Department of Ophthalmology
Mahatma Gandhi Mission's Medical College and Hospital
Aurangabad, Maharashtra, India
tsnehal73@gmail.com

Ramesh S Bajaj
Director
Pediatric Surgery
Ganga Hospital
Aurangabad, Maharashtra, India
drrlarbajaj@rediffmail.com

Naveen Bajaj
Deep Hospital
Ludhiana, Punjab, India
bajajneo@yahoo.com

Pradeep Suryawanshi
NICU Incharge and Consultant Neonatologist
Associate Professor
Division of Neonatology
Department of Pediatrics
Bharati Vidyapeeth University Medical College
Pune, Maharashtra, India
docpsurya@hotmail.com

Rajib Chatterjee
Professor and Unit Head
Department of Pediatrics
Incharge Neonatology
Rural Medical College
Pravara Institute of Medical Sciences
Ahmednagar, Maharashtra, India
drrajibchatterjees@yahoo.co.in

SECTION 2: FEVER WITH RASH

Editors

Arun Shah
Associate Professor
Nalanda Medical College and Hospital
Consultant Pediatrician
Muzaffarpur, Bihar, India
drarunshah@hotmail.com

Ketan H Shah
Private Practitioner
Ketan Children Hospital
Surat, Gujarat, India
ketanhet@gmail.com
ketanhet@yahoo.co.in

Contributors

Sanjata Roy Chaudhary
Head
Department of Pediatrics
Patna Medical College and Hospital
Patna, Bihar, India
drsre@hotmail.com

Utpal Kant Singh
Ex-Professor and Head
Department of Pediatrics
Nalanda Medical College and Hospital
Patna, Bihar, India
utpalkant.singh@yahoo.co.in

Vijay Kumar Jain
Consultant Pediatrician
Gaya, Bihar, India
drvijaymanjujain@rediffmail.com

Yugal Kishore Prasad
Consultant Pediatrician
Sitamarhi, Bihar, India

Braj Mohan
Professor and Head
Department of Pediatrics
Sri Krishna Medical College
and Hospital
Muzaffarpur, Bihar, India

RK Sinha
Professor and Head
Department of Pediatrics
Jawahar Lal Nehru Medical College
and Hospital
Bhagalpur, Bihar, India

Shyam Bihari
Consultant Pediatrician
Nalanda, Bihar, India
drs_bihari@yahoo.co.uk

SA Krishna
Retd Professor and Head
Department of Pediatrics
Nalanda Medical College and Hospital
Patna, Bihar, India
drsakrishna@gmail.com

SBP Singh
Consultant Pediatrican
Begusarai, Bihar, India
sbpsingh@rediffmail.com

Atul Kulkarni
Consultant Pediatrician
Venkatesh Hospital
Solapur, Maharashtra, India
dratulkulkarni@rediffmail.com

Ananda Kesavan
Associate Professor
Government Medical College
Thrissur, Kerala, India
dranandiap@gmail.com

SECTION 3: RESPIRATORY TRACT INFECTIONS

Editors

Devaraj Raichur
Professor of Pediatrics
Karnataka Institute of Medical
Sciences
Hubli, Karnataka, India
drdevaraj@rediffmail.com

S Nagabhushana
Clinical Associate
CSI Hospital, Bengaluru
Visiting Consultant
Columbia Asia Hospital
Bengaluru, Karnataka, India
nagabhushana59@gmail.com

Contributors

Rajendra V Naidu
Professor of Pediatrics
Karnataka Institute of Medical Sciences
Hubli, Karnataka, India
rajnaidu57@yahoo.co.in

NC Gowrishankar
Consultant Pediatrician
Mehta Children's Hospital
Chennai, Tamil Nadu, India
cugowri@yahoo.com

Shaila M Sankeshwar
Postgraduate Pediatric Resident
Karnataka Institute of Medical Sciences
Hubli, Karnataka, India
drshailams@gmail.com

Bhavna Koppad
Postgraduate Pediatric Resident
Karnataka Institute of Medical Sciences
Hubli, Karnataka, India
bhavna.d23@gmail.com

Suvarna P Reddy
Postgraduate Pediatric Resident
Karnataka Institute of Medical Sciences
Hubli, Karnataka, India
suvarna.p.reddy@gmail.com

Prakash Wari
Professor of Pediatrics
Karnataka Institute of Medical Sciences
Hubli, Karnataka, India
pkwari@rediffmail.com

Sudhindrashayana R Fattepur
Assistant Professor
Department of Pediatrics
Karnataka Institute of Medical Sciences
Hubli, Karnataka, India
sshayan26@gmail.com

Maniramakrishna
Postgraduate Radiology Resident
Kanchi Kamakoti Child Trust Hospital
Chennai, Tamil Nadu, India
mann_comp@hotmail.com

S Muralinath
Consultant Pediatric Radiologist
Kanchi Kamakoti Child Trust Hospital
Chennai, Tamil Nadu, India
muralinath_sonic@yahoo.co.in

CR Femine
Consultant Pediatrician
Department of Pediatrics
Church of South India Hospital
Bengaluru, Karnataka, India
drfeminecraj@yahoo.com

KB Shashikiran
Postgraduate Pediatric Resident
Karnataka Institute of Medical Sciences
Hubli, Karnataka, India
kbshashikiran@gmail.com

Vinod H Ratageri
Associate Professor
Department of Pediatrics
Karnataka Institute of Medical Sciences
Hubli, Karnataka, India
ratageri@rediffmail.com

Pramod G Shanbhag
Consultant Pediatrician
Shanbhag Hospital
Bengaluru, Karnataka, India
drpramod1947@gmail.com

TA Shepur
Professor and Head
Department of Pediatrics
Karnataka Institute of Medical Sciences
Hubli, Karnataka, India
drtashepur@rediffmail.com

Sujatha Thyagarajan
Consultant Pediatric Intensivist
Shanbhag Hospital
Bengaluru, Karnataka, India
suja_raghu@yahoo.com

H Paramesh
Pediatric Pulmonologist and Environmentalist
Lake Side Hospital
Bengaluru, Karnataka, India
dr_paramesh1@yahoo.com

SECTION 4: GASTROINTESTINAL INFECTIONS

Editors

Neelam Mohan
Director
Department of Pediatrics
Gastroenterology Hepatology and Liver Transplantation
Medanta: The Medicity Hospital
Gurgaon, Haryana, India
drneelammohan@yahoo.com
drneelam@yahoo.com

Yogesh Waikar
Consultant
(Pediatrics Gastroenterology and Liver Transplantation)
Department of Pediatrics
Gastroenterology and Hepatology
Care Hospital
Nagpur, Maharashtra, India
www.pedgihep.jigsy.com
pedgihep@yahoo.com

SECTION 5: URINARY TRACT INFECTIONS

Editors

Brigadier Madhuri Kanitkar
Consultant Pediatric Nephrologist
Base Hospital Delhi and
Army College of Medical Sciences
Department of Pediatrics, Base Hospital
Delhi Cantt, New Delhi, India
mkanitkar15@gmail.com

Pankaj V Deshpande
Consultant Pediatric Nephrologist
Hinduja Hospital, Bethany Hospital
Mahatma Gandhi Mission's Medical College and Hospital, Vashi
Navi Mumbai, Maharashtra, India
ajinkyapl@hotmail.com
drpankajdeshpande@gmail.com

SECTION 6: INFECTIONS IN CENTRAL NERVOUS SYSTEM

Editors

Ritesh C Shah
Consultant Pediatric Neurologist
Child Neurology and Epilepsy Center
Surat, Gujarat, India
drriteshcshah@yahoo.co.in

Shekhar Patil
Consultant Pediatric Neurologist
Dr Yewale's Hospital for Children
Navi Mumbai, Maharashtra, India
spatil74@rediffmail.com

Contributors

Vrajesh Udani
Consultant Pediatric Neurologist
PD Hinduja Hospital
Mahim, Mumbai, Maharashtra, India
vrajeshudani@yahoo.co.in

Ananda Kesavan
Associate Professor
Government Medical College
Thrissur, Kerala, India
dranandiap@gmail.com

SECTION 7: SKIN AND SOFT TISSUE INFECTIONS

Editor

C Vijayabhaskar Chandran
Consultant Pediatric Dermatologist
Vijaya Health Centre, Vadapalani
Chennai, Tamil Nadu, India
Assistant Professor
Department of Dermatology
Madras Medical College
Chennai, Tamil Nadu, India
buskii@yahoo.com

Contributors

R Madhu
Senior Assistant Professor
Department of Dermatology (Mycology)
Madras Medical College
Chennai, Tamil Nadu, India
renmadhu08@gmail.com

V Anandan
Professor and Head
Department of Dermatology
Government Stanley Medical College and Hospital
Chennai, Tamil Nadu, India
dermanandan@gmail.com

V Suganthy
Postgraduate Resident in Dermatology
Madras Medical College
Vanarapet, Puducherry, India
suganthyvalavan@yahoo.com

R Akila
Postgraduate Resident in Dermatology
Madras Medical College and
Rajiv Gandhi Government
General Hospital
Chennai, Tamil Nadu, India
drakilaarivu@yahoo.com

SECTION 8: OPHTHALMIC INFECTIONS

Editor

Atul Seth
Consultant
(Squint and Pediatric Ophthalmology)
Medical Director
Eyemax Superspeciality Eye Center
Nerul-Seawoods (West)
Navi Mumbai, Maharashtra, India
dratulseth@yahoo.com

Contributors

Parul M Deshpande
Consultant Ophthalmologist
Sarvodaya Eye Hospital and
Cornea Clinic
Santa Cruz, Mumbai (West)
Maharashtra, India
parul72@yahoo.com

Hrishikesh Tadwalkar
Consultant Ophthalmologist
Sankalp Eye Clinic, Nerul
Navi Mumbai, Maharashtra, India
drtadwalkar@gmail.com

Vishram A Sangit
Consultant Ophthalmologist
Department of Cornea and
Ocular Immunology
Laxmi Eye Institute
Raigad, Maharashtra, India
vishramsangit@rediffmail.com

Mamta V Manglani
Professor and Head
Department of Pediatrics
Program Director
Pediatric Center of Excellence for HIV Care
Lokmanya Tilak Municipal Medical College and General Hospital
Mumbai, Maharashtra, India
mmanglani@hotmail.com

Mihir Kothari
Consultant Pediatric Ophthalmologist
Jyotirmay Eye Clinic
Thane (West), Maharashtra, India
drmihirkothari@jyotirmay.com
drmihirkothari@gmail.com

SECTION 9: EAR, NOSE AND THROAT INFECTIONS

Editor

Pradip Uppal
Consultant ENT Surgeon
Dr Uppal ENT Hospital
Thane (West), Maharashtra, India
pradipuppal@yahoo.co.in

Contributors

Amol S Khale
Rajiv Gandhi Medical College and Chhatrapati Shivaji Maharaj Hospital
Thane, Maharashtra, India
khalemeister@gmail.com

Kamal Ghanshamnani
Consultant ENT Specialist
Senses Eye and ENT Hospital
Jupiter Hospital
Thane, Maharashtra, India
kamalpg@hotmail.com

SECTION 10: INFECTIONS IN MUSCULOSKELETAL SYSTEM

Editor

Alaric Aroojis
Consultant
Pediatric Orthopedics
Kokilaben Dhirubhai Ambani Hospital
Bai Jerbai Wadia Hospital for Children
Mumbai, Maharashtra, India
alaric.aroojis@relianceada.com

Contributors

Rujuta Mehta
Head
Department of Pediatrics
Bai Jerbai Wadia Hospital for Children
Consultant
Dr Balabhai Nanavati Hospital,
Shushrusha Hospital, Jaslok Hopsital
Mumbai, Maharashtra, India
rujutabos@gmail.com

John Mukhopadhaya
Consultant Orthopedician
Mukhopadhaya Orthopedic Clinic
Patna, Bihar, India
mukhoj@gmail.com

SECTION 11: INFECTIONS REQUIRING SURGICAL CARE

Editor

Arbinder Kumar Singal
Pediatric Urologist and Hypospadiologist
Mahatma Gandhi Mission's Medical College and Hospital
Navi Mumbai, Maharashtra, India
Minimaly Invasive Therapeutic Referral Urology Center and
Hypospadias Foundation, Kharghar
Navi Mumbai, Maharashtra, India
arbinders@gmail.com

SECTION 12: INFECTIONS IN THE IMMUNOCOMPROMISED CHILD

Editor

Anita Shet
Associate Professor
Department of Pediatrics
St. John's Medical College Hospital
Bengaluru, Karnataka, India
anitashet@gmail.com

Contributors

Ira Shah
Consultant Pediatrician
Bai Jerbai Wadia Hospital for Children
Mumbai, Maharashtra, India
irashah@pediatriconcall.com

Mukesh M Desai
Chief of Immunology and Professor of Pediatric Hematology (DNB)
Bai Jerbai Wadia Hospital for Children
Honorary Hematologist
Dr Balabhai Nanavati Hospital
Sir HN Hospital, Saiffee Hospital
Borivali (West)
Mumbai, Maharashtra, India
mmdesai007@gmail.com

Preethy Harrison
Assistant Professor
Department of Dermatology
St John's Medical College Hospital
Bengaluru, Karnataka, India
preethyh@gmail.com

Anand Prakash
Associate Professor
Department of Pediatrics
St John's Medical College Hospital
Sarjapur Road
Bengaluru, Karnataka, India
anand94@rediffmail.com

Foreword

It gives me the immense pleasure and privilege to write this foreword for one more innovative creation *Atlas of Pediatric Infectious Diseases* on the footprints of *Color Atlas of Pediatrics,* which was published a year back. Infectious Diseases Chapter, one of the biggest and best chapters in the folds of Indian Academy of Pediatrics has taken the mantle of compiling collection of some excellent and rare pictures of pediatric infectious diseases commonly and uncommonly seen in the office practice. The initiative taken by the Chairperson Dr Ritabrata Kundu is applaudable. The editorial board comprising of Dr Ritabrata Kundu, Dr Vijay N Yewale, Dr Digant D Shastri, Dr Abhay K Shah, Dr Jaydeep Choudhury and Dr Dhanya Dharmapalan under the leadership of Dr A Parthasarathy, has done a commendable job of collecting illustrious images and pictures through 12 Section Editors and crafting them into a beautiful atlas, which indeed will serve as a ready-reckoner for a practitioner in his busy schedule. It is said that 'brain remembers what the eyes see better than what they read'.

I compliment and congratulate the entire editorial board, the section editors and all the contributors, for sharing the lovely images (though a suffering for the tiny tots), for the composition of this state-of-the-art creation.

Rohit C Agrawal
President
Indian Academy of Pediatrics, 2012
Chairperson
Committee of Immunization
Immediate Past Chairperson IAP-ID Chapter

Foreword

It gives me a great pleasure to write the foreword for *Atlas of Pediatric Infectious Diseases*, a publication of Indian Academy of Pediatrics Infectious Diseases Chapter.

Indian Academy of Pediatrics and its Chapters have published many books in the last 7 years. Infectious diseases constitute a major bulk of child health problems in our country. The Chapter has also published a textbook on infectious diseases recently. The diagnosis in many infectious diseases is clinical. Hence, a need for the atlas was felt. I appreciate the efforts put in by Indian Academy of Pediatrics Infectious Diseases Chapter to publish the atlas, a comprehensive coverage of day-to-day problems, encountered in pediatric infectious diseases, with precise management guidelines to the extent possible.

I congratulate the editorial board led by Dr A Parthasarathy, Editor-in-Chief, for bringing out this wonderful atlas. The atlas covers all aspects of infections divided under 12 Sections, viz. Infections in Neonates, Fever with Rash, Systemic Infections, Ophthalmic Infections, and Ear, Nose and Throat Infections. It also covers Infections Requiring Surgical Care and Infections in the Immunocompromised Child. I appreciate the efforts put in by Dr Dhanya Dharmapalan, Publication Editor, and other members of editorial board, Dr A Parthasarathy, Dr Ritabrata Kundu, Dr Rohit C Agrawal, Dr Jaydeep Choudhury, Dr Abhay K Shah, Dr Digant D Shastri and Dr Vijay N Yewale. I thank authors from across the country who contributed articles in the atlas.

I am sure that readers will find this atlas very informative and useful. I hope, this IAP publication becomes a desktop ready-reckoner, for all practicing pediatricians and also postgraduate students.

CP Bansal
President
Indian Academy of Pediatrics, 2013

Prologue

It is a matter of great honor and pleasure for us to write the prologue for *Atlas of Pediatric Infectious Diseases*, a publication of Indian Academy of Pediatrics Infectious Diseases Chapter.

Academics and advocacy are two important wings of Indian Academy of Pediatrics. It has always been an endeavor of Indian Academy of Pediatrics to update the skill and knowledge of its members by various scientific programs and publications related to child health. Infectious Diseases Chapter of Indian Academy of Pediatrics is also committed and focused to the noble mission. It is one of the most active Chapters known for its various scientific publications and other activities. Such type of publications has definitely made a positive impact as far as the rational management and prevention of the infectious diseases are concerned.

Infectious diseases contribute a major chunk of cases in our day-to-day practice. It also contributes tremendously to child mortality and morbidity. In spite of availability of modern therapeutic and preventive modalities, thousands of children die in our resource poor country because of various infections. Infectious Diseases Chapter of Indian Academy of Pediatrics has decided to come out with an important publications *Atlas of Pediatric Infectious Diseases*. Experts and stalwarts with national and international reputation have contributed to this noble cause initiated by Infectious Diseases Chapter of Indian Academy of Pediatrics. We are sure that the book will have a phenomenal impact in our understanding of various aspects of childhood infections, such as rational diagnostic approach, and management and prevention. We express our gratitude to all the contributors, editors and office bearers of Indian Academy of Pediatrics for their cooperation and contribution. We also take this opportunity to thank Dr A Parthasarathy, Editor-in-Chief, for his constant guidance and encouragement.

We are sure that the book will be very useful for clinicians in their day-to-day practice and will serve as a ready-reckoner for the readers.

Ritabrata Kundu
Chairman 2012
Infectious Diseases Chapter

Digant D Shastri
Chairman 2013
Infectious Diseases Chapter

Abhay K Shah
Secretary 2012-2013
Infectious Diseases Chapter

Preface

The Infectious Diseases Chapter of the Indian Academy of Pediatrics is proud to present the first edition of *Atlas of Pediatric Infectious Diseases*. The publication of the book was encouraged by the instant popularity and wide acceptance gained by the release of the *IAP Color Atlas of Pediatrics*, a brainchild of Dr A Parthasarathy, Editor-in-Chief, in the year 2012. This book exclusively focuses on the pediatric infectious diseases in contrast to *IAP Color Atlas of Pediatrics*, which covered all the pediatrics subspecialties from neonatology to adolescent health.

Infectious diseases in children remain the leading cause of morbidity and mortality. Considering the ever-changing trends of infectious diseases, atypical presentations of diseases, and new emerging infectious diseases, an early clinical diagnosis can be challenging. The book offers a pictorial ready-reckoner for infections, both common and uncommon, encountered by the health care provider in day-to-day practice.

There is no known publication, such as *Atlas of Pediatric Infectious Diseases* in children from a developing country. It provides a rich gallery of spotters in various infectious diseases prevalent in the tropical countries. The infections have been classified as per the organ systems: Infections in Neonates, Fever with Rash and Infections in the Immunocompromised Child, have been discussed separately. Each image is accompanied by a brief and precise description of the clinical feature as well as suggested management for the same.

We appreciate the efforts taken by the office bearers of the Indian Academy of Pediatrics and IAP Infectious Diseases Chapter. It is the product of sincere hard work put in by all the Section Editors and various contributors in spite of their extremely busy schedules. We also thank the team of publishers for producing the book with flawless and top class quality print.

Your feedback, either as appreciation or criticism, will help us to improvise and strive harder for several such academic endeavors in future.

—Editorial Board

Acknowledgments

We acknowledge with a gratitude the office bearers of Indian Academy of Pediatrics and Infectious Diseases Chapter for the motivation, encouragement, commitment and support due to which the publication has seen the light of the day.

A special thanks and appreciation to all the Section Editors for having compiled their sections meticulously in spite of their extremely busy schedules.

We are thankful to all the contributors for providing the high-quality images and relevant text matter.

Our acknowledgment to Shri Jitendar P Vij (Group Chairman) and Mr Ankit Vij (Managing Director) of M/s Jaypee Brothers Medical Publishers (P) Ltd, New Delhi, India, for their kind acceptance and assurance to bring out the book with world class quality in a short span of time; and Mr Tarun Duneja (Director-Publishing), Mr KK Raman (Production Manager), Mrs Samina Khan (PA to the Director-Publishing), Dr Richa Saxena (Editor-in-Chief), Mr Rajnish Kumar and Mr Nitish Kumar Dubey (Medical Editors), Mrs Yashu Kapoor (Typesetter), Anil Sharma (Graphic Designer) and Dr Mohd Naved (Sr Proofreader) and other members, for their untiring coordination efforts in the publication.

We appreciate the help rendered by Dr Rajendra Saoji (Consultant Pediatric Surgeon), Nagpur, Maharashtra, India, for compilation of the section Gastrointestinal Infections. We also thank Mr Somashekhar, for secretarial help provided for compilation of the section Respiratory Tract Infections.

We also place on record our sincere appreciation of the help rendered by the local branch managers of the Jaypee Brothers—Mr Mukherjee (Branch Manager), Mr Jayanandan (Senior Commissioning Editor), Chennai Branch Office, for the help rendered as well as to Mr R Janardhanan, Dr (Mrs) Prathibha, Mrs Nirmala, Mr P Balaji, Mrs Kavitha, Ms Shruthi Pavana, Ms Swathi Pavana, Ms Kavya, Ms Mahiya, Mr D Prakash, Mrs Umadevi Sathish, Mr Ajay Kumar and Mr Shukla, and to Mr Sathiyathassan for secretarial and correspondence assistance at Chennai to the Editor-in-Chief.

—Editorial Board

Contents

Section 1

Infections in Neonates

Section Editors

Rhishikesh Thakre, Sandeep Kadam

Contributors

Naveen Bajaj, Ramesh S Bajaj, Rajeeb Chatterjee,
Sandeep Kadam, Pradeep Suryawanshi,
Snehal Thakre, Rhishikesh Thakre

Section Outline

1.1 Superficial Infections

- Acute Otitis Media
- Bacille Calmette-Guérin Abscess
- Breast Abscess
- Cellulitis
- Conjunctivitis
- Gangrene
- Impetigo
- Neonatal Scabies
- Oral Thrush
- Pustules
- Umbilical Sepsis

1.2 Systemic Infections

- Brain Abscess
- Necrotizing Enterocolitis
- Neonatal Candidiasis
- Neonatal Osteomyelitis
- Neonatal Meningitis
- Pneumonia with Pneumatoceles
- Sclerema Neonatorum
- Septic Shock
- Staphylococcal Scalded Skin Syndrome

1.3 Congenital Infections

- Congenital Cytomegalovirus
- Congenital HIV
- Congenital Rubella Syndrome
- Congenital Syphilis
- Congenital Toxoplasmosis
- Congenital Tuberculosis
- Neonatal Chickenpox
- Neonatal Tetanus

1.4 Miscellaneous

- Hand Washing
- Sepsis Screen

Picture	Note	Management

1.1 SUPERFICIAL INFECTIONS

Acute Otitis Media

Picture	Note	Management
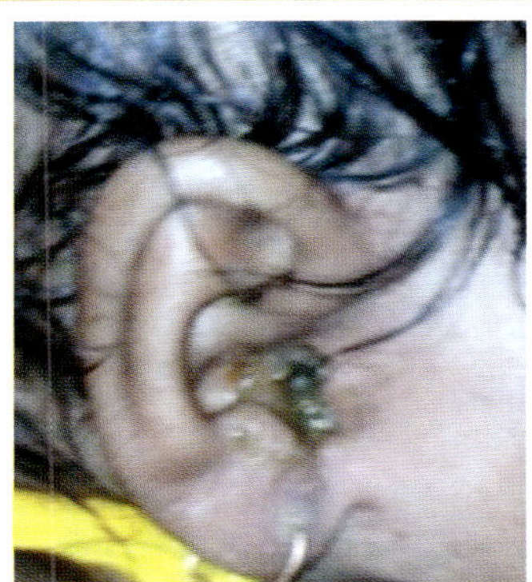 **Figure 1.1.1:** Acute otitis media *Photo Courtesy*: Rhishikesh Thakre, Aurangabad	Note the purulent discharge in the external ear. It may be isolated or part of sepsis syndrome. Irritability, incessant crying, and feeding difficulty may be the only manifestations. Fever may or may not be there (Fig. 1.1.1).	• Otoscopy is diagnostic. Sepsis workup is required. • Analgesics, antipyretics and parenteral antibiotics with hospitalization is necessary. • Decongestants and antihistamines do not appear to have efficacy. Instillation of eardrops or oil drops is not required.

Bacille Calmette-Guérin Abscess

Picture	Note	Management
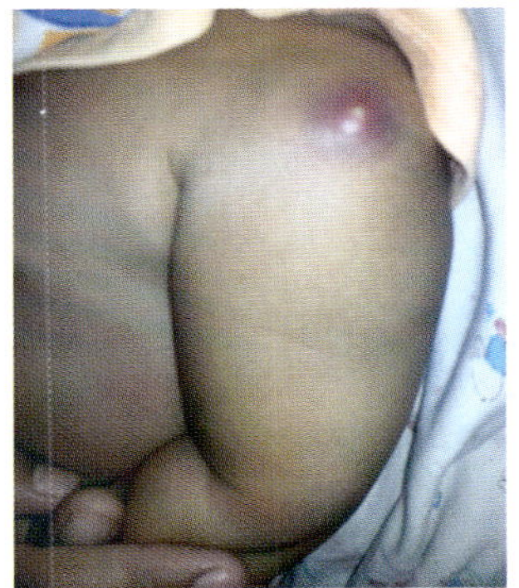 **Figure 1.1.2:** BCG abscess *Photo Courtesy*: Rhishikesh Thakre, Aurangabad	Note the pus formation at Bacille Calmette-Guérin (BCG) site. There is no erythema, discharge or local warmth. The newborn is otherwise well and manifests 1–5 months post vaccination (Fig. 1.1.2). At times there may be ulceration and lymphadenopathy.	• Localized complications—hypersensitivity reactions, abscesses at the injection site, and localized lymphadenopathy are usually self limiting post BCG vaccination. • There is no role of drainage, needle aspiration, topical or systemic isoniazid, or systemic erythromycin therapy. • Early accelerated and exaggerated BCG response may indicate immune compromised state.

Breast Abscess

Picture	Note	Management
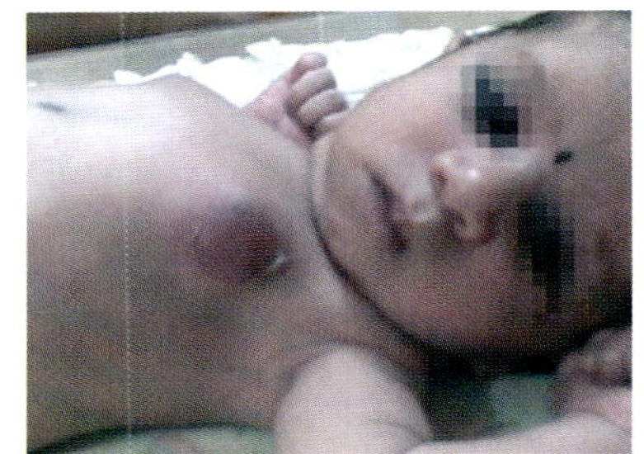 **Figure 1.1.3:** Breast abscess *Photo Courtesy*: Rhishikesh Thakre, Aurangabad	Note the redness and fullness of the left breast (Fig. 1.1.3). This is usually associated with warmth, local tenderness and fluctuation with no discharge. History of squeezing milk from the nipple is often present.	Incision and drainage, analgesics and antibiotic therapy is required.

Picture	Note	Management

Cellulitis

Picture	Note	Management
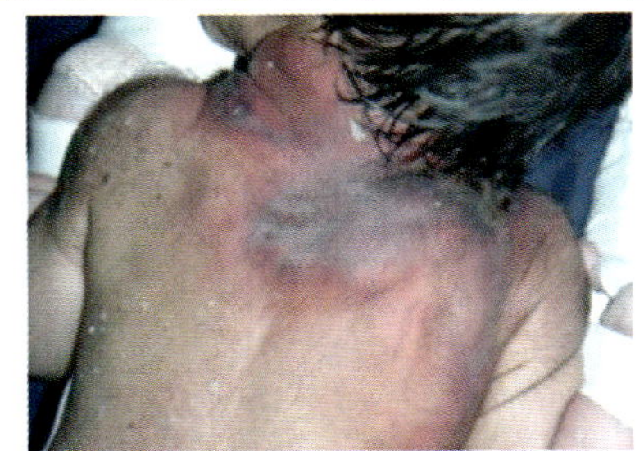 **Figure 1.1.4:** Cellulitis *Photo Courtesy*: Ramesh S Bajaj, Aurangabad	Note the bluish blackish discoloration of skin over the back with adjoining erythema, edema and skin induration extending on to neck with patchy areas of ulceration and necrosis (Fig. 1.1.4). Signs of worsening such as increasing redness or swelling or foul-smelling drainage from the affected area warrant surgical consult.	• Workup should include sepsis screen and blood culture. • Broad spectrum antibiotics may be started empirically pending culture reports. Antibiotic should cover streptococci and staphylococci.

Conjunctivitis

Picture	Note	Management
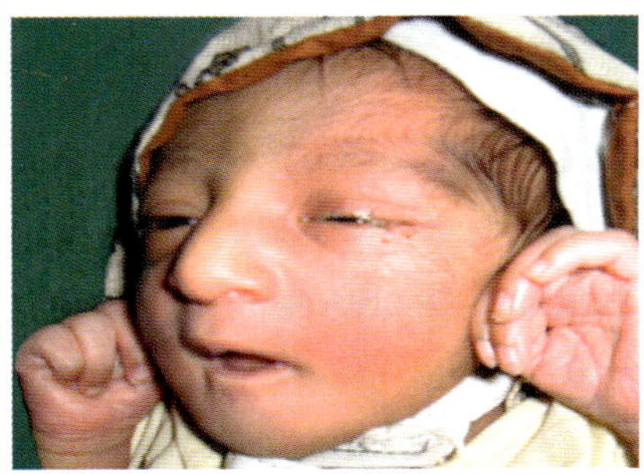 **Figure 1.1.5:** Conjuncitivis *Photo Courtesy*: Sandeep Kadam, Pune	Note the bilateral purulent eye discharge with partial ability to open the eyes. This is usually associated with conjunctival congestion. Watery discharge with no conjunctival congestions is seen in dacrocystitis. Gonococcal conjunctivitis tends to be more severe than any other causes of ophthalmia neonatorum (Fig. 1.1.5).	• To define the exact etiology, conjunctival scraping for Gram stain, Giemsa stain, culture on chocolate agar and/or Thayer-Martin for *N. gonorrhea* and culture on blood agar for other bacteria is required. • Pending lab results, topical erythromycin ointment and IV or IM third-generation cephalosporin (if gonococcal infection suspected) should be initiated. Treatment may be modified later as per culture results. • Thorough eye cleaning with sterile saline swab, each separate for each eye is most important. Eye should be cleaned from medial to lateral side.

Gangrene

Picture	Note	Management
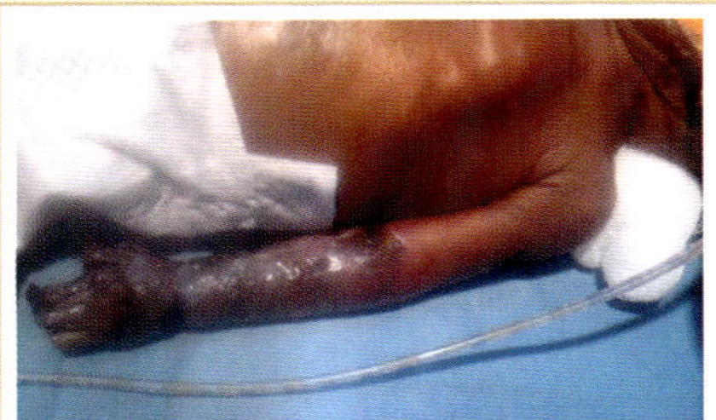 **Figure 1.1.6:** Gangrene *Photo Courtesy*: Sandeep Kadam, Pune	Note bluish blackish discoloration of fingers, palms, hands extending up to the elbow. There is overlying induration, hardening and necrosis with clear line of demarcation with healthy skin (Fig. 1.1.6). With underlying severe sepsis embolus, thrombosis and/or coagulopathy predispose to gangrene formation. Arterial thrombosis, emboli, trauma, congenital heart disease, coagulopathy, polycythemia, congenital bands, and birth trauma are some of the causes which should be considered.	• Sepsis workup, early prompt surgical reference along with prompt IV antibiotics, flow enhancers, (heparin, vasodilators, lomodex, hyper baric oxygen, etc.) blood transfusions, wound cleansing (hydrogen peroxide), local ointments (betadine, soframicin), slough removal (eusol, salutyl ointment) and regular dressings are required. • Dry dressing is applied over gangrenous area. Appearance of line of demarcation needs amputation.

Picture	Note	Management

Impetigo

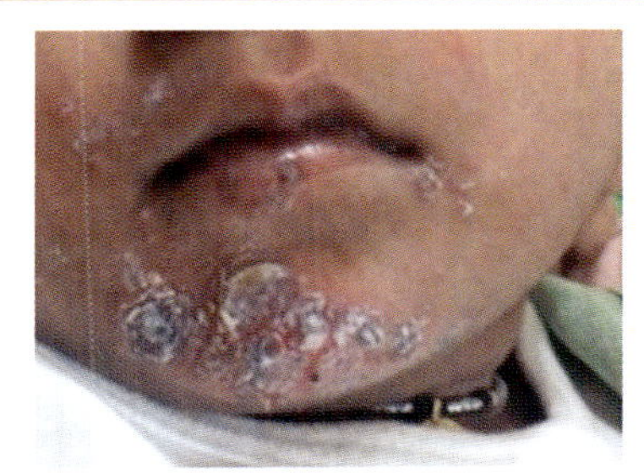 **Figure 1.1.7:** Impetigo *Photo Courtesy*: Rhishikesh Thakre, Aurangabad	Note multiple superficial lesions over the chin with adjoining erythema and crust formation (Fig. 1.1.7). It is highly contagious and is primarily caused by *Staphylococcus aureus*.	• Treatment involves washing with soap and water and letting the impetigo dry in the air. • Mild cases may be treated with bactericidal ointment, such as mupirocin. • More severe cases require oral antibiotics, such as amoxicillin or first generation cephalosporin.

Neonatal Scabies

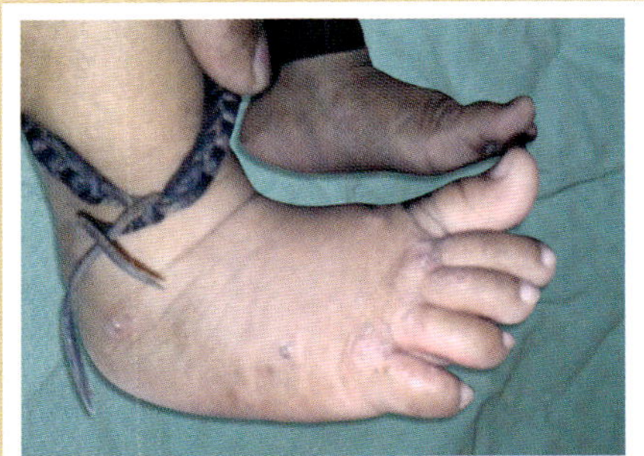 **Figure 1.1.8:** Neonatal scabies *Photo Courtesy*: Rhishikesh Thakre, Aurangabad	Note the macules, papules and vesicles over the foot and the web spaces (Fig. 1.1.8). There is a tendency to form pustules early in the course of illness. Such lesions are also seen over the face, neck, scalp, and palms. Eczematization and impetiginization are common. History of scabies in one of the family member or care taker is often present.	• Examination of close contacts and a careful history should lead to the correct diagnosis. Microscopic examination of scrapings of the vesicles reveals mites, eggs, and feces. • Treatment of the infant and family members with 5% permethrin cream successfully eradicates the infestation.

Oral Thrush

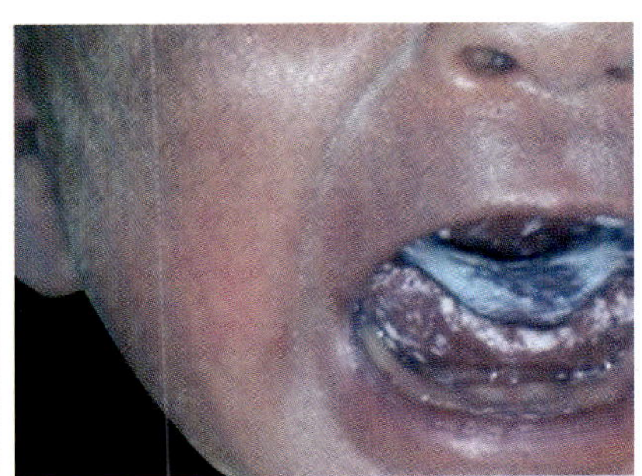 **Figure 1.1.9:** Oral thrush *Photo Courtesy*: Rhishikesh Thakre, Aurangabad	Note the whitish, curdy plaques over the tongue, buccal mucosa and the soft palate (Fig. 1.1.9). These lesions bleed on scrapping and cannot be removed easily. The newborn presents with feeding difficulty.	• Oral thrush is a common fungal infection caused by *Candida albicans*. The diagnosis is clinical. • Oral nystatin suspension is used. Simultaneous treatment of the mother's nipple is must. • Recurrent oral thrush is an indicator of immunocompromised state like HIV.

Picture	Note	Management

Pustules

Picture	Note	Management
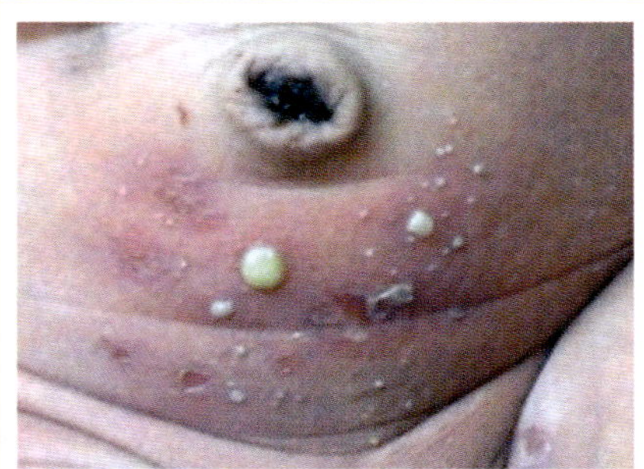 **Figure 1.1.10:** Pustules *Photo Courtesy*: Rhishikesh Thakre, Aurangabad	Note multiple pustules in the peri-umbilical area. There is surrounding erythema (Fig. 1.1.10). They may also be present over the trunk, axilla, and groins. At times, there may be induration, hardening of the adjoining skin with pus discharge. Many a times the newborn is asymptomatic.	• Few lesions in a healthy term infant may be treated with topical antibiotic and oral therapy. • More extensive lesions, systemic illness, or pustulosis occurring in the premature infant requires IV therapy. • Most common causative organism is *Staphylococcus aureus*.

Umbilical Sepsis

Picture	Note	Management
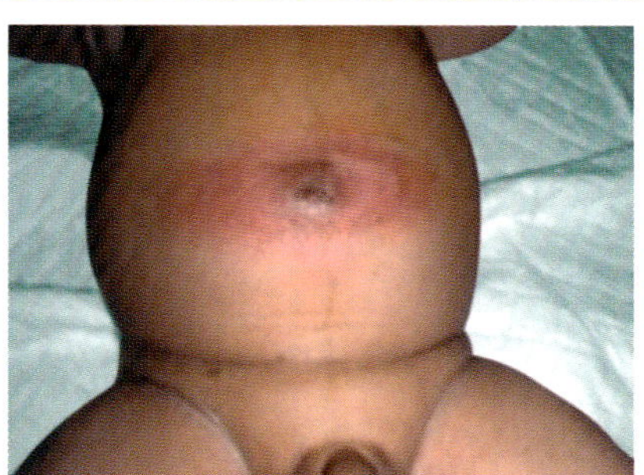 **Figure 1.1.11:** Umbilical sepsis *Photo Courtesy*: Ramesh S Bajaj, Aurangabad	Note the visible periumbilical erythema and induration. These are suggestive of umbilical sepsis. This is usually associated with local warmth, pus discharge and foul smell (Fig. 1.1.11). There may be nonspecific signs such as fever, irritability, feeding difficulty or respiratory distress. It may remain localized or can quickly progress to sepsis and present as a potentially life threatening condition. Underlying umbilical polyp should be looked for.	• Diagnosis is made clinically with supportive history and physical examination. • Treatment consists of antibiotic therapy (penicillin + aminoglycoside) in addition to supportive care for any complications which might result from the infection itself.

1.2 SYSTEMIC INFECTIONS

Brain Abscess

Picture	Note	Management
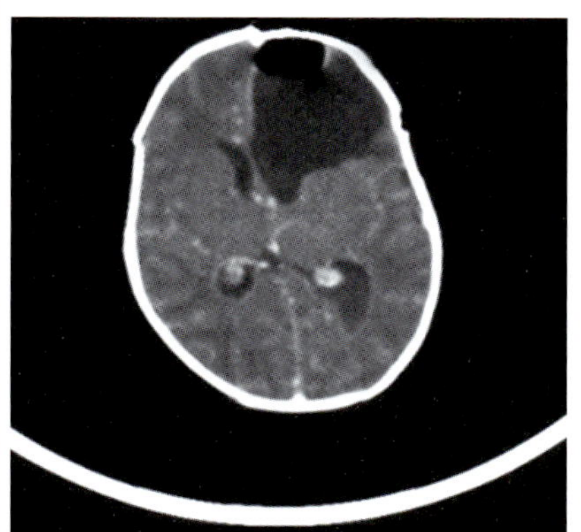 **Figure 1.2.1:** Brain abscess *Photo Courtesy*: Pradeep Suryawanshi, Pune	Note a single, large space occupying lesion in frontal lobe with surrounding edema with minimal shift of midline with no dilatation of ventricles (Fig. 1.2.1). These arise as a complication of septicemia, meningitis or underlying systemic cause for thrombosis or embolism. Presence of unexplained high fever, lethargy, seizures, focal deficit, worsening sensorium should raise suspicion of brain abscess. Any new born baby with acute pyogenic meningitis who is not responding to routine treatment should be screened for complication like subdural empyema, brain abscess, etc.	• Sepsis screen, cerebrospinal fluid (CSF) study including culture, blood culture, CT brain or MRI confirm brain abscess. • USG/CT guided aspiration, antibiotics (4–8 weeks) and if non-responsive, surgery may be needed. • Abscesses larger than 2.5 cm are excised or aspirated, while those smaller than 2.5 cm or which are at the cerebritis stage are aspirated for diagnostic purposes only.

Picture	Note	Management

Necrotizing Enterocolitis

Picture	Note	Management
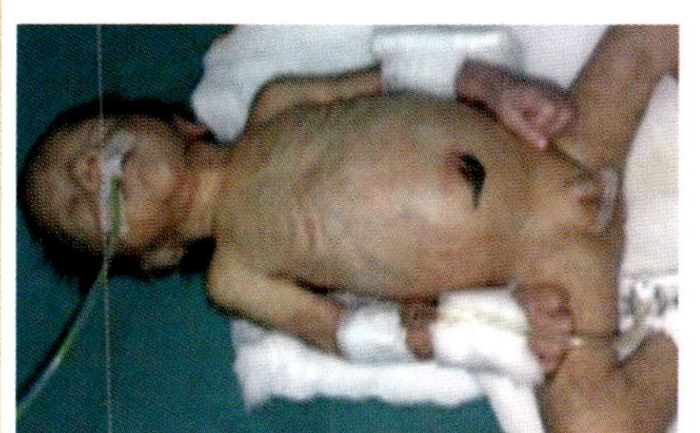 **Figure 1.2.2:** Necrotizing enterocolitis *Photo Courtesy*: Naveen Bajaj, Ludhiana	Note the preterm baby has abdominal distension which is tense with overlying shiny abdominal skin. There are yellowish brown gastrointestinal (GI) aspirates (Fig. 1.2.2). These features suggest necrotizing enterocolitis (NEC). The NEC is primarily a disease process of the GI tract of preterm that results in inflammation and bacterial invasion of the bowel wall.	• Management includes fluid restriction, gastric decompression, nil by mouth, antibiotics, inotropic support, correction of anemia, thrombocytopenia and acidosis as required. • Surgery may be required in some patients.

Neonatal Candidiasis

Picture	Note	Management
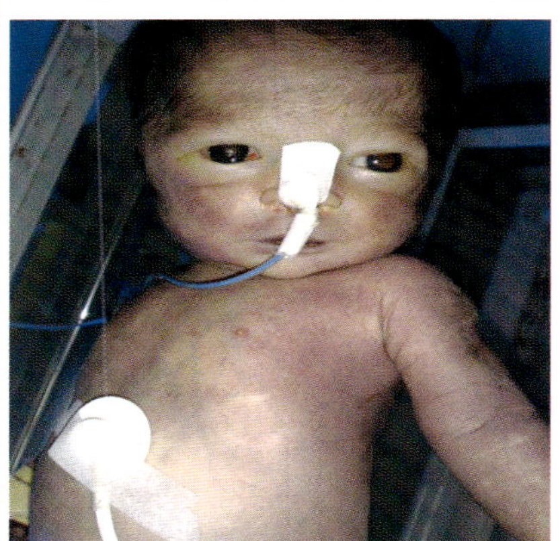 **Figure 1.2.3:** Neonatal candidiasis *Photo Courtesy*: Sandeep Kadam, Pune	Note the ashen gray complexion in a sick, preterm baby. A slow evolving infection with risk factors like prolonged antibiotics, ventilation, prolonged ICU stay, total parenteral nutrition (TPN), invasive lines and procedures predispose to *Candida* infection (Fig. 1.2.3). Unexplained thrombocytopenia, cholestasis, oliguria, nonresponsive to antibiotics warrants screening for *Candida*.	• Fungal infections should be suspected whenever, in the presence of a predisposing host conditions, despite seemingly appropriate antibacterial therapy, the illness continues to have a smoldering and persistent course. • Blood culture is diagnostic. Screening for end organ damage is recommended (USG liver, kidney, brain, 2D echo, fundus) once candidiasis is diagnosed. • Amphotericin B (4–6 weeks) is drug of choice. • Removal of catheter is justified in case of catheter related blood stream infection.

Neonatal Osteomyelitis

Picture	Note	Management
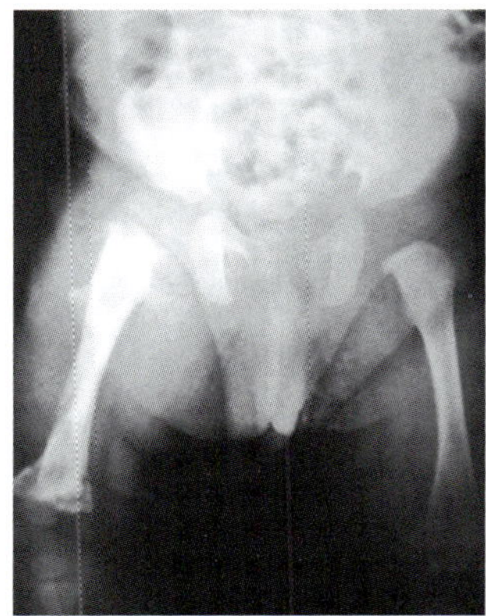 **Figure 1.2.4:** Neonatal osteomyelitis *Photo Courtesy*: Sandeep Kadam, Pune	Note the metaphyseal irregularity, radiolucency, periosteal reaction of proximal end of femur. There is also soft tissue swelling. There may be associated widening of the joint space, subluxation or dislocation (Fig. 1.2.4). Clinical symptoms include poor feeding and/or irritability. There may be a history of swelling or failure to move the affected limb (pseudoparalysis).	• A high index of suspicion, coupled with careful physical examination, is important for early identification and treatment. • Ultrasound allows the detection of subperiosteal collections and joint effusions. Note that a normal ultrasound scan does not exclude osteomyelitis. • Surgical debridement or drainage, as required, and antibiotic therapy (4–8 weeks) are the pillars of therapy. Antistaphylococcal coverage is needed.

Picture	Note	Management

Neonatal Meningitis

Picture	Note	Management
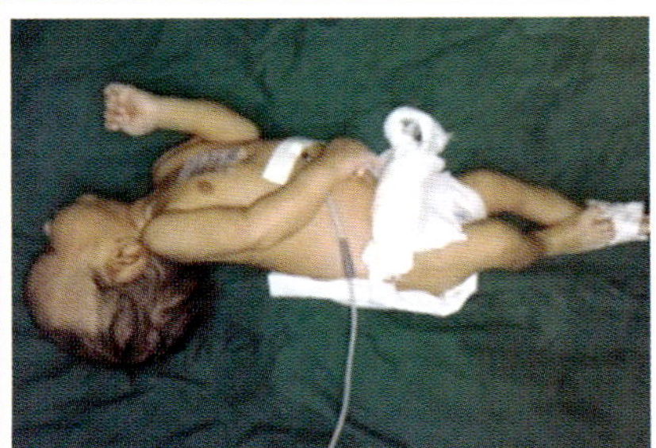 **Figure 1.2.5:** Neonatal meningitis *Photo Courtesy*: Rajeeb Chatterjee, Loni	Note the extensor posturing with retraction of neck. Accompanying features include seizures, temperature instability, episodes of apnea or bradycardia, hypotension, feeding difficulty, tense fontanelle and irritability alternating with lethargy (Fig. 1.2.5). Constellation of these signs should raise suspicion of meningitis.	• The diagnosis is confirmed on CSF examination (microscopy, chemistry and culture) obtained by lumbar puncture. • Management includes appropriate antibiotics (14–21 days), meticulous fluid therapy, supportive care and use of anticonvulsants for seizures. There is no role of steroids or mannitol.

Pneumonia with Pneumatoceles

Picture	Note	Management
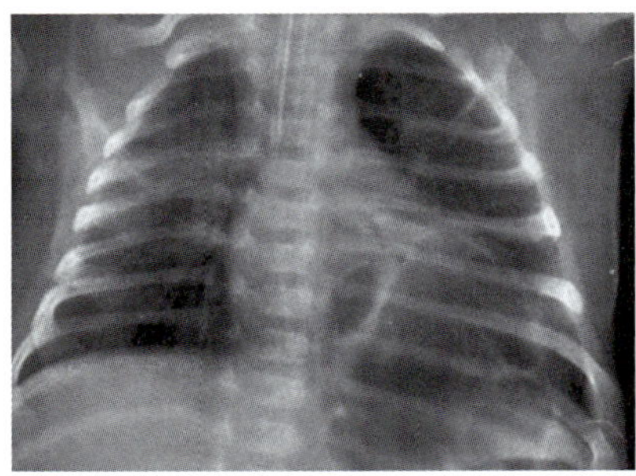 **Figure 1.2.6:** Pneumonia with pneumatoceles *Photo Courtesy*: Naveen Bajaj, Ludhiana	Radiograph shows bilateral patchy infiltration of both lung fields more so in the right lung. Multiple air filled cavities of different sizes are seen in the left lower lobe suggestive of pneumatoceles (Fig. 1.2.6). Pneumonia complicated by pneumatocele formation is commonly due to staphylococci, *Klebsiella* and *E. coli*.	• Ensuring adequacy of oxygen, aggressive supportive care, antibiotics (usually cloxacillin, oxacillin or vancomycin with a aminoglycoside) and meticulous clinical monitoring is the key. • Respiratory support needs to be anticipated. • Rarely surgical intervention is required.

Sclerema Neonatorum

Picture	Note	Management
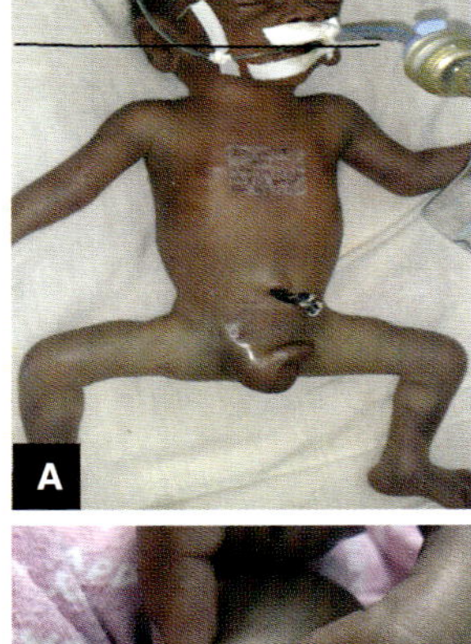 **Figures 1.2.7A and B:** Sclerema neonatorum *Photo Courtesy*: Rajeeb Chatterjee, Loni	Note the newborn is sick, ventilated with ET *in situ*, with signs of poor perfusion. The skin appears shiny, taut with fullness of extremities (Fig. 1.2.7A). On pinching the skin there is hardness with inability to lift the skin between fingers due to edema and thickening of subcutaneous tissue suggestive of sclerema (Fig. 1.2.7B). The signs initially appear over the thigh and may progress to mask like facies, diffuse woody to stony hard induration of extremities, with restricted joint mobility, temperature instability and poor respiratory efforts. Onset of sclerema heralds poor prognosis.	• Aggressive management with resuscitation, strict attention to fluid, electrolyte and acid-base balance, ventilatory support, inotropes and broad spectrum antibiotics is needed. • Steroid and exchange transfusion are reserved for refractory cases. • The prognosis is guarded.

Picture	Note	Management

Septic Shock

Picture	Note	Management
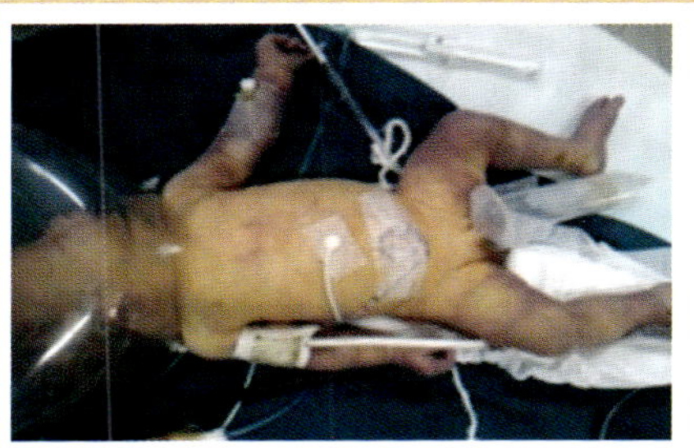 **Figure 1.2.8:** Septic shock *Photo Courtesy*: Rhishikesh Thakre, Aurangabad	Note the dusky palms and soles, with patchy bluish discoloration of both hands and legs. There is associated tachycardia, drowsiness, prolonged capillary refill time (CRT), cold extremities with warm trunk, oliguria and hypotension suggestive of septic shock on clinical examination (Fig. 1.2.8).	• History and clinical course is suggestive. Confirmation is by blood culture and sepsis screen. • Aggressive fluid resuscitation, inotropes, meticulous monitoring of vitals, fluids, electrolytes and sugars is the mainstay of management.

Staphylococcal Scalded Skin Syndrome

Picture	Note	Management
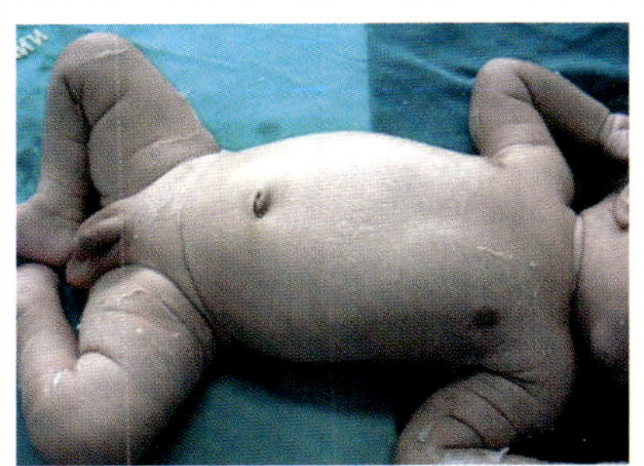 **Figure 1.2.9:** Staphylococcal scalded skin syndrome (SSSS) *Photo Courtesy*: Sandeep Kadam, Pune	Note the generalized exfoliation of skin. Manifestations include erythematous, bullous skin lesions over face, back and extremities with peeling of skin on contact (Nikolsky sign) (Fig. 1.2.9). Desquamation subsides by 48 hours of appropriate therapy. Skin lesions heal without scarring. Such exfoliation is most commonly seen due to staphylococcal infection.	• Diagnosis is clinical with isolation of staphylococci in blood culture or pharyngeal swab or gastric aspirate. • Skin culture and skin biopsy is useful. • The complications include fluid loss, septic arthritis, cellulitis, pneumonia, sepsis, and osteomyelitis. • Adequate hydration, meticulous skin care with antistaphylococcal antibiotics are the main stay of therapy.

1.3 CONGENITAL INFECTIONS

Congenital Cytomegalovirus

Picture	Note	Management
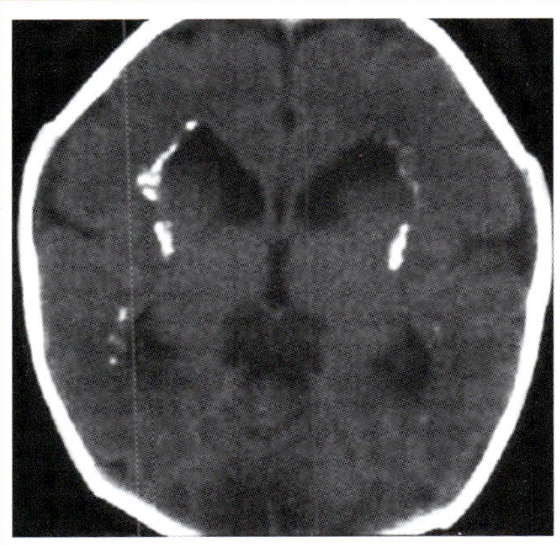 **Figure 1.3.1:** Congenital cytomegalovirus *Photo Courtesy*: Rhishikesh Thakre, Aurangabad	Note the CT brain shows calcification which are along the subependymal ventricular region (Fig. 1.3.1). Periventricular calcifications with small head are a clinical clue to cytomegalovirus (CMV) infection. Clinical features include growth retardation, thrombocytopenia, anemia, hepatosplenomegaly, neurological problems such as poor tone and seizures.	• Diagnosis is confirmed by presence of IgM antibody, IgG with fourfold rising antibody titers, PCR or viral cultures. • Maternal testing for CMV is required. • Ganciclovir is indicated if there is life threatening or sight threatening CMV infection.

Picture	Note	Management

Congenital HIV

Picture	Note	Management
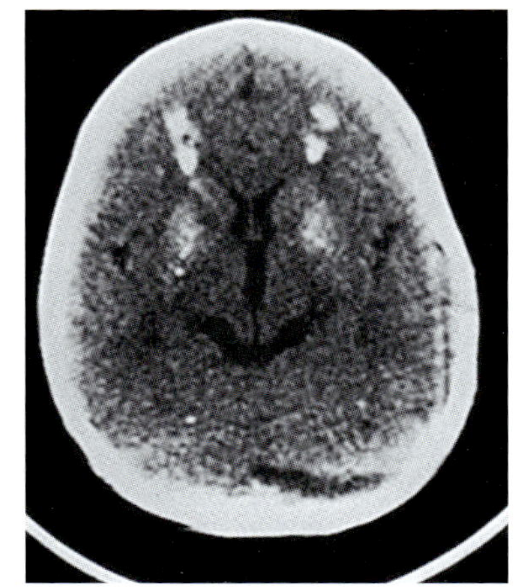 **Figure 1.3.2:** Congenital HIV *Photo Courtesy*: Rhishikesh Thakre, Aurangabad	Note the CT brain study shows discrete calcifications in the basal ganglia. There is no evidence of loss of gray-white matter differentiation or ventricular dilatation. Progressive leukoencephalopathy with atrophy of brain is characteristic of congenital HIV infection (Fig. 1.3.2). Clinical manifestation includes failure to thrive, hepatosplenomegaly, chronic diarrhea, thrush and recurrent bacterial infections.	• Confirmation is done by HIV PCR or using two different sets of enzyme-linked immunosorbent assay (ELISA) and/or western blot. • Anti-retroviral drugs are the mainstay of treatment.

Congenital Rubella Syndrome

Picture	Note	Management
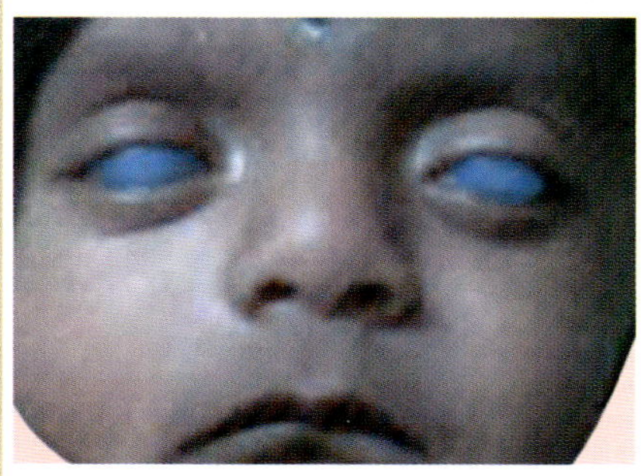 **Figure 1.3.3:** Congenital rubella syndrome *Photo Courtesy*: Snehal Thakre, Aurangabad	Note that both eyes are hazy with enlarged cornea. Intraocular pressure is increased suggesting buphthalmos. Presence of microcephaly, congenital heart defect such as PDA, growth retardation, sensorineural hearing loss is hallmark of rubella infection (Fig. 1.3.3).	• Fourfold rise in IgG antibody titers or positive IgM antibody or isolation of rubella virus is diagnostic. • There is no specific treatment.

Congenital Syphilis

Picture	Note	Management
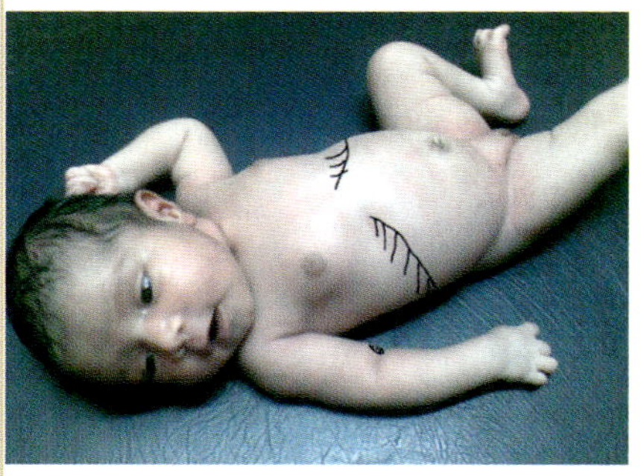 **Figure 1.3.4:** Congenital Syphilis *Photo Courtesy*: Rhishikesh Thakre, Aurangabad	Note the right upper limb in extended posture with paucity of spontaneous movement suggestive of pseudoparalysis (Fig. 1.3.4). Associated hepatosplenomegaly, epitrochlear lymph node and irritability should raise suspicion of congenital syphilis. Clavicle fracture (swelling or palpable break) or brachial plexus injury (absent grasp) also present with monoparesis.	• Maternal venereal disease research laboratory (VDRL) status, newborn VDRL testing or specific anti-treponemal antibody is diagnostic. X-ray changes are suggestive. • Treatment involves penicillin with simultaneous screening/treatment of parents. • Long-term follow-up is mandatory.

Picture	Note	Management

Congenital Toxoplasmosis

Picture	Note	Management
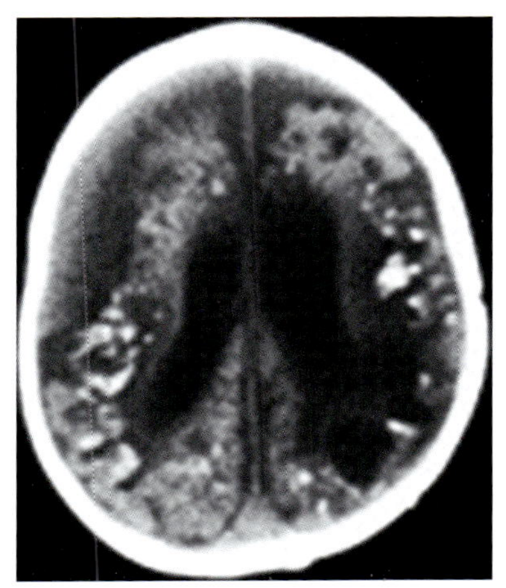 **Figure 1.3.5:** Congenital toxoplasmosis *Photo Courtesy*: Rhishikesh Thakre, Aurangabad	Note the CT brain showing evidence of diffuse calcification in the periventricular region and adjacent brain parenchyma (Fig. 1.3.5). Congenital toxoplasmosis is more likely with diffuse calcification and large head. Associated features include hydrocephalus, chorioretinitis, convulsions, hepatosplenomegaly, anemia and rash.	• A double sandwich IgM EIA and IgM immunosorbent would help in diagnosis. • Agglutination assay (ISAGA) is more specific than commercial IgM EIAs. • IgG avidity is now the standard "confirmatory" test. • Treatment includes pyrimethamine (1 mg/kg orally daily), sulphadiazine (50 mg/kg orally, twice daily) and folinic acid (1 ml/kg, orally twice weekly).

Congenital Tuberculosis

Picture	Note	Management
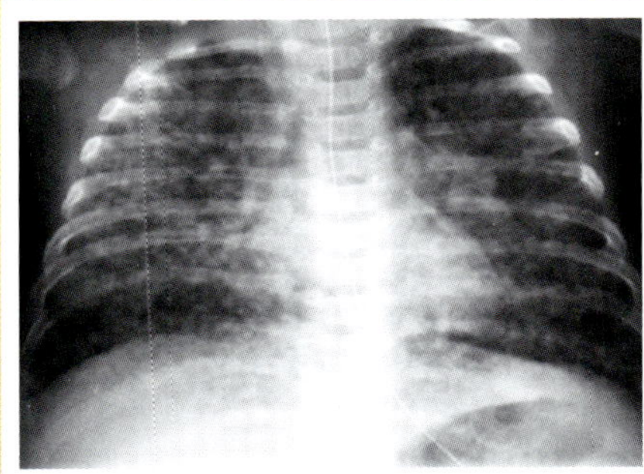 **Figure 1.3.6:** Congenital tuberculosis *Photo Courtesy*: Rhishikesh Thakre, Aurangabad	Note the chest X-ray shows diffuse miliary shadows all over the lung fields (Fig. 1.3.6). Clinically respiratory distress with hepatosplenomegaly should raise suspicion of congenital tuberculosis.	• History of contact, documentation of primary lesion in the placenta or liver confirms the diagnosis. • Anti-tubercular treatment is the main stay of treatment. Immunocompromised state should be ruled out.

Neonatal Chickenpox

Picture	Note	Management
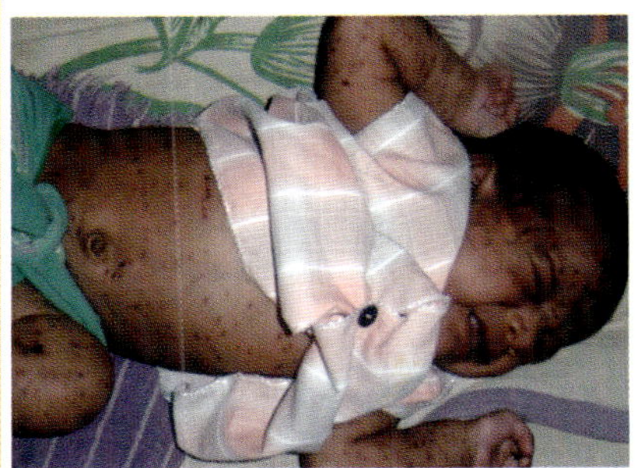 **Figure 1.3.7:** Neonatal chickenpox *Photo Courtesy*: Rhishikesh Thakre, Aurangabad	Note the erythematous rash on face and trunk. The rash assumes vesicular form on red base and spread over trunk and limbs. There is evidence of crusting in some lesions with pleomorphism which is diagnostic of chickenpox (Fig. 1.3.7).	• Treatment with varicella zoster immunoglobulin (VZIg) is indicated prophylactically in preterm, newborn born to mother with chickenpox 5 days before or 2 days after delivery. • If VZIg not available or affordable IV Ig can be used. • Acyclovir is indicated with clinical manifestation.

Picture	Note	Management

Neonatal Tetanus

Picture	Note	Management
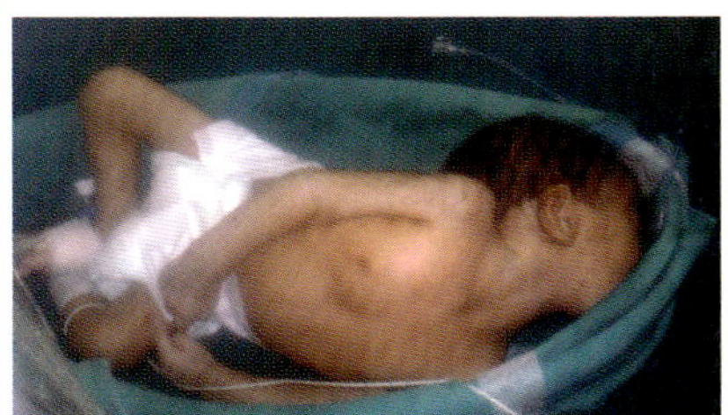 **Figure 1.3.8:** Neonatal tetanus *Photo Courtesy*: Sandeep Kadam, Pune	Note the neonate has retracted neck (retrocollis) and complete arching of the back (opisthotonus).There is associated mask like facies with inability to open mouth (trismus). Opisthotonus and stimulus induced spasms with intact sensorium is hallmark of tetanus (Fig. 1.3.8).	Treatment is essentially supportive, minimal stimulation, sedatives, muscle relaxants, anticonvulsants, penicillin and tetanus immunoglobulin.

1.4 MISCELLANEOUS

Hand Washing

Picture	Note	Management
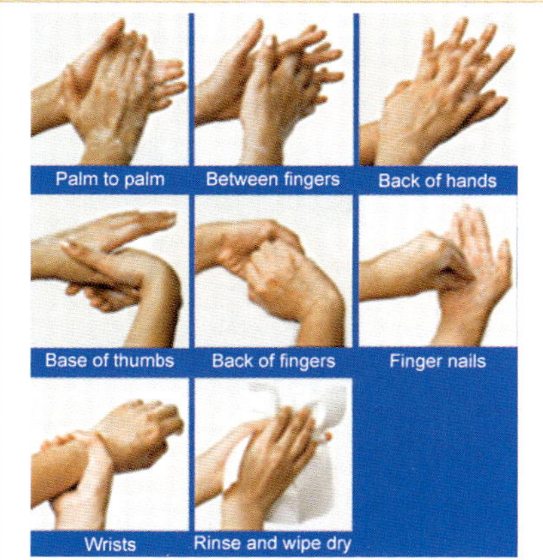 **Figure 1.4.1:** Hand washing *Photo Courtesy*: Rhishikesh Thakre, Aurangabad	The picture depicts cleaning of the hands with the use of water and soap under an elbow operated tap. Hand washing involves systematic hand motions in six steps to done before entering the nursery (2 min) and after each contact with the patient (Fig. 1.4.1). The purpose is to remove soil, dirt, and/or microorganisms from hand surfaces. Center for Disease Control (CDC) recommends it as one of the most important measures for preventing the spread of pathogens.	• Use of alcohol based hand rub is not a substitute for hand washing. • Medicated hand rubs are indicated only in epidemic situations. • Hand drying may be done by sterile cloth or hand dryers.

Sepsis Screen

Picture	Note	Management
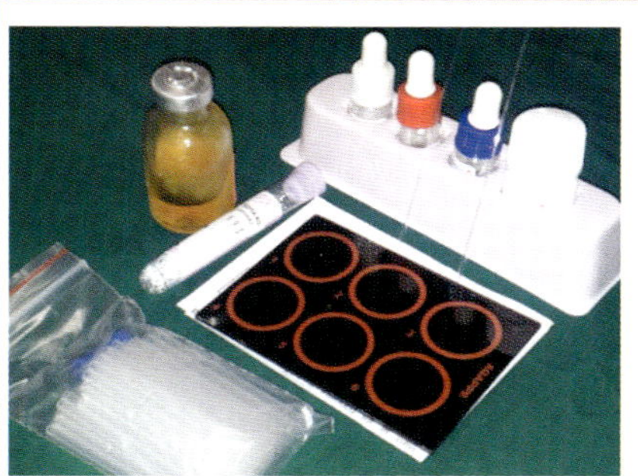 **Figure 1.4.2:** Sepsis screen *Photo Courtesy*: Rhishikesh Thakre, Aurangabad	Picture depicts commonly used kits for screening for neonatal infection–EDTA (For CBC, ANC, I:T ratio, platelet count), micro tubes (uESR), plain bulb (CRP) or qualitative CRP kit and blood culture broth (Fig. 1.4.2).	• The utility of sepsis screen is more in "ruling out" sepsis than "ruling in" sepsis. • Blood culture is considered to be the gold standard for confirming the diagnosis of sepsis. • For maximum utility, interpret taking into consideration the clinical course, risk factors and results of sepsis screen. • Adequate blood volume, proper storage and transport of the sample will improve the yield of blood culture.

Section 2

Fever with Rash

Section Editors

Arun Shah, Ketan H Shah

Contributors

Arun Shah, Ketan H Shah, Vijay Jain, RK Sinha, SBP Singh, Utpal Kant Singh, Shyam Bihari, Yugal Kishor Prasad, Braj Mohan, SA Krishna, Sanjata Roy Chaudhary, Ananda Kesavan, Atul Kulkarni

Section Outline

- Impetigo
- Erythema Nodosum
- Necrotizing Fasciitis
- Erythema Marginatum
- Hand-Foot-and-Mouth Disease
- Henoch-Schönlein Purpura
- Herpes Zoster
- Janeway Lesion
- Meningococcal Lesion
- Staphylococcal Scalded Skin Syndrome
- Toxic Epidermal Necrolysis
- Toxic Shock Syndrome
- Urticaria
- Herpetic Gingivostomatitis
- Systemic Lupus Erythematosus
- Aplastic Anemia
- Post Kala-Azar Dermal Leishmaniasis
- Conjunctivitis with Coryza
- Classical Rash of Dengue Fever
- Petechial Spots on Lower Limb with Occasional Macules
- Measles Rash
- Black Discoloration and Hyperpigmentation
- Erythematous Changes on Sole and Tip of the Toe
- Red Ear due to Chikungunya Fever
- Freckle-like Pigmentation at Recovery
- Multiple Purpurae with Blueberry Muffin Rash
- Pale Rose Red Blanching Macules and Papules on the Palm
- Vasculitis with Gangrenous Changes in Same Patient of Rickettsia

Picture	Note	Management

Impetigo

Picture	Note	Management
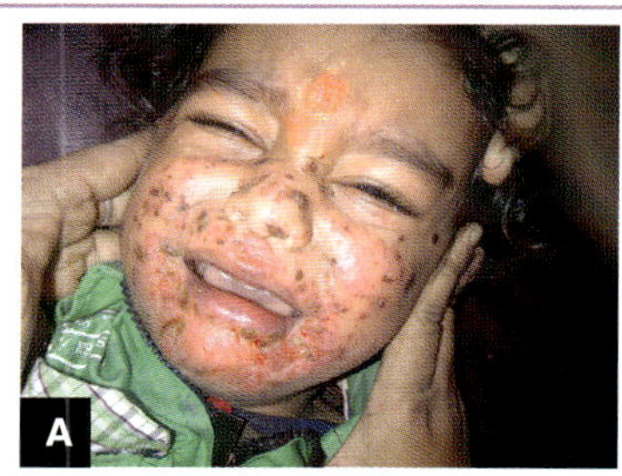 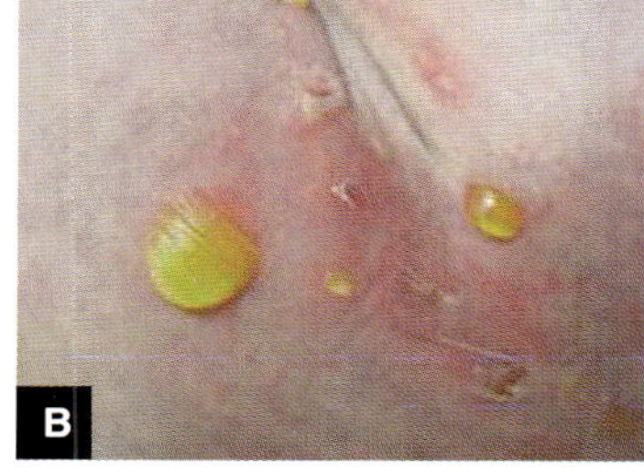 **Figures 2.1.1A and B:** Impetigo *Photo Courtesy*: Arun Shah, Muzaffarpur	Note lesion with honey colored crust over face (Fig. 2.1.1A). While the other shows bullae with serous fluid (Fig. 2.1.1B). Impetigo is superficial bacterial infection of the skin caused primarily by *Staphylococcus aureus*. Lesions tend to be located in exposed areas especially the face and extremities. Lesions often spread due to autoinoculation. The diagnosis is most often made based on the clinical findings. Bacterial culture can assist in identifying the specific etiologic agent and antibiotic sensitivities.	• For milder, localized cases, topical mupirocin ointment can be applied 2 times daily for 5–7 days. • When there is more widespread involvement, 7–10 days course of a systemic antibiotic (e.g. cephalexin) may be necessary with attention to resistance patterns for each geographic location.

Erythema Nodosum

Picture	Note	Management
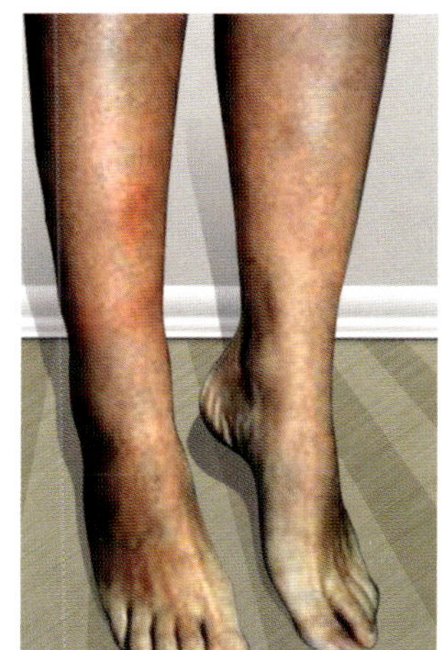 **Figure 2.1.2:** Erythema nodosum *Photo Courtesy*: Arun Shah, Muzaffarpur	Note erythematous nodular lesion on pretibial surface of lower extremities. Erythema nodosum (EN) is acute inflammatory condition characterized by bilateral symmetrical painful subcutaneous nodules (Fig. 2.1.2). EN is presumed to be hypersensitivity reaction to infections most commonly streptococcal infection and tuberculosis, inflammatory bowel diseases, sarcoidosis and drugs. It may be idiopathic also. It is also seen with rheumatic fever. The erythematous nodules usually begin on lower legs (shin of tibia) that evolve into bruise like lesions which disappear within 4–6 weeks.	• Evaluation includes complete blood count (CBC), erythrocyte sedimentation rate (ESR), C-reactive protein (CRP), throat swab, anti-streptolysin O (ASO) titer estimation, tuberculin test and chest X-ray. • It is self-limiting condition in most of the cases and also responds to treatment of underlying etiology. • To alleviate pain symptomatic treatment includes use of NSAID (non-steroidal anti-inflammatory drugs), bed rest, leg elevation and cool wet compresses.

Picture	Note	Management

Necrotizing Fasciitis

Picture	Note	Management
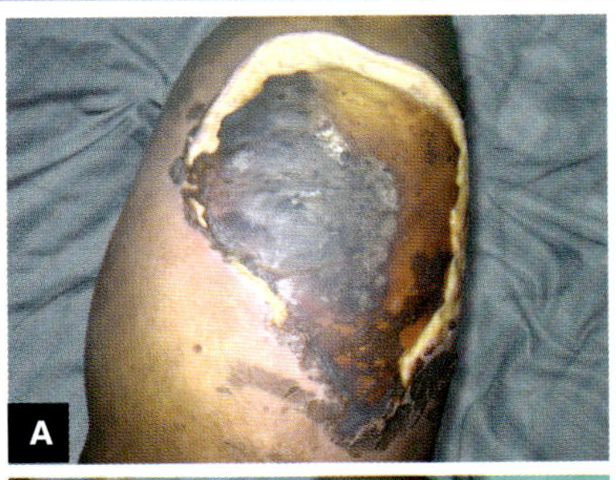 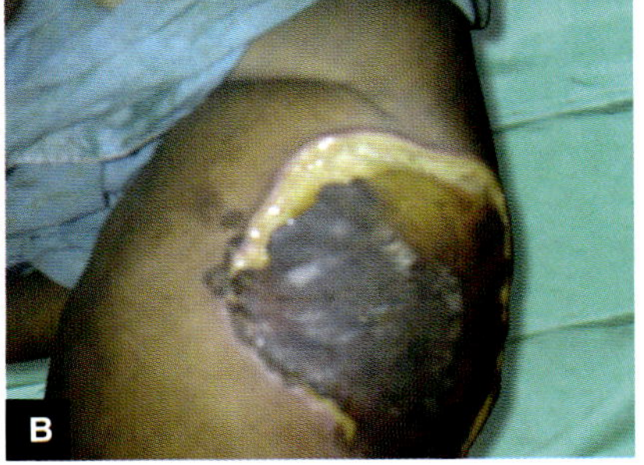 **Figures 2.1.3A and B:** Necrotizing fasciitis *Photo Courtesy*: Arun Shah, Muzaffarpur	Note gangrene and slough in upper part of trunk in a 2-year-old child. Necrotizing fasciitis is subcutaneous tissue infection involving layer of superficial fascia. Most commonly caused by *S. pyogens* and staphylococci (Figs 2.1.3A and B). It may be polymicrobial infection. Aerobic and anaerobic bacteria act together to cause tissue necrosis. The incidence is higher in immune-compromised status. It begins with fever, local swelling, erythema, tenderness and heat. The infection spreads along the superficial fascial plane with few cutaneous signs. Later frank tissue gangrene and slough develop due to ischemia and necrosis. Of late community-associated MRSA infections (CA MRSA) with PVL toxin are associated with deep soft tissue infections including fasciitis.	• Definitive diagnosis is made by surgical exploration. • Early supportive care, surgical debridement to remove devitalized tissue and parenteral administration of broad spectrum antibiotics with antistaphylococcal cover are sheet anchor in management. • Clindamycin has added advantage of anaerobic coverage.

Erythema Marginatum

Picture	Note	Management
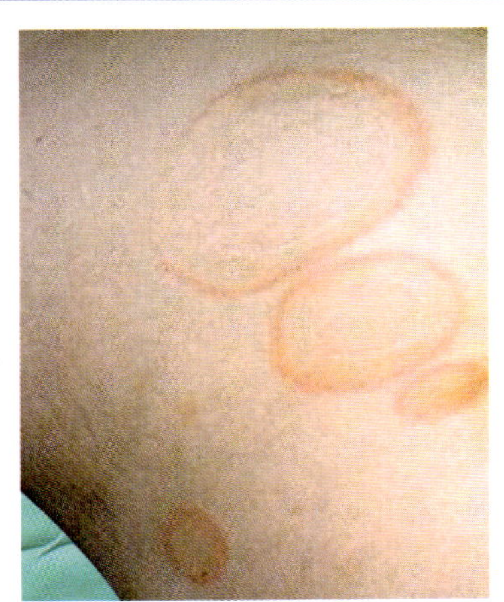 **Figure 2.1.4:** Erythema marginatum *Photo Courtesy*: Vijay Jain, Gaya	Note erythematous macular lesion involving trunk. Erythema marginatum is one of the major zone's criteria for clinical diagnosis of acute rheumatic fever (Fig. 2.1.4). It is rare, occurs in less than 5% of patients with rheumatic fever. The lesion is characterized by erythematous, serpeginous, macular, non-pruritic lesion with pale center primarily involving trunk and extremities but never affecting face. It is difficult to detect the lesion in dark skinned person. The lesion can fade and reappear within hours and may persist intermittently for weeks to months.	• Erythema marginatum is associated with either one major or two minor criteria with evidence of preceding Group A Streptococcal infection. • It indicates a high probability of acute rheumatic fever and should be treated with penicillin in recommended dosage and duration.

Picture	Note	Management

Hand-Foot-and-Mouth Disease

Picture	Note	Management
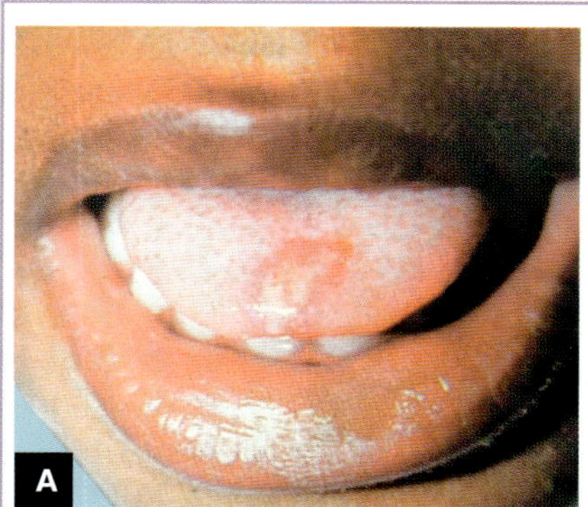 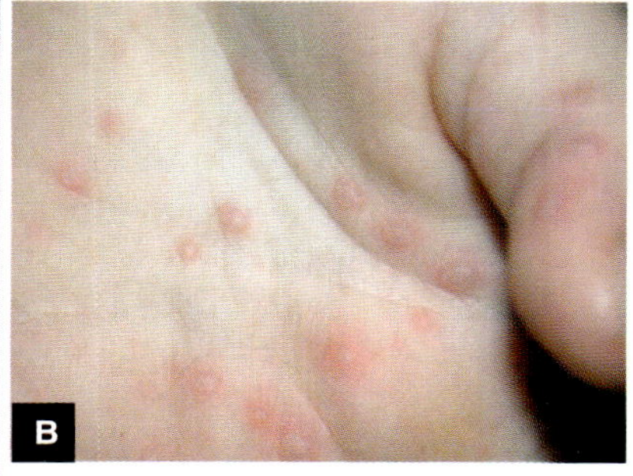 **Figures 2.1.5A and B:** Hand-foot-and-mouth disease *Photo Courtesy*: RK Sinha, Bhagalpur	Note the ulcer with erythematous base on tongue and oval eruptions with surrounding erythema on palm (Figs 2.1.5A and B). Hand-foot-and-mouth disease (HFMD) is most distinctive enteroviral exanthema affecting infants and children between 1 and 4 year of age. Most often caused by coxsackievirus A16 and less frequently by enterovirus 71. Highly contagious, the eruption is preceded by mild constitutional symptoms like fever and malaise. An enanthem develops first and subsequently the characteristic exanthema. Enanthem is characterized by vesicles that erode to form ulcers on a red base most commonly on buccal mucosa and tongue. Lesions are often quite painful. Exanthema characterized by vesiculopustules or oval vesicles with surrounding erythema. Typically lesions are limited to the palm and sole. The disease affects more than one member of the family and often takes a toll of epidemic situation.	• Hand-foot-and-mouth disease caused by enterovirus 71 is more severe and is associated with neurological diseases like aseptic meningitis and encephalitis. • The typical appearance and distribution of lesion is characteristic of HFMD. It is a self-limiting condition. • Symptomatic treatment with use of NSAID is adequate for pain relief.

Henoch-Schönlein Purpura

Picture	Note	Management
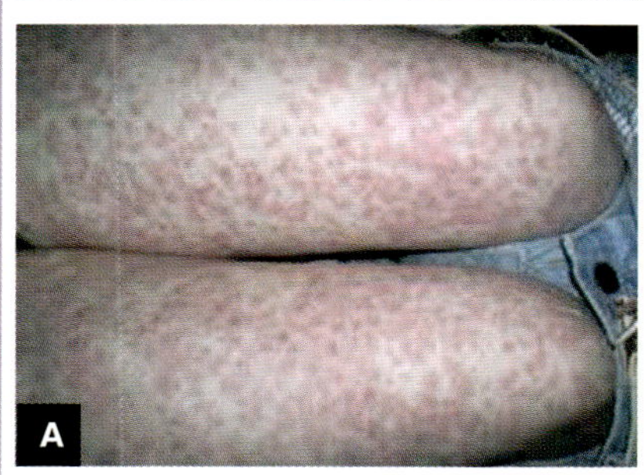 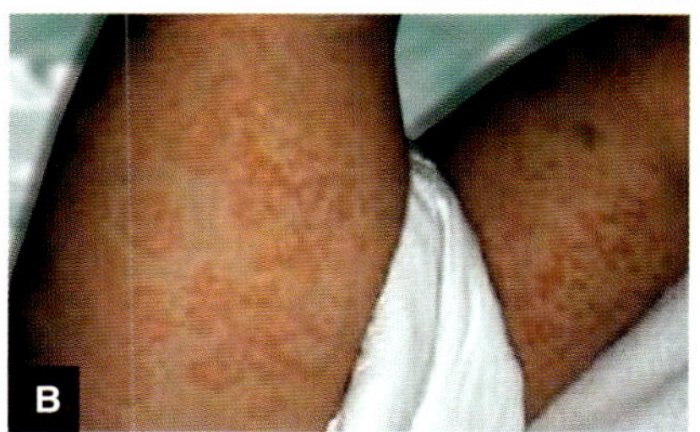 **Figures 2.1.6A and B:** Henoch-Schönlein purpura *Photo Courtesy*: SBP Singh, Begusarai	Note extensive purpuric spots over lower extremities (Figs 2.1.6A and B). Henoch-Schönlein purpura (HSP) is small vessel systemic vasculitis. Exact cause is not known. Palpable purpura, arthritis and abdominal pain are classic triad of HSP. Purpura typically appears on legs and buttock. There may be associated renal involvement in 40% cases. The disease is often preceded by viral infection such as pharyngitis.	• The diagnosis is usually clinical. Platelet count is normal. Rarely skin biopsy is required in doubtful cases. • The disease is self-limiting and requires no specific treatment apart from symptom control such as pain abdomen and joint pain. Steroids are generally avoided.

Picture	Note	Management

Herpes Zoster

Picture	Note	Management
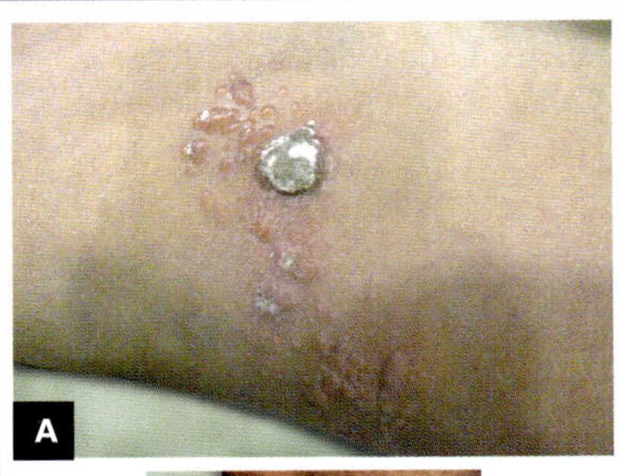 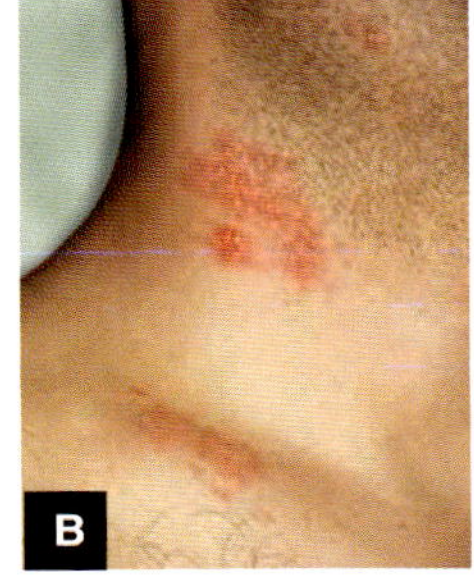 **Figures 2.1.7A and B:** Herpes zoster *Photo Courtesy*: Utpal Kant Singh, Patna	Note vesicular eruption and drying of rash with crust formation in chest and neck limited to one dermatome. Herpes zoster represents reactivation of latent varicella-zoster virus infection in the sensory nerve root ganglia, which persists after preceding varicella infection. Pain, itching, or paresthesia in a localized distribution may precede the skin eruption. Malaise, headache, and fever may precede and/or accompany the eruption. Individual lesions may appear as grouped erythematous papules or circumscribed erythematous patches that evolve to discreet grouped vesicles on an erythematous base. Vesicles may become cloudy pustules before rupturing and forming crusts (Figs 2.1.7A and B).	• The eruption is characteristically unilateral, following the distribution of 1–3 dermatomes. Thoracic dermatomes are most commonly involved in children followed by the ophthalmic branch of the trigeminal nerve. • Specific therapy is unnecessary in patients with mild symptoms and limited involvement. Topical antipruritics (menthol/camphor lotions) and oral antihistamines are useful for symptomatic relief of itching. • Antiviral therapy with acyclovir (oral or intravenous) is justified in any patient with more severe disease in immune compromised patients. • Ophthalmic zoster carries poor prognosis.

Janeway Lesion

Picture	Note	Management
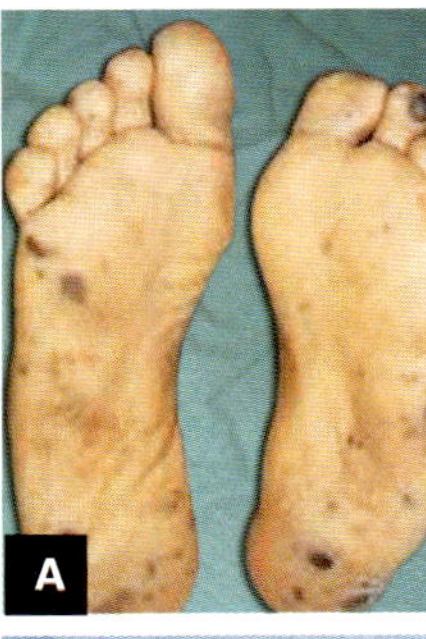 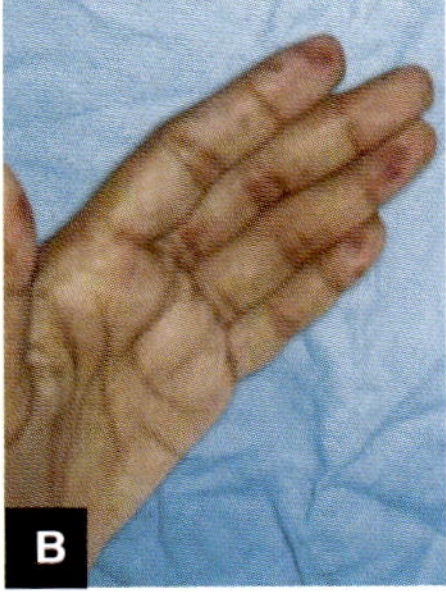 **Figures 2.1.8A and B:** Janeway lesion *Photo Courtesy*: Shyam Bihari, Biharsarif	Note erythematous and hemorrhagic rashes on palm and soles characteristic of infective endocarditis (Figs 2.1.8A and B). Infective endocarditis (IE) is often a complication of congenital or rheumatic heart disease but can occur in children without any abnormal valves or cardiac malformations. The lesions are painless. Bicuspid aortic valve is the common site for endocarditis to occur.	• Persistent fever with unexplained tachycardia and refractory cardiac failure are the pointer to the suspicion of IE. • Identification of IE is most often based on high index of suspicion during evolution of an infection in a child with an underlying contributory factor. • Appropriate antibiotic therapy based upon blood culture and sensitivity for 4–16 weeks is recommended.

Picture	Note	Management

Meningococcal Lesion

Picture	Note	Management
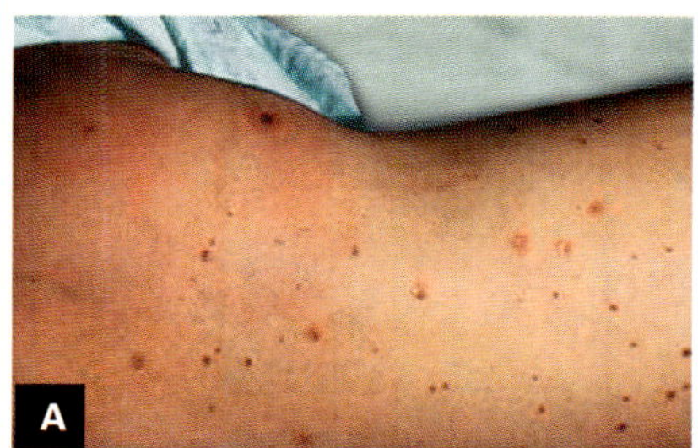 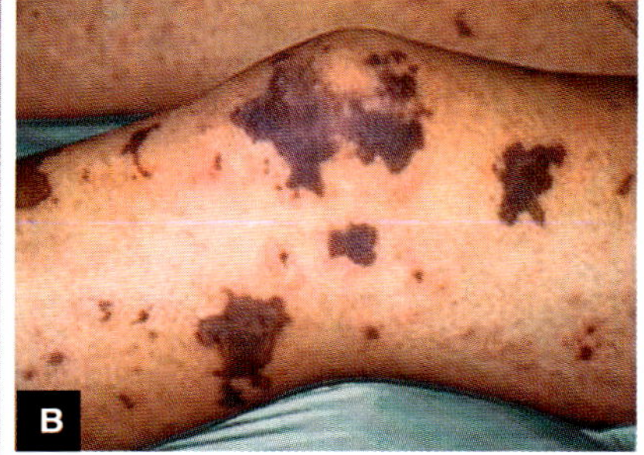 **Figures 2.1.9A and B:** Meningococcal lesion *Photo Courtesy*: Yugal Kishore Prasad, Sitamarhi	Note purpuric lesion with jagged edges in lower extremities is meningococcal lesion caused by *Neisseria meningitidis* (Figs 2.1.9A and B). Leading cause of bacterial meningitis in children, particularly infants younger than 12 months of age. Approximately two-thirds of patients with meningococcemia will develop cutaneous manifestations. At the outset, symptoms may mimic a viral illness (e.g. fever, myalgia, headache, malaise). Early finding in young children may include leg pain, cold hands and feet, and abnormal skin color. May have associated meningitis with headache, photophobia, vomiting, and nuchal rigidity with bulging fontanelle. Cutaneous findings initially are erythematous, urticarial, or morbilliform macules and papules, petechiae, pustules, and vesicles often develop along with purpuric lesions. Patients may develop profound hypotension and shock with overwhelming meningococcemia.	• Diagnosis is based on clinical finding and confirmed by culture of the blood and cerebrospinal fluid. • Supportive therapy including fluids and vasoactive agents is needed. Intravenous penicillin G is recommended at a dose of 250,000 U/kg per day up to a maximum of 12 million units per day divided every 4–6 hours. • Cefotaxime, ceftriaxone and ampicillin are acceptable alternatives.

Staphylococcal Scalded Skin Syndrome

Picture	Note	Management
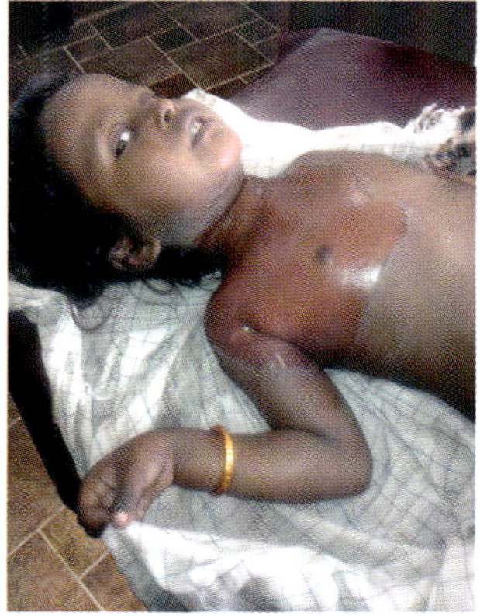 **Figure 2.1.10:** Staphylococcal scalded skin syndrome *Photo Courtesy*: Arun Shah, Muzaffarpur	Note large denuded area on upper part of trunk with erythematous base in a 5-year-old child (Fig. 2.1.10). Involvement of oral mucous membrane is absent. Staphylococcal scalded skin syndrome is caused by an exfoliative toxin produced by *Staphylococcus aureus*, most often from phage group II. The toxin is spread hematogenously from the primary site of infection; it causes a cleavage in the epidermis that leads to blister formation. Most often seen in children younger than 5 years of age. Patients present with generalized erythema, tender skin and irritability. Fever is occasionally, but not always present. Flaccid bullae form, bullae rapture easily and produce large eroded areas. Nikolsky sign is present.	• Treatment is systemic anti-staphylococcal antibiotic orally for mild cases. • Children with severe disease or who are toxic in appearance should receive parenteral antibiotics adequate to cover methicillin resistant *S. aureus* (e.g. clindamycin, vancomycin). • Proper hydration, nutrition and meticulous skin care along with anti-staphyloccal antibiotic are most important aspects of its successful treatment.

Picture	Note	Management

Toxic Epidermal Necrolysis

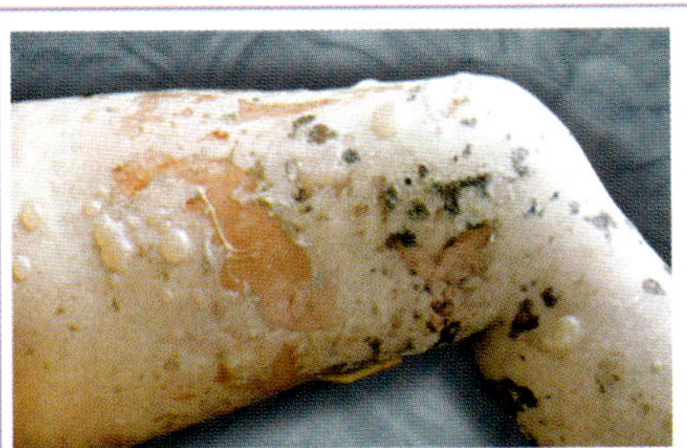 **Figure 2.1.11:** Toxic epidermal necrolysis *Photo Courtesy*: Braj Mohan, Muzaffarpur	Note wide spread bulla formation along with sloughing of skin in a 3-year-old child (Fig. 2.1.11). Toxic epidermal necrolysis (TEN), like Steven-Johnson syndrome and erythema multiforme are characterized by confluent epidermal necrosis with minimal associated inflammation. TEN is a severe potentially life threatening multisystem illness of sudden onset characterized by generalized tender erythematous skin with extensive bulla formation and loss of epidermis. More than 30% of body surface is affected. Most cases are due to drugs like antibiotics, anti-epileptics, sulfonamides and NSAID and antimetabolites like methotrexate.	• The first-line of treatment is early withdrawal of culprit drugs, early referral and management in burn or intensive care unit with supportive management, and nutritional support. • Treatment is symptomatic and supportive that includes maintenance of fluid and electrolyte balance, infection control, emollient over denuded area, topical antibiotics, parenteral antibiotics and intravenous immunotherapy may be considered. • Role of steroid is controversial. Intravenous immunoglobulin, plasmapheresis, cyclosporine, etc. are also suggested. • In severe leukopenia granulocyte colony stimulating factor is also used.

Picture	Note	Management

Toxic Shock Syndrome

Picture	Note	Management
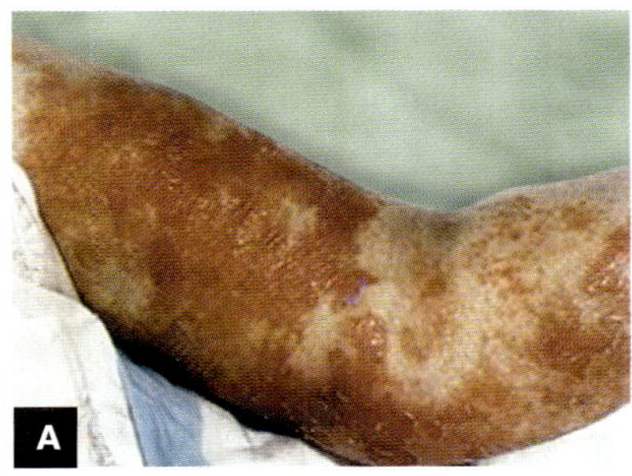 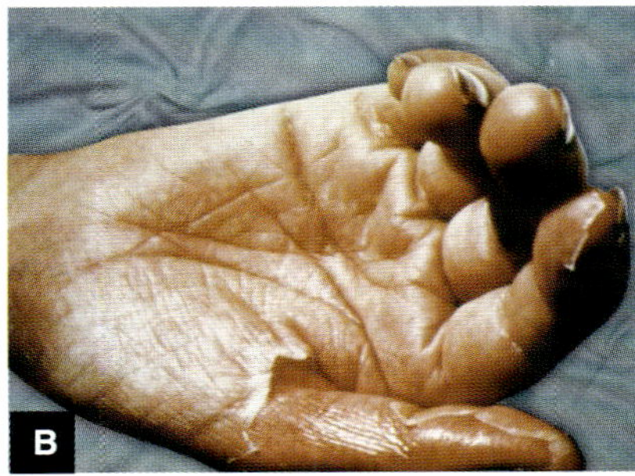 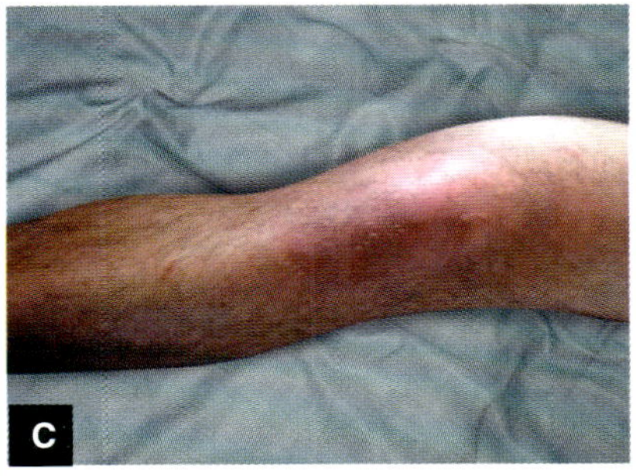 **Figures 2.1.12A to C:** Toxic shock syndrome *Photo Courtesy:* SA Krishna, Patna	Note diffuse macular erythematous lesions and exfoliation in hand and leg (Figs 2.1.12A to C). Toxic shock syndrome (TSS) is a constellation of symptoms including fever, rash, hypotension and multiorgan dysfunction. Caused by toxin-producing *S. aureus* or *S. pyogenes*. Case definition of TSS: definite diagnosis if all 6 criteria are present; probable diagnosis if 5 criteria are present. Fever, erythema (usually diffuse macular erythroderma), desquamation 1–2 weeks after the onset of the illness, particularly of the palms, soles, and digits, hypotension. Involvement of 3 or more of the following systems: gastrointestinal: vomiting or diarrhea, muscular: severe myalgia or CPK greater than twice normal, renal: sterile pyuria, blood urea nitrogen or creatinine greater than twice normal, hepatic: bilirubin, hepatic enzymes greater than twice the upper limit of normal, hematological: platelet count $\leq 100,000/mm^3$, central nervous system (disorientation, altered consciousness without focal neurologic signs). Mucocutaneous finding in TSS: erythema, conjunctival injection, necrolysis (necrosis with exfoliation), multiple pustules and desquamation. Symptoms of TSS vary depending on the underlying cause. TSS resulting from infection with the bacterium *S. aureus* typically manifests in otherwise healthy individuals. The characteristic rash, often seen early in the course of illness, resembles sunburn, and can involve any region of the body, including the lips, mouth, eyes, palms and soles. In patients who survive the initial phase of the infection, the rash desquamates, or peels off, after 10–14 days. In contrast, TSS caused by the bacterium *S. pyogenes,* or TSLS, typically presents in people with pre-existing skin infections with the bacteria. These individuals often experience severe pain at the site of the skin infection, followed by rapid progression of symptoms as described above for TSS. In contrast to TSS caused by *Staphylococcus*, streptococcal TSS less often involves a sunburn-like rash.	• Diagnosis is clinical and confirmed by a positive culture for *S. aureus* or other causative organism. • Supportive therapy including maintaining fluid status and use of vasoactive agents as necessary. Adequate drainage of suppurative sites or surgery with debridement for streptococcal TSS. • Specific therapy with antistaphylococcal antibiotic adequate to inhibit methicillin resistant *S. aureus* (e.g. vancomycin). Addition of clindamycin (which inhibits toxin synthesis) often is recommended. Use of immune globulin (intravenous) should be considered.

Picture	Note	Management

Urticaria

Picture	Note	Management
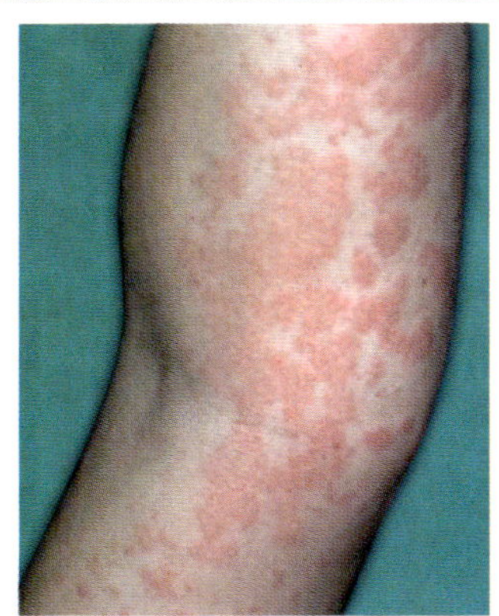 **Figure 2.1.13:** Urticaria *Photo Courtesy*: Arun Shah, Muzaffarpur	Note pink to red raised wheals of various size and shape (Fig. 2.1.13). Urticaria is common dermatological condition of childhood. It has abrupt onset following exposure to specific triggers of histamine release like infections, drugs, foods and physical factors like heat, cold, sun or water. The lesions appears pink to red raised wheals of variable size and shape. Lesions are transient usually resolving in few hours before reappearing in other locations. The rashes are associated with intense itching.	• Oral H_1 antihistamine is effective in symptomatic management of urticaria. Systemic corticosteroid represents second-line therapy for severe disease.

Herpetic Gingivostomatitis

Picture	Note	Management
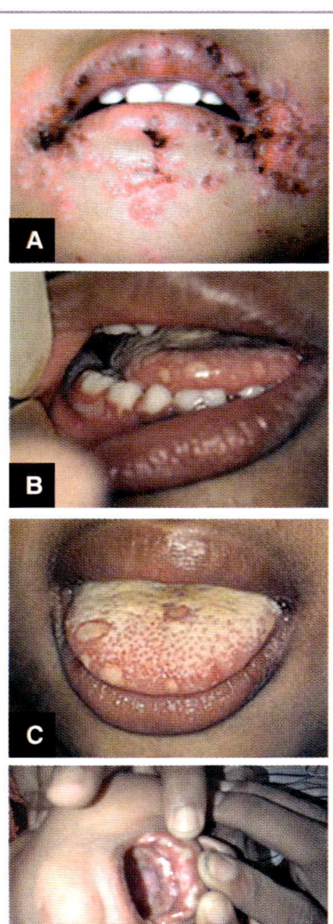 **Figures 2.1.14A to D:** Herpetic gingivostomatitis *Photo Courtesy*: Arun Shah, Muzaffarpur	Note vesiculo-pustular lesion covered with yellowish gray membrane affecting tongue, gum and perioral region (Figs 2.1.14A to D). Herpetic gingivostomatits is probably most common cause of stomatitis caused by herpes simplex virus (HSV) in children 1–3 years of age. It may occur in older children also. Symptoms start abruptly with pain in mouth, salivation, fetor oris, refusal to eat and high grade fever. Lesion primarily affects the anterior part of mouth. Fever and irritability may precede oral lesion by 1–2 days. Submaxillary lymphadenitis is common.	• It is a self-limited condition and requires only symptomatic and supportive treatment.

Picture	Note	Management

Systemic Lupus Erythematosus

Picture	Note	Management
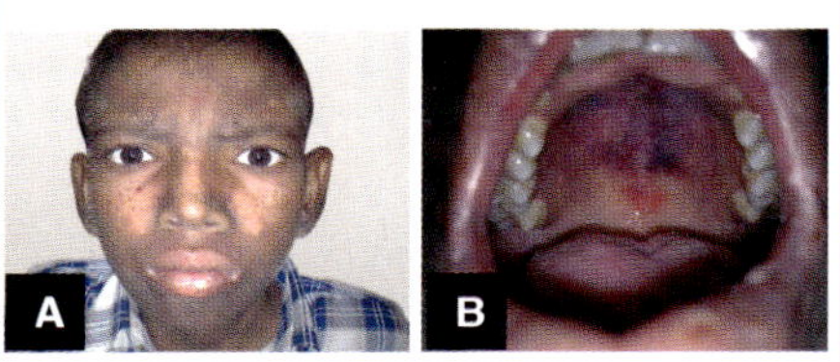 **Figures 2.1.15A and B:** Systemic lupus erythematosus *Photo Courtesy*: Sanjata Roy Chaudhary, Patna	Note hypopigmented lesion over face and ulcer with erythematous rash over hard palate and soft palate (Figs 2.1.15A and B). Systemic lupus erythematosus (SLE) is an autoimmune connective tissue disease characterized by unpredictable course with periods of flares and remission. More common in girls between 3–15 years of age. The exact cause is not known. Environmental triggers have been implicated along with genetic predisposition. The disease affects predominantly skin, joint, kidney, heart, lung and nervous system.	• Diagnosis is usually made by criteria's laid down by American College of Rheumatology. Positive antinuclear antibody test has 99% sensitivity and 49% specificity. • The treatment aims to induce remission, prevent flare ups and reduce the severity and duration of symptoms when they occur. Drugs include NSAID, steroids, hydroxychloroquine and immunosuppressives.

Aplastic Anemia

Picture	Note	Management
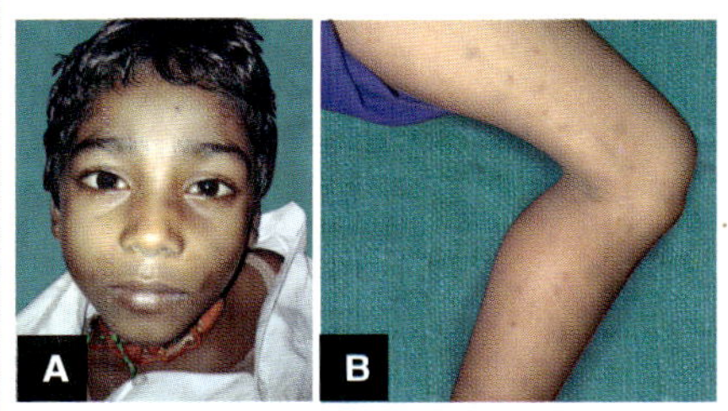 **Figures 2.1.16A and B:** Aplastic anemia *Photo Courtesy*: Arun Shah, Muzaffarpur	Note marked pallor and petechial spots on face and legs in a 8-year-old child (Figs 2.1.16A and B). The child presented with prolonged fever, pallor, petechial spots and bleeding from nose. Most cases of aplastic anemia are idiopathic. The disease may be caused by exposure to various drugs, insecticides and infectious agents. Clinical examination showed severe anemia, cutaneous bleeding, no organomegaly and no lymphadenopathy. Peripheral blood smear exam demonstrated pancytopenia with reticulocytopenia. Bone marrow examination revealed hypoplasia of marrow.	• Supportive care with repeated blood transfusion, control of infection with broad spectrum antibiotics. • Bone marrow transplantation offers 90% chance of long-term survival with incorporation of antithymocyte globulin, cyclophosphamide and hematopoietic colony stimulating factor.

Post Kala-Azar Dermal Leishmaniasis

Picture	Note	Management
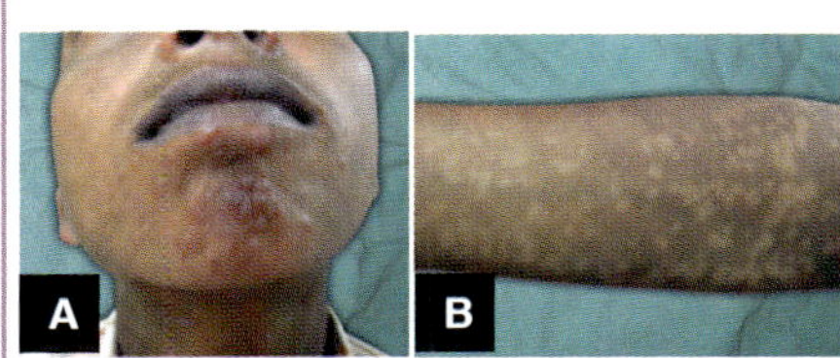 **Figures 2.1.17A and B:** Post kala-azar dermal leishmaniasis *Photo Ccurtesy*: Arun Shah, Muzaffarpur	Note nodular eruptions on face of a patient and hypopigmented macular lesion in hand in another patient (Figs 2.1.17A and B). Post kala-azar dermal leishmaniasis (PKDL) is late onset complication of visceral leishmaniasis characterized by macular, maculopapular or nodular eruption in a patient who has recovered from kala-azar. It occurs in 5–10% treated cases of VL. These patients act as reservoir for parasites. The pathogenesis of the disease is due to persistence of parasites (LD bodies) in skin and largely immune mediated.	• Diagnosis is made by history of kala-azar in past, positive rapid immunochromatographic test rK 39, and confirmed by demonstration of LD bodies in skin scrap. • Treatment is with parenteral administration of sodium stibogluconate for 3 months. Alternatively Amphotericin B is recommended in resistant cases.

Picture	Note	Management

Conjunctivitis with Coryza

Picture	Note	Management
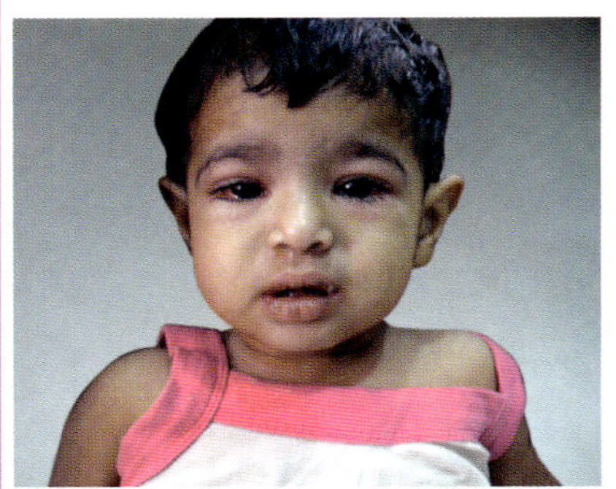 **Figure 2.1.18A:** Conjunctivitis with coryza *Photo Courtesy*: Ketan H Shah, Surat	A one-and-half-year-old female with history of cough, cold and fever (Fig. 2.1.18A). She had respiratory distress. Photo shows conjunctivitis with coryza.	• The features are nonspecific for any viral disease, but looking to respiratory distress and high fever, with normal count, it likely represents adenoviral disease. • X-ray chest shown in Figure 2.1.18B.
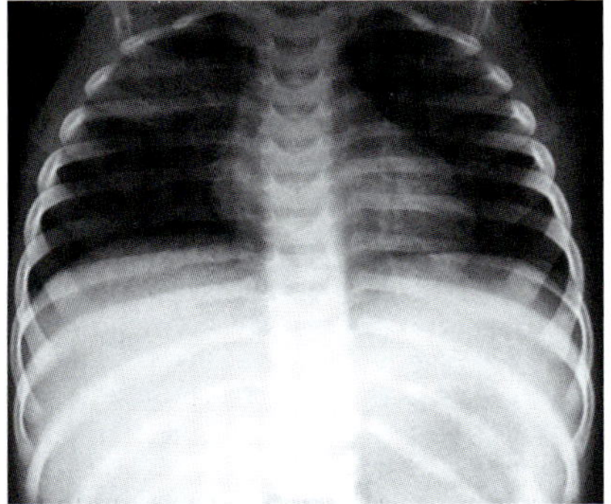 **Figure 2.1.18B:** Lobar consolidation *Photo Courtesy*: Ketan H Shah, Surat	X-ray of same child showing lobar consolidation (Fig. 2.1.18B).	• Lobar consolidation with conjunctivitis and coryza likely represent adenoviral disease. • Management includes symptomatic treatment.

Classical Rash of Dengue Fever

Picture	Note	Management
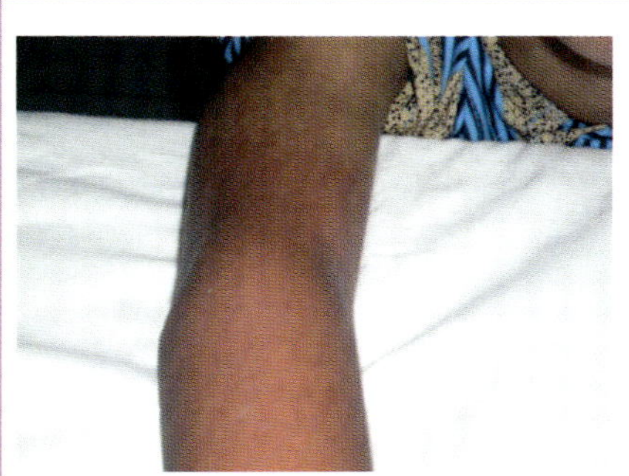 **Figure 2.1.19:** Classical rash of dengue fever *Photo Courtesy*: Ketan H Shah, Surat	It shows red flushing of upper limb (Fig. 2.1.19). With occasional white area. These are classical rash of dengue fever, called as "isles of white in the sea of red".	• Dengue fever is very common entity. Its clinical features are fever, headache, bodyache and rash. Rash usually appears on 3rd–5th days of disease. • Different types of rash can be seen. Macular, flush, petechial and morbilliform. It may be pruritic rash.

Picture	Note	Management

Petechial Spots on Lower Limb with Occasional Macules

Picture	Note	Management
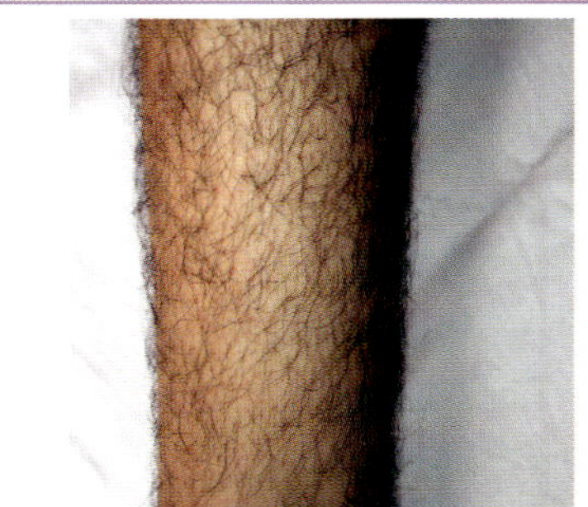 **Figure 2.1.20:** Petechial spots on lower limb with occasional macules *Photo Courtesy*: Ketan H Shah, Surat	It shows petechial spots on lower limb with occasional macules (Fig. 2.1.20). Child had fever for 5–6 days and bodyache. On 6th day of fever blood reports show low platelet count. Rash and petechial spots developed on 6th day of disease.	These are findings of dengue fever. Low platelet count needs attention. Child may go for shock or may not. These findings are seen in critical phase of the disease.

Measles Rash

Picture	Note	Management
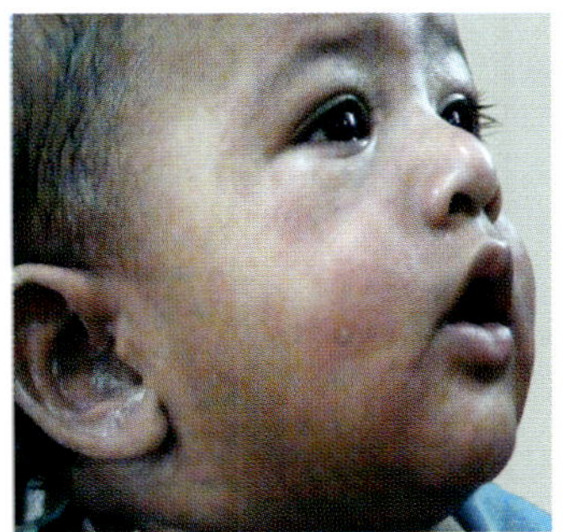 **Figure 2.1.21:** Measles rash *Photo Courtesy*: Ketan H Shah, Surat	A 10-month-old child with fever and rash, cough, coryza and Koplik spot. Figure 2.1.21 shows macular eruption with flush and occasional dry area on ears. Conjunctival congestion is also seen.	These are rash of measles. Measles is highly contagious. Child was not vaccinated. All three siblings in family developed measles. It needs symptomatic treatment and vitamin A supplement. We need to watch for complications, like secondary pneumonia and flaring of underlying Koch's.

Black Discoloration and Hyperpigmentation

Picture	Note	Management
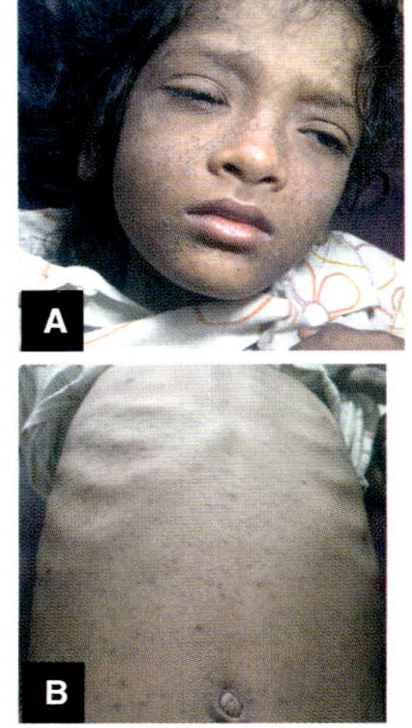 **Figures 2.1.22A and B:** Black discoloration and hyperpigmentation *Photo Courtesy*: Arun Shah, Muzaffarpur	It shows black discoloration and hyperpigmentation (Figs 2.1.22A and B). It usually occurs after 10–12 days of disease and may persist for long time.	Measles in recovery phase can leave behind black discoloration and hyperpigmentation. Recovery starts with disappearance of fever and gradually subsiding rash. It leaves behind black discoloration.

Picture	Note	Management

Erythematous Changes on Sole and Tip of the Toe

Picture	Note	Management
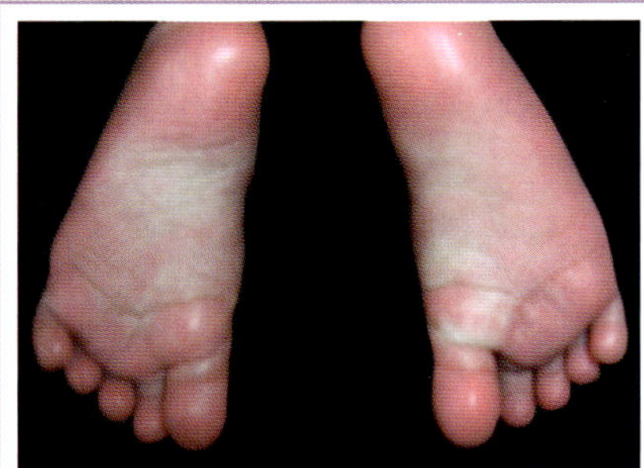 **Figure 2.1.23:** Erythematous changes on sole and tip of the toe *Photo Courtesy*: Ananda Kesavan, Thrissur	Child had fever with rash on body during monsoon season. Figure 2.1.23 shows erythematous changes on sole and tip of the toe. Edema of the foot is also seen.	In monsoon season, it likely represents chikungunya fever. At the onset of the disease, child will have high fever and toxic look. Rash appears with fever and it may persist for 3–5 days. Different types of rashes may develop.

Red Ear Due to Chikungunya Fever

Picture	Note	Management
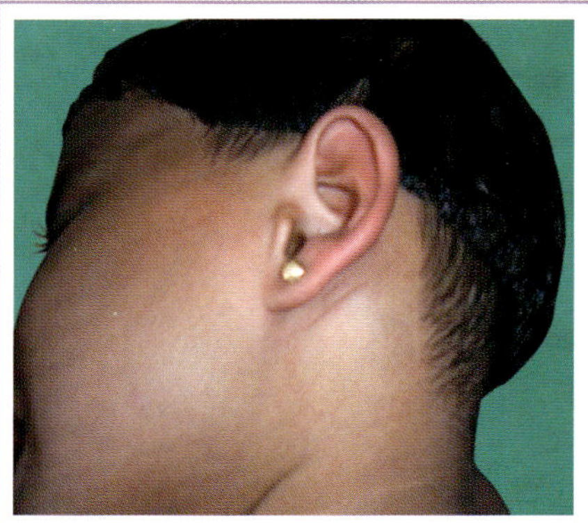 **Figure 2.1.24:** Red ear due to chikungunya fever *Photo Courtesy*: Ananda Kesavan, Thrissur	Figure 2.1.24 shows red ear.	This is also one important finding of chikungunya fever. However not specific, but along with other manifestation, it can be pointer toward the disease.

Freckle-like Pigmentation at Recovery

Picture	Note	Management
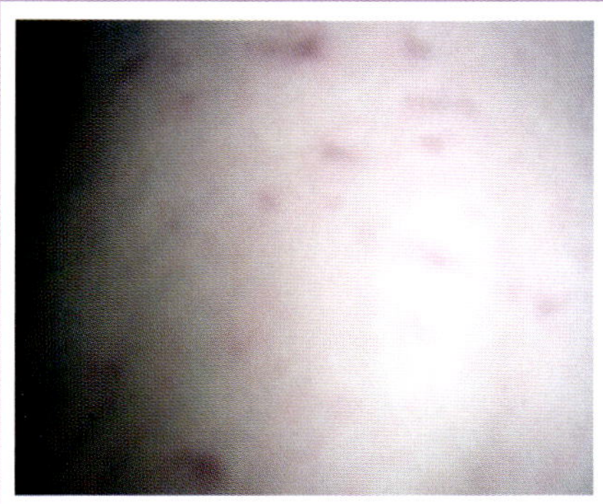 **Figure 2.1.25:** Freckle-like pigmentation at recovery *Photo Courtesy*: Ananda Kesavan, Thrissur	Same patient had developed Freckle-like pigmentation at recovery (Fig. 2.1.25).	This is also seen in chikungunya disease. It may persist for 3–4 months. It is sometimes pruritic.

Picture	Note	Management

Multiple Purpurae with Blueberry Muffin Rash

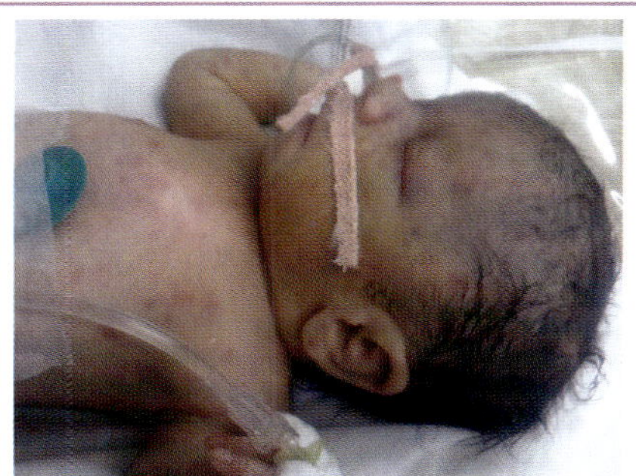 **Figure 2.1.26:** Multiple purpurae with blueberry muffin rash *Photo Courtesy*: Ananda Kesavan, Thrissur	Figure 2.1.26 shows multiple purpurae with blueberry muffin rash. Child is 2 months old. Child had recurrent cough cold and respiratory distress. Child had cataract and murmur.	These are findings of congenital rubella syndrome. Mother had history of fever with rash at 6 weeks of pregnancy. Congenital rubella syndrome (CRS) needs symptomatic treatment and it leaves behind life-long sequel.

Pale Rose Red Blanching Macules and Papules on the Palm

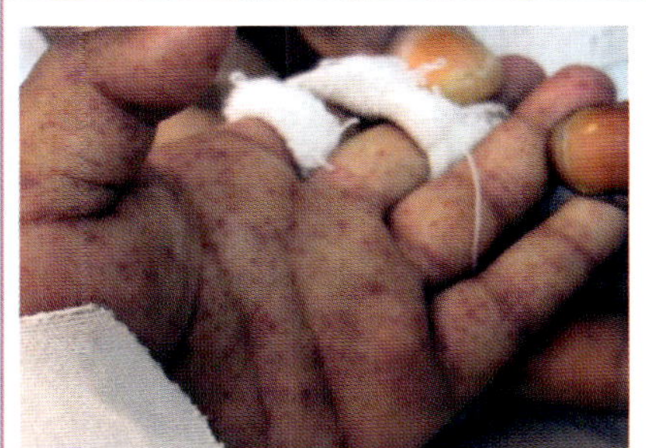 **Figure 2.1.27:** Pale rose red blanching macules and papules on the palm *Photo Courtesy*: Atul Kulkarni, Solapur	Figure 2.1.27 shows pale rose red blanching macules and papules on the palm. Rash appeared on 3rd–4th day of fever. It has affected ankle, wrist and lower limbs. Later, rash spreads rapidly to involve the entire body including palms and soles. After several days, the rash has become more petechial, sometimes with palpable purpura. Petechiae may enlarge into ecchymosis.	These are features of rickettsial disease. Initially the illness appears to be nonspecific. It may present with headache, fever, anorexia, myalgia and restlessness. Calf muscle pain and tenderness are common in children. Gastrointestinal symptoms include nausea, vomiting, and diarrhea may be present. Skin rash is usually not present until after 2–4 days of illness. The typical triad of fever, headache and rash is observed in 44% of patients. Headache is severe, unremitting and usually unresponsive to analgesics.

Vasculitis with Gangrenous Changes in Same Patient of Rickettsia

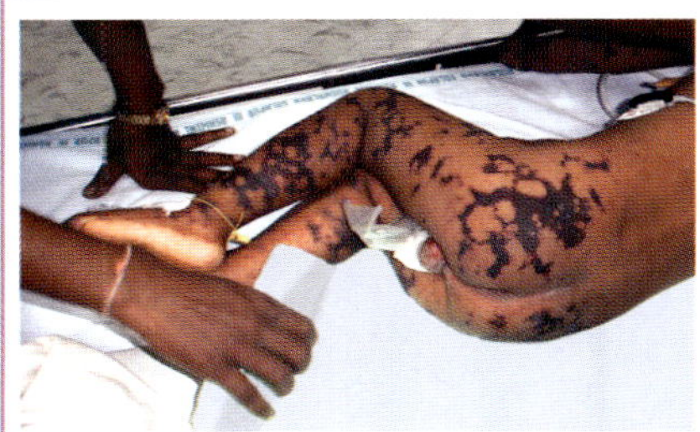 **Figure 2.1.28:** Vasculitis with gangrenous changes in same patient of rickettsia *Photo Courtesy*: Atul Kulkarni, Solapur	Figure 2.1.28 shows vasculitis with gangrenous changes in same patient of rickettsia.	Severe vaso-occlusive disease secondary to rickettsial vasculitis and thrombosis is infrequent but can result in gangrene of the digits, toes, earlobes, scrotum, nose or entire limbs. Painless eschar, the tache noire, may be seen at the initial site of tick attachment and regional lymphadenopathy.

Section 3

Respiratory Tract Infections

Section Editors

S Nagabhushana, Devaraj Raichur

Contributors

H Paramesh, Pramod G Shanbagh, T Sujatha, CR Femine, TA Shepur, Devaraj Raichur, Rajendra V Naidu, Prakash Wari, Vinod H Ratageri, SR Fattepur, Bhavna Koppad, Shaila M Sankeshwar, Suvarna P Reddy, KB Shashikiran, NC Gowrishankar, Muralinath, Maniramakrishna

Section Outline

3.1 Upper Respiratory Tract Infections

- Membranous Tonsillopharyngitis due to *Klebsiella Pneumoniae*
- Pansinusitis—Sphenoidal, Frontal, Maxillary Sinusitis—CT Paranasal Sinuses
- Oral Candidiasis
- Croup Syndrome
- Retropharyngeal Abscess
- Epiglottitis
- Pertussis with Subconjunctival Hemorrhage

3.2 Lower Respiratory Tract Infections

- Round Pneumonia
- Thymus
- Consolidation: Left Lower Lobe
- Consolidation: Right Upper Lobe
- Unilateral Hilar Lymphadenopathy
- Chest Indrawing
- Acute Bronchiolitis
- Acute Bronchiolitis with Segmental Collapse of the Left Lower Lobe
- Bronchiolitis with Multiple Atelectatic/ Pneumonic Patches
- Wheeze Associated Lower Respiratory Infection
- Viral Croup with WALRI
- Pneumomediastinum with Surgical Emphysema in WALRI
- Pneumomediastinum with Surgical Emphysema in WALRI-Clinical Profile
- Collapse-Consolidation RUL
- Collapse-Consolidation RUL in GB Syndrome with Palatopharyngeal Paralysis
- Parapneumonic Effusion—Left
- Dengue Fever with Right Pleural Effusion
- Empyema Left Side—Soft Tissue Bulge
- Empyema Right Side
- Measles with Right-Sided Empyema
- Pulmonary Tuberculosis
- Cavitary Tuberculosis with Necrotizing Bronchopneumonia
- HIV with Tuberculosis
- HIV with *Pneumocystis jiroveci (carinii)* Pneumonia—Early
- HIV with *Pneumocystis jiroveci (carinii)* Pneumonia—Late
- Lung Abscess with Bronchopneumonia
- Lung Abscess with Right-Middle-Lobe Consolidation
- Staphylococcal Pneumonia
- Congenital Pneumonia
- Calcified Hilar Node—Tuberculosis
- Multiple Cysts Left Side
- Mass Lesion in Right Hemithorax
- Pneumonia both Lower Lobes
- Pneumonia with Parapneumonic Effusion
- Tension Pneumothorax with Pneumatoceles with Subcutaneous Emphysema
- Postcardiac Repair State—Atelectasis both Lower Lobes Endobronchial Tuberculosis

3.1 UPPER RESPIRATORY TRACT INFECTIONS

Membranous Tonsillopharyngitis due to *Klebsiella Pneumoniae*

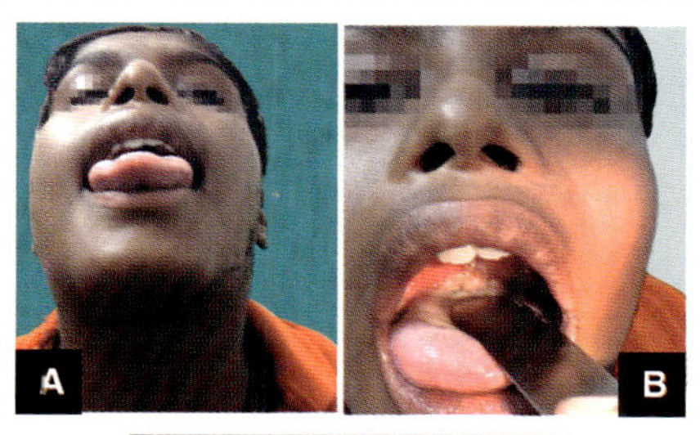

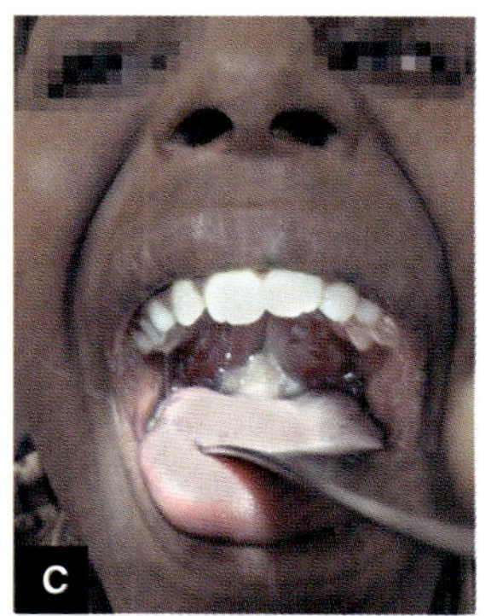

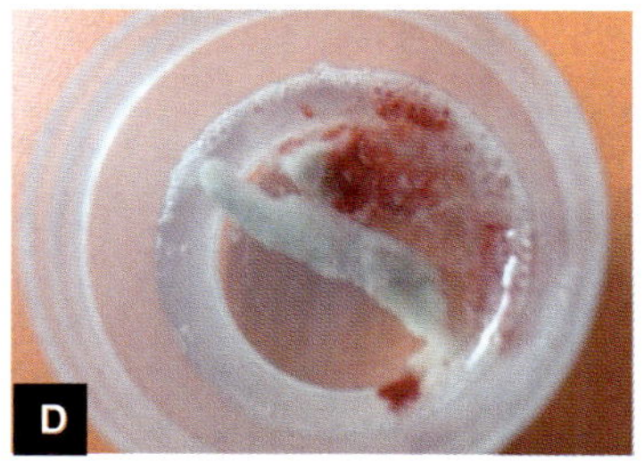

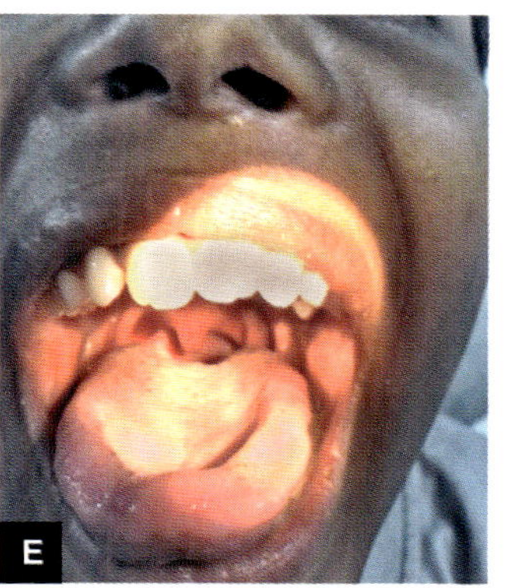

Figures 3.1.1A to E: (A) Bull neck with cervical lymphadenopathy; (B) Membranous tonsillopharyngitis; (C) Membranous tonsillopharyngitis; (D) Coughed up membranes; (E) Complete recovery
Photo Courtesy: Pramod G Shanbagh, T Sujatha, Bengaluru

Membranous tonsillopharyngitis due to *Klebsiella pneumoniae*, associated with bull neck and cervical lymphadenopathy, in a previously immunocompetent and fully immunized child is rare and can cause severe obstructive breathing or respiratory arrest (Figs 3.1.1A to E).

Investigations should rule out diphtheria, HIV/immunodeficiency. Throat swab helps to identify the pathogen and treatment may be optimized based on sensitivity. Early recognition of risk of obstructive breathing is vital. Tracheostomy may be required to relieve severe obstructive symptoms. Treatment includes steroids to relieve inflammatory swelling of upper airways and a prolonged course of antibiotics based on sensitivity. Elective tonsillectomy must be done at a later date.

Picture	Note	Management

Pansinusitis—Sphenoidal, Frontal, Maxillary Sinusitis—CT Paranasal Sinuses

Picture	Note	Management
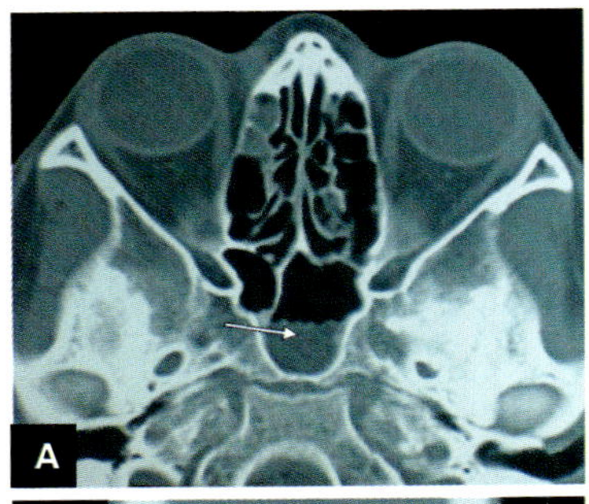 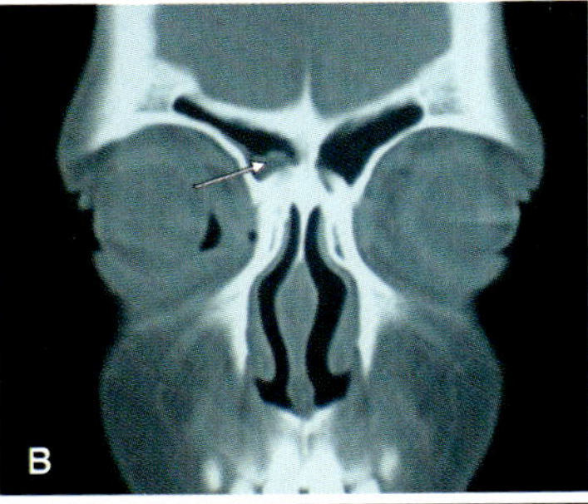 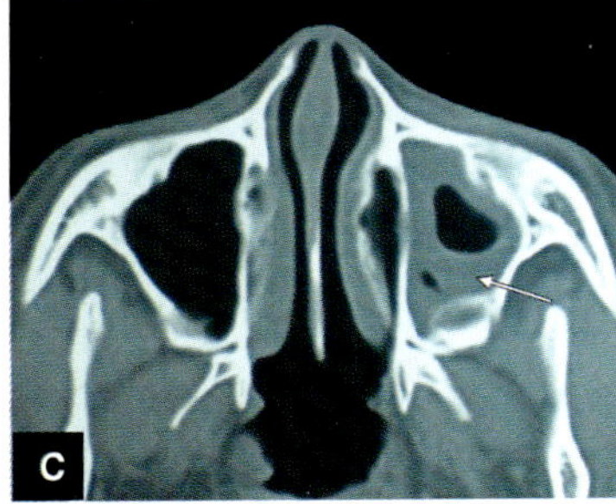 **Figures 3.1.2A to C:** Pansinusitis—sphenoidal, frontal, maxillary sinusitis—CT paranasal sinuses *Photo Courtesy*: NC Gowrishankar, Chennai	Most often the diagnosis is clinical and should be suspected when the "usual" viral cold does not subside, instead worsens by the end of first week. Occasionally, the onset may be dramatic and explosive. CT is a reliable tool for confirmation (Figs 3.1.2A to C).	Symptomatic treatment, appropriate antibiotics and care of precipitating factor is the mainstay of therapy.

Oral Candidiasis

Picture	Note	Management
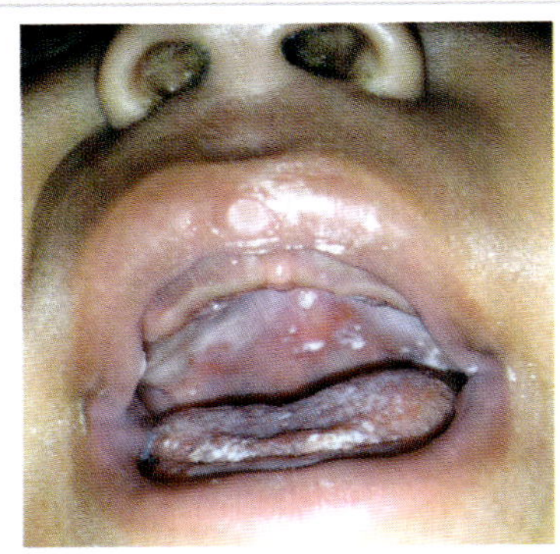 **Figure 3.1.3:** Oral candidiasis *Photo Courtesy*: CR Femine, Bengaluru	• White patches on mucous membrane of tongue and palate are seen. • Removal of the patches may lead to punctuate bleeding. • Common after prolonged antibiotic therapy and in immunodeficiency (Fig. 3.1.3).	Treatment is with local antifungal agents like clotrimazole, miconazole, nystatin or gentian violet.

Picture	Note	Management

Croup Syndrome

Picture	Note	Management
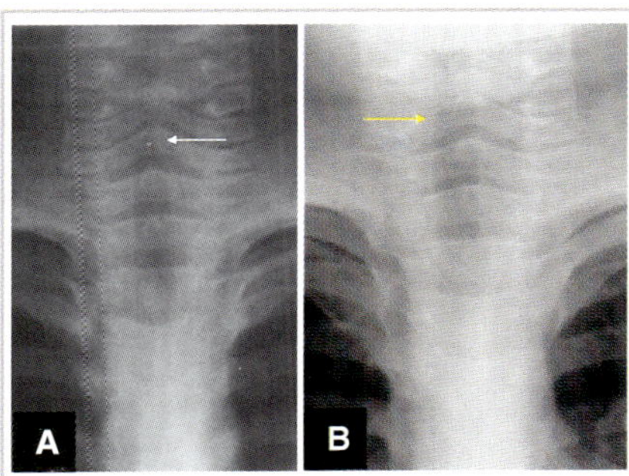 **Figures 3.1.4A and B:** "Steeple Sign" of viral croup (white arrow) and its disappearance 24 hours after (yellow arrow) treatment with nebulized adrenaline and budesonide *Photo Courtesy*: Devaraj Raichur, Shaila M Sankeshwar, Hubli	Diagnosed by barking cough with inspiratory stridor and hoarse voice preceded by cold with fever. In the X-ray, narrowing of the airway in the subglottic region is seen. After one dose of nebulized adrenaline, symptomatic relief was obtained and in the X-ray taken after 24 hours, the subglottic airway has normal width (Fig. 3.1.4A). Nebulized budesonide is often effective in viral croup (Fig. 3.1.4B).	• Comfortable position • Humidified oxygen • Mist therapy • Nebulized adrenaline (5 mL, 1:1,000 solution) in moderate to severe respiratory distress • Dexamethasone [0.6 mg/kg PO (preferred), IV or IM; single dose] • Nebulized budesonide

Retropharyngeal Abscess

Picture	Note	Management
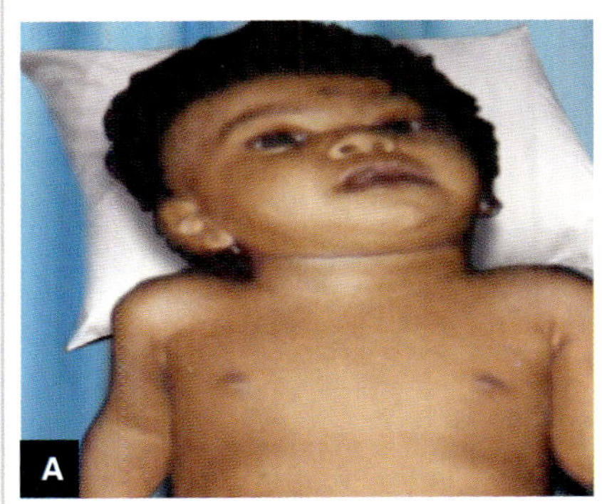 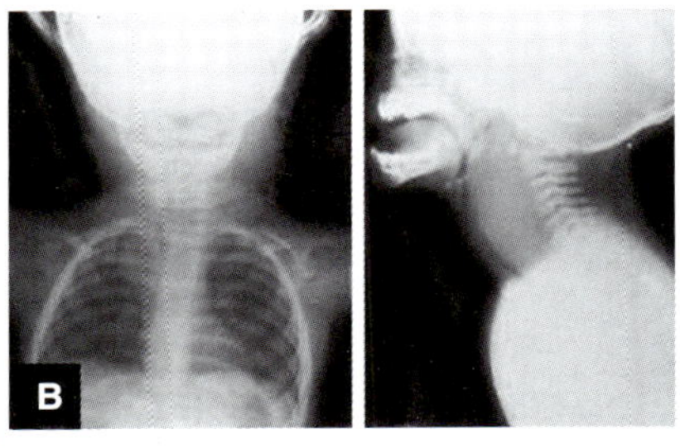 **Figures 3.1.5A and B:** (A) Retropharyngeal abscess; (B) X-ray neck (AP and lateral) *Photo Courtesy*: H Paramesh, Bengaluru	Note the extended neck with widening and opening of the mouth (Fig. 3.1.5A). Clinically child will have inspiratory stridor and drooling of saliva. Lateral neck X-ray shows widening of the retropharyngeal space. Acute retropharyngeal abscess common in young children. AP view of X-ray shows widening of the neck and extending to superior mediastinum on the right side (Fig. 3.1.5B). Lateral view shows widening of retropharyngeal space and bowing of tracheal air column. Note normal retropharyngeal space and thumb sign at epiglottic area.	Treatment is IV antibiotics and surgical drainage.

Picture	Note	Management

Epiglottitis

Picture	Note	Management
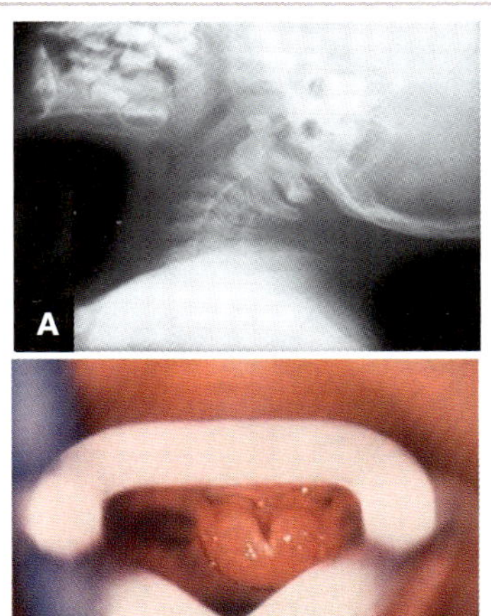 **Figures 3.1.6A and B:** (A) Lateral neck X-ray; (B) Cherry red swollen epiglottis *Photo Courtesy*: H Paramesh, Bengaluru	Note, cherry red swollen epiglottis (Fig. 3.1.6B).	When epiglottitis is suspected please take the lateral neck X-ray in an extended neck position while keeping things ready for an artificial airway (Fig. 3.1.6A). Do not disturb the quiet child. *Treatment*: Antibiotics and artificial airway for 2–3 days.

Pertussis with Subconjunctival Hemorrhage

Picture	Note	Management
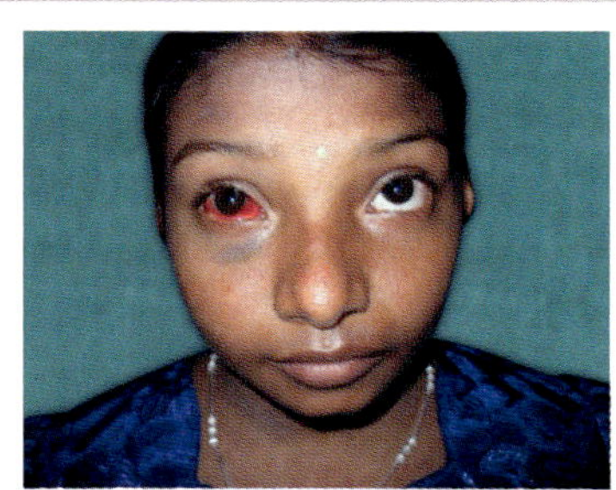 **Figure 3.1.7:** Pertussis with subconjunctival hemorrhage *Photo Courtesy*: NC Gowrishankar, Chennai	Subconjunctival hemorrhage is a complication in pertussis due to venous pressure changes occurring during the violent coughs (Fig. 3.1.7).	Macrolides are given mainly to limit the spread of the infection and for possible clinical benefit. Isolation may help to limit the spread of the infection.

3.2 LOWER RESPIRATORY TRACT INFECTIONS

Round Pneumonia

Picture	Note	Management
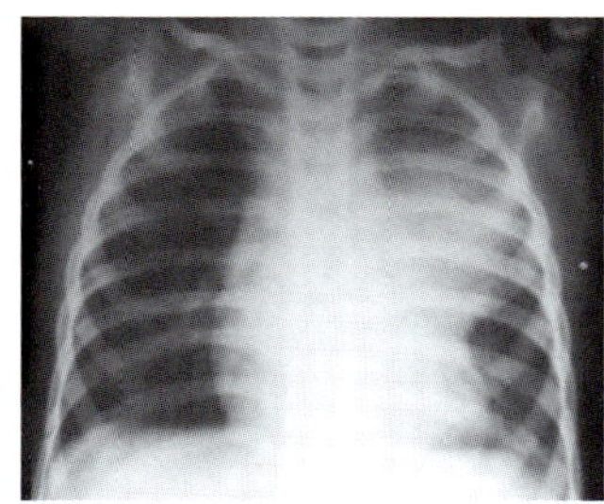 **Figure 3.2.1:** Round pneumonia *Photo Courtesy*: Muralinath, Maniramakrishna, Chennai	The chest radiograph demonstrates a round pneumonia of the left upper zone (Fig. 3.2.1). Most children present with typical features of pneumonia (high-grade fever, chest pain and cough with bronchial breathing and leukocytosis with elevated acute phase reactants). Most round pneumonias are believed to be caused by *Pneumococcus*.	Most children with round pneumonia respond dramatically to antibiotics. Amoxicillin is the drug of choice. Radiological clearance typically occurs by 2–3 weeks.

Picture	Note	Management

Thymus

Picture	Note	Management
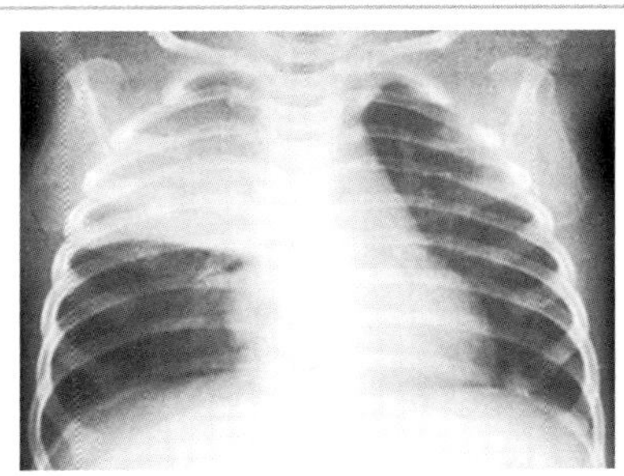 **Figure 3.2.2:** Thymus *Photo Courtesy*: Muralinath, Chennai	A 4-month-old child had fever and cough for 2 days. Clinical examination showed mild tachypnea with no respiratory distress and occasional crepitations bilaterally. SpO_2 was 94% in room air. The X-ray shows normal heart, lungs and thymic shadow on the right side. The thymus is notorious for mimicking pathology. It can assume any size or shape and can be present even in older children (Fig. 3.2.2). One should be alert to the absence of thymus as it might indicate a T-cell immunodeficiency.	Thymus can be differentiated by the characteristic sail sign caused by the interdigitation of the soft thymic shadow in the intercostal spaces. A lateral X-ray may help to identify the scalloped thymus outline. Most often, the diagnosis is clinical; in case of doubt, an ultrasound will settle the issue.

Consolidation: Left Lower Lobe

Picture	Note	Management
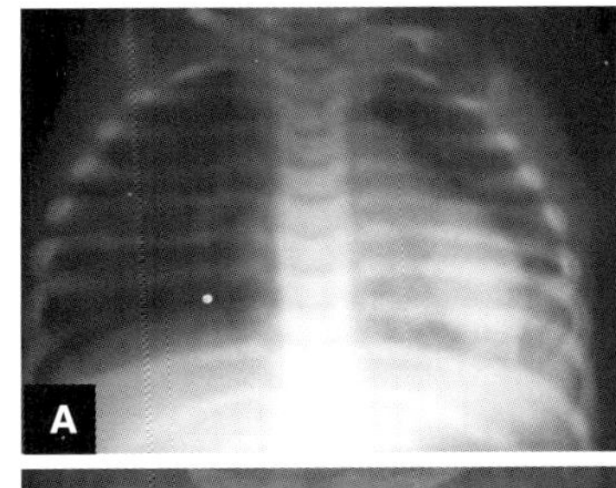 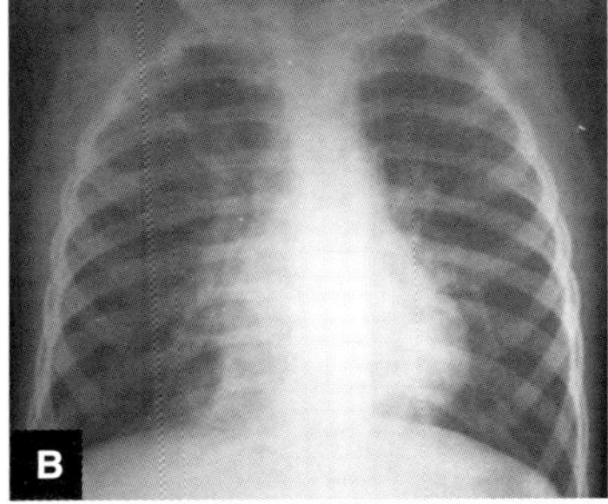 **Figures 3.2.3A and B:** (A) Left lower lobe consolidation; (B) Para-hilar, peri-bronchial infiltrates and subsegmental atelectasis *Photo Courtesy*: Muralinath, Chennai	The first picture shows consolidation of the left lower lobe (Fig. 3.2.3A). Lobar consolidation is typical of air-space pathogens (usually bacteria). The second picture shows parahilar, peribronchial infiltrates and subsegmental atelectasis (Fig. 3.2.3B). Such a picture is consistent with airway pathogens such as viruses and atypical organisms including *Mycoplasma*.	The treatment will depend on the clinical correlation. The choice of the antibiotic in lobar consolidation will depend on the age of the child and the severity of presentation as well as the presence or absence of risk factors. Atypical organisms are more common after the age of 5 years. It would be prudent to look out for extrapulmonary manifestations which will strengthen the clinical suspicion. Serology to diagnose *Mycoplasma* may be helpful. Macrolides are the drug of choice in *Mycoplasma* pneumonia.

Picture	Note	Management

Consolidation: Right Upper Lobe

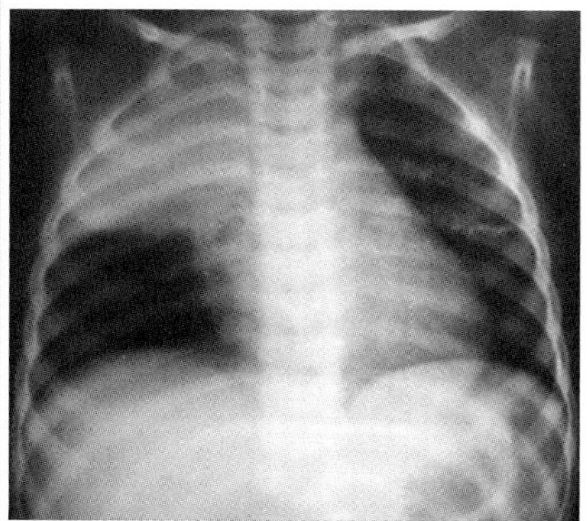 **Figure 3.2.4:** Consolidation of the right upper lobe *Photo Courtesy*: Muralinath, Chennai	The X-ray shows a child with consolidation of the right upper lobe taken (Fig. 3.2.4).	The child was initially treated with IV antibiotics and later with oral antibiotics for a period of 14 days. Clinical improvement precedes radiological clearance. It usually takes 3–4 weeks for radiological normalization. Repeat X-rays are not usually indicated unless warranted clinically.

Unilateral Hilar Lymphadenopathy

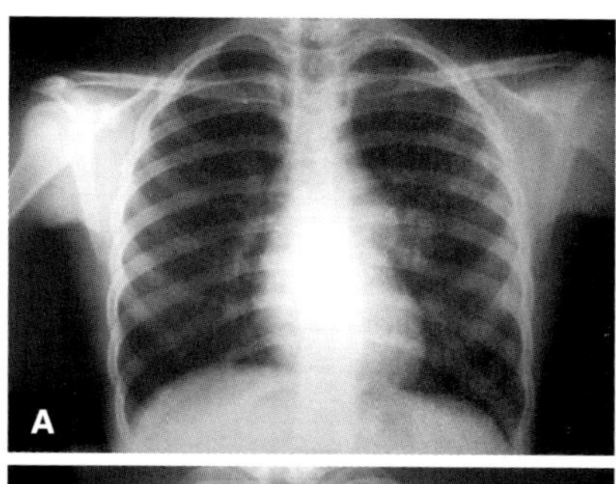 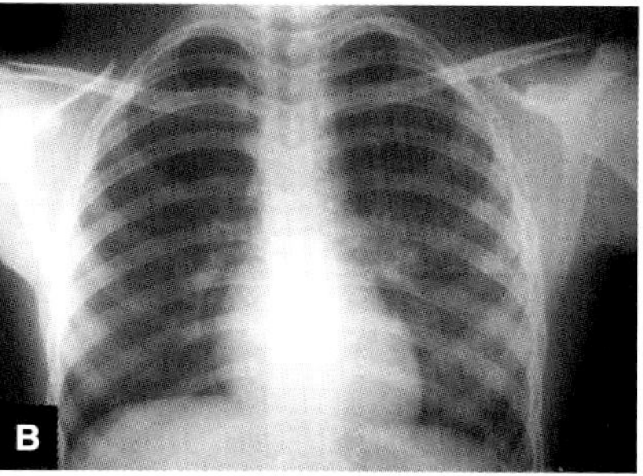 **Figures 3.2.5A and B:** Unilateral hilar lymphadenopathy *Photo Courtesy*: Muralinath, Maniramakrishna, Chennai	The X-ray on the left shows left hilar adenopathy which has regressed in size following treatment for 2 months. Unilateral hilar adenopathy in our country is primary pulmonary tuberculosis unless proved otherwise. It is usually smooth and discrete. Occasionally hilar lymphadenopathy may have other causes like lymphoma, sarcoidosis or histiocytosis (Figs 3.2.5A and B).	Confirmation of the diagnosis of tuberculosis is important before starting antituberculous treatment. In the RNTCP, sputum microscopy is the primary tool for detection of the infectious agent. For childhood TB, under the RNTCP, the diagnosis is based on a combination of clinical presentation, sputum examination wherever possible, chest X-ray (PA view), Mantoux test (1 TU PPD RT23 with Tween 80, positive if induration more than 10 mm after 48-72 hours) and history of contact. All efforts should be made to demonstrate bacteriological evidence in the diagnosis of pediatric TB. In cases where sputum is not available for examination or sputum microscopy fails to demonstrate AFB, alternative specimens (gastric lavage, induced sputum, bronchoalveolar lavage) should be collected, depending upon the feasibility, under the supervision of a pediatrician.

Picture	Note	Management

Chest Indrawing

Picture	Note	Management
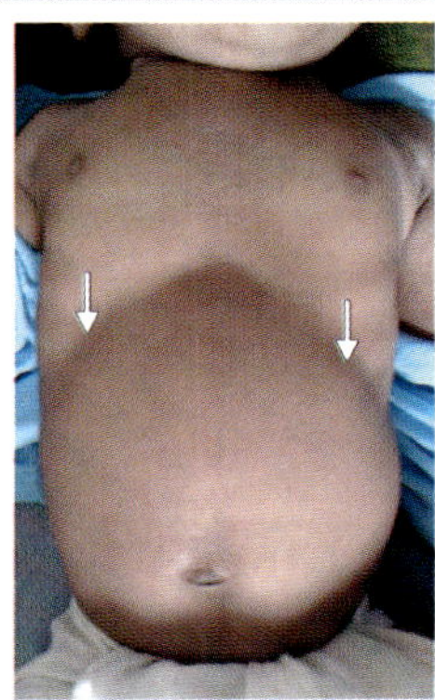 **Figure 3.2.6:** Chest indrawing *Photo Courtesy*: Devaraj Raichur, Hubli	Chest indrawing (subcostal retractions) is seen [arrows (Fig. 3.2.6)]. As of WHO criteria for the management of acute respiratory infections, in the presence of fast-breathing, chest indrawing indicates severe pneumonia.	• Assess airway, breathing and circulations (ABCs). • Warm, humidified oxygen inhalation. • Assisted ventilation if needed. • An effort should be made to find the cause of the respiratory distress. • Broad spectrum antibacterials for pneumonia, till culture and sensitivity reports allow specific antibacterials.

Acute Bronchiolitis

Picture	Note	Management
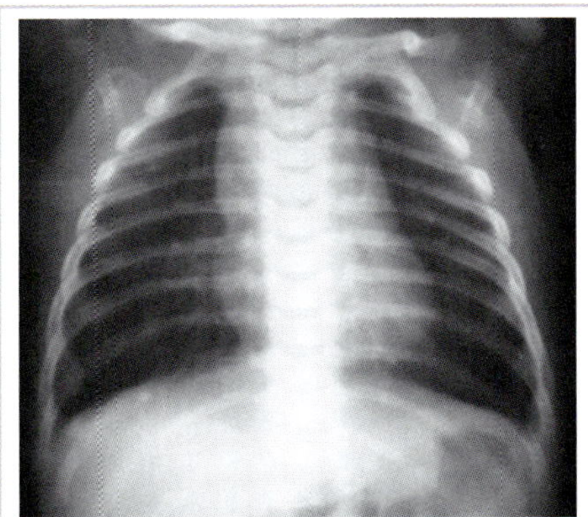 **Figure 3.2.7:** Acute bronchiolitis *Photo Courtesy*: Devaraj Raichur, Hubli	Hyperinflated lungs, with flattening of diaphragm and air below the level of heart, are evident (Fig. 3.2.7). Prominent thymus seen in such cases as this should not be mistaken for a "mediastinal tumor."	• *O_2 therapy*: When SpO_2 is less than 94% or in the presence of clinically significant respiratory distress. • *IV fluids*: Maintain hydration. • *Bronchodilators and steroids*: Their role is debatable. • Inhaled adrenaline may be better than β-agonists. • *Hypertonic saline nebulization* may have some benefit but this is yet to be established.

Acute Bronchiolitis with Segmental Collapse of the Left Lower Lobe

Picture	Note	Management
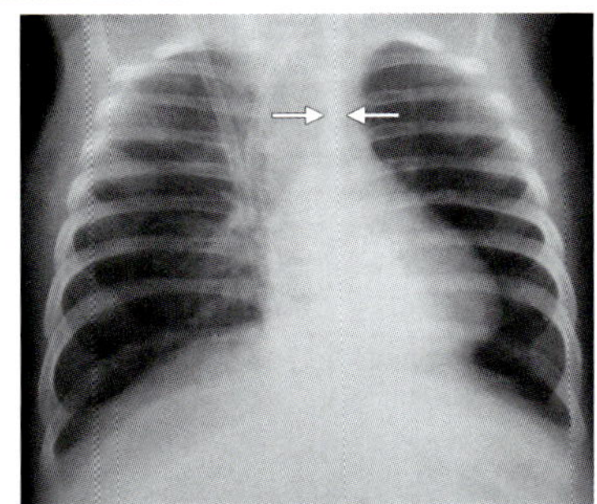 **Figure 3.2.8:** Acute bronchiolitis with segmental collapse of the left lower lobe *Courtesy*: Devaraj Raichur, Suvarna P Reddy, Hubli	Note the hyperinflated lungs depressing both domes of diaphragm and narrowing of the mediastinal structures with impinging right (white arrow) and left (yellow arrow) lungs (Fig. 3.2.8). There is segmental collapse of the left lower lobe.	See above.

Picture	Note	Management

Bronchiolitis with Multiple Atelectatic/Pneumonic Patches

Picture	Note	Management
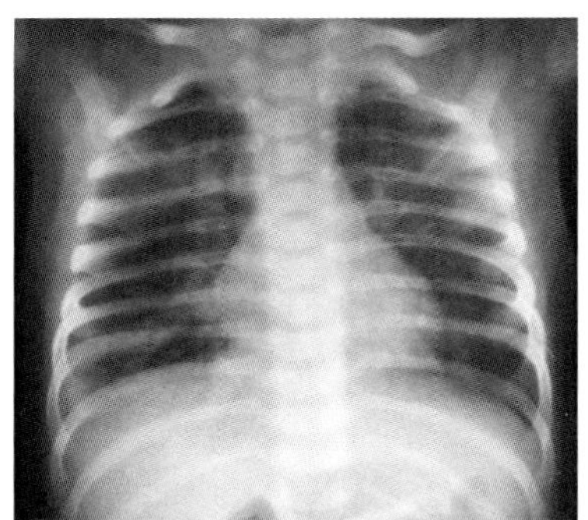 **Figure 3.2.9:** Bronchiolitis with multiple atelectatic/pneumonic patches *Courtesy*: Devaraj Raichur, Hubli	Hyperinflated lungs with patchy opacities in both lung-fields. The opacities may represent patchy consolidation or atelectasis (Fig. 3.2.9). This child improved without antibiotics.	See above.

Wheeze Associated Lower Respiratory Infection

Picture	Note	Management
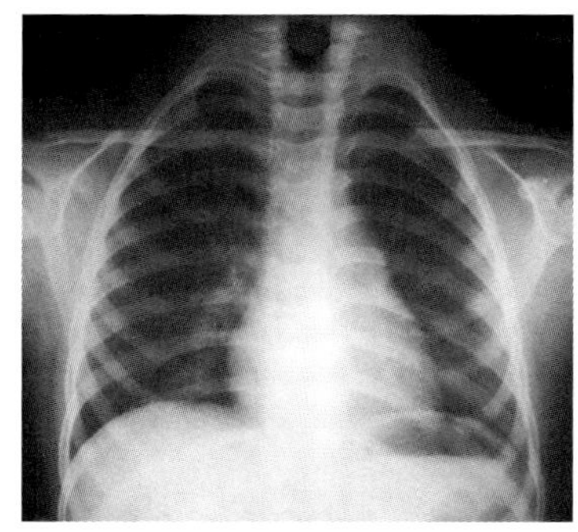 **Figure 3.2.10:** Wheeze associated lower respiratory infection (WALRI) *Photo Courtesy*: Devaraj Raichur, Hubli	Note the hyperinflated lungs (Fig. 3.2.10). In this case, peribronchial patches are also present in both lower zones.	• Inhaled or oral bronchodilators • Inhaled steroids in severe cases • Other symptomatic therapy • Oxygen as and when needed.

Viral Croup with WALRI

Picture	Note	Management
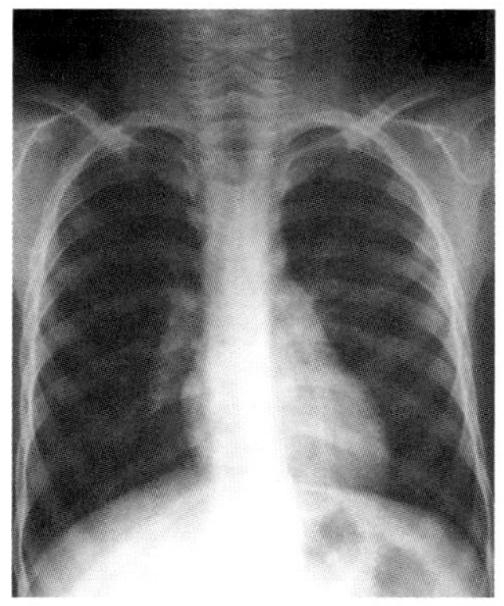 **Figure 3.2.11:** Viral croup with WALRI *Photo Courtesy*: Devaraj Raichur, Shaila M Sankeshwar, Hubli	Hyperinflated lungs (depressed and flattened domes of diaphragm) with subglottic narrowing of the airway (steeple sign) are seen (Fig. 3.2.11). This child had both stridor and wheeze. Stridor responded dramatically to adrenaline inhalation whereas wheeze took a few days to improve. Such extensive involvement of respiratory tract highlights the fact that viruses causing croup can also produce bronchitis, bronchiolitis and pneumonia.	• For viral croup: See above. • For WALRI: See above.

Picture	Note	Management

Pneumomediastinum with Surgical Emphysema in WALRI

Picture	Note	Management
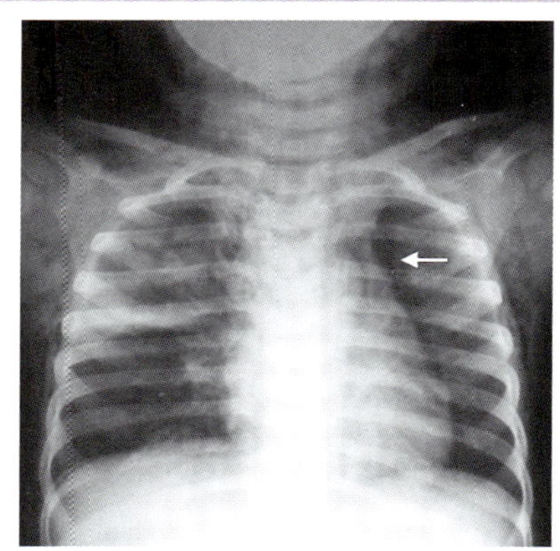 **Figure 3.2.12:** Pneumomediastinum with surgical emphysema in WALRI *Photo Courtesy*: Rajendra V Naidu, KB Shashikiran, Hubli	Note the presence of gas in the chest outside the rib cage, extending into neck and face. Pneumomediastinum is conspicuous by gas in the mediastinum pushing the pleura laterally [arrow (Fig. 3.2.12)]. Gas in the anterior wall overlaps the lung to produce apparent shadows of "bronchopneumonia".	Administering 100% oxygen may quicken resolution. The cause of the air leak (in this case, WALRI) must be managed appropriately.

Pneumomediastinum with Surgical Emphysema in WALRI-Clinical Profile

Picture	Note	Management
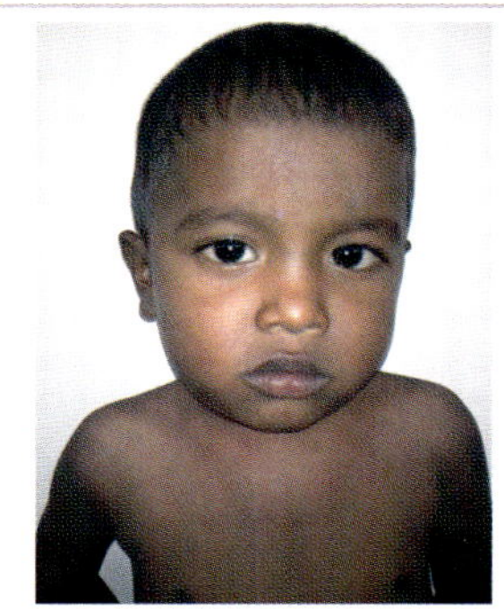 **Figure 3.2.13:** Pneumomediastinum with surgical emphysema in WALRI-clinical profile *Photo Courtesy*: Devaraj Raichur, Rajendra V Naidu, Hubli	Same child as above. Note the surgical emphysema manifesting as bulge in the axillae, fullness in deltopectoral groove and puffy cheeks (Fig. 3.2.13).	See above.

Collapse-Consolidation RUL

Picture	Note	Management
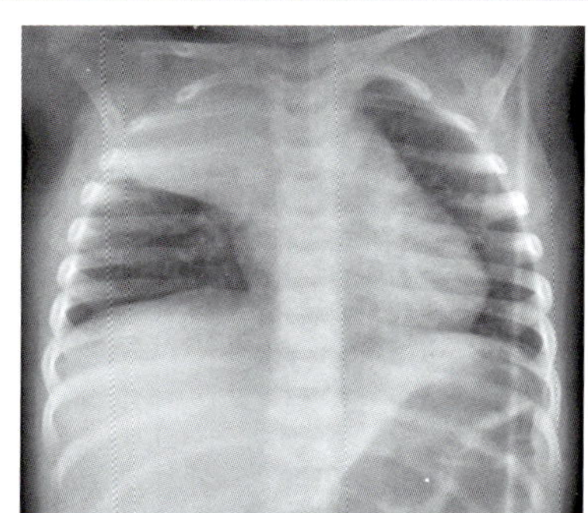 **Figure 3.2.14:** Collapse-consolidation RUL *Photo Courtesy*: Devaraj Raichur, Hubli	Right upper lobe (RUL) collapse—consolidation is evident by the right upper zone haziness limited below by the horizontal fissure and hyperinflated other parts of the right lung (Fig. 3.2.14). *Pneumococcus* is a common cause for such lobar distribution of pneumonia; *Klebsiella pneumoniae* and *S. aureus* are other likely causes.	• Management of respiratory distress (see above) • Antibiotic therapy • Symptomatic therapy

Picture	Note	Management

Collapse-Consolidation RUL in GB Syndrome with Palatopharyngeal Paralysis

Picture	Note	Management
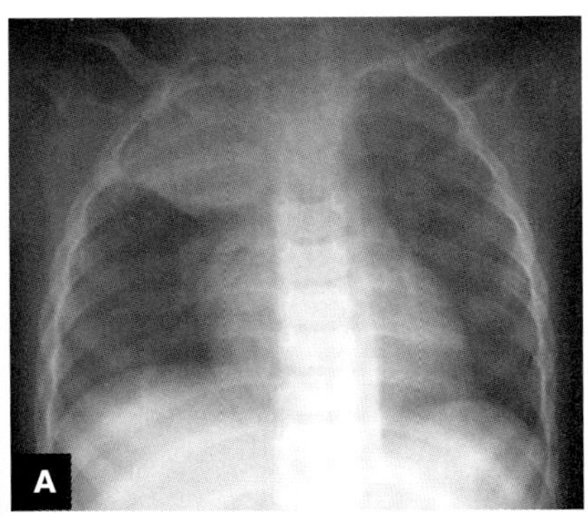	Aspiration pneumonia manifesting as right upper lobe collapse-consolidation (Fig. 3.2.15A). This child had palatopharyngeal paralysis due to GB syndrome.	Broad spectrum antibiotics, in this case covering anaerobes also. *Treatment of GB syndrome*: IVIG, plasmapheresis.
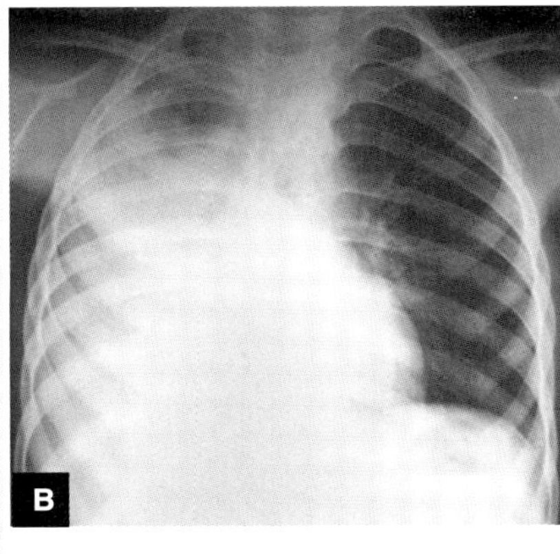	Same child as above; while the upper lobe lesion has partially cleared, the lower and middle lobe collapse consolidation is evident by: • Tracheal pull towards right • Positive cardiac silhouette sign on right side (obliteration of cardiac border) Ultrasonography in this child showed a small right-sided pleural effusion (Fig. 3.2.15B).	See above.
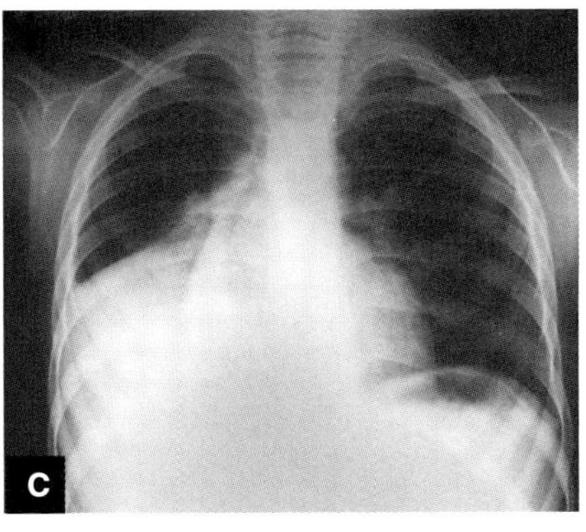 **Figures 3.2.15A to C:** (A) Collapse-consolidation RUL in GB syndrome with palatopharyngeal paralysis; (B) Collapse-consolidation of right lung in the same child as above (GB syndrome with palatopharyngeal paralysis); (C) Collapse-consolidation of right middle and lower lobes during recovery in the same child as above (GB syndrome with palatopharyngeal paralysis) *Photo Courtesy*: Devaraj Raichur, Suvarna P Reddy, Hubli	Same child as above; further during the clinical course the collapse consolidation of the lung improved. Note the complete clearance of the right upper zone opacities, which are replaced now by compensatory hyperinflation (Fig. 3.2.15C).	See above.

Picture	Note	Management

Parapneumonic Effusion—Left

Picture	Note	Management
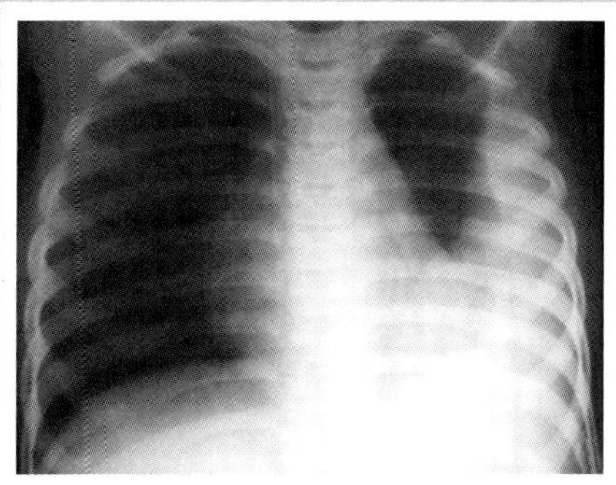 **Figure 3.2.16:** Parapneumonic effusion—Left *Photo Courtesy*: NC Gowrishankar, Chennai	• X-ray in a sick febrile child with respiratory distress (Fig. 3.2.16) • Opaque right hemithorax • Absent bronchovascular markings • Mediastinal shift to opposite side	Pleural tapping and drainage, biochemical and microbial examination of fluid and culture, sensitivity will decide the antimicrobial to be used.

Dengue Fever with Right Pleural Effusion

Picture	Note	Management
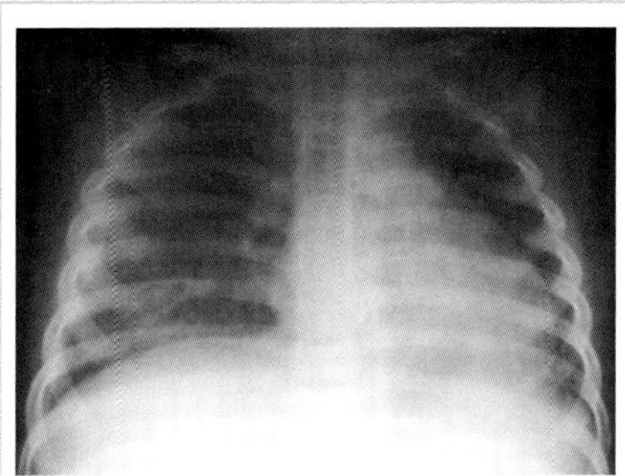 **Figure 3.2.17:** Dengue fever with right pleural effusion *Photo Courtesy*: Devaraj Raichur, Hubli	Note the lamellar pleural effusion on right side (Fig. 3.2.17). Pleural effusions and ascites are common in severe dengue fever.	Symptomatic and supportive therapy. Follow-up CBC, serial hematocrit, urine output chart and meticulous fluid management is the key.

Empyema Left Side—Soft Tissue Bulge

Picture	Note	Management
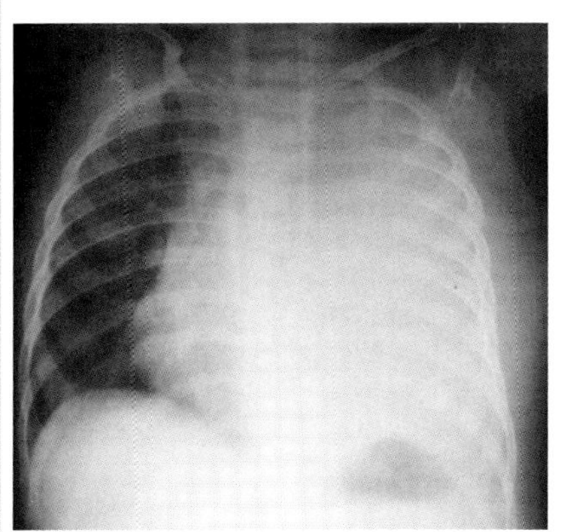 **Figure 3.2.18A:** Empyema left side—soft tissue bulge *Photo Courtesy*: Prakash Wari, Hubli	Note the evidence of massive pleural effusion (opacification of whole left side of chest *without* air-bronchogram, tracheal and mediastinal shift to opposite side) combined with soft tissue swelling on the left-side, indicating empyema (Fig. 3.2.18A).	• Treat the underlying disease and the respiratory distress • Proper antibiotics (for as long as 3–4 weeks) • Chest tube drainage with fibrinolytic therapy (with streptokinase or urokinase) • Video-assisted thoracoscopic surgery (VATS) • Open decortication

Picture	Note	Management

Empyema Right Side

Picture	Note	Management
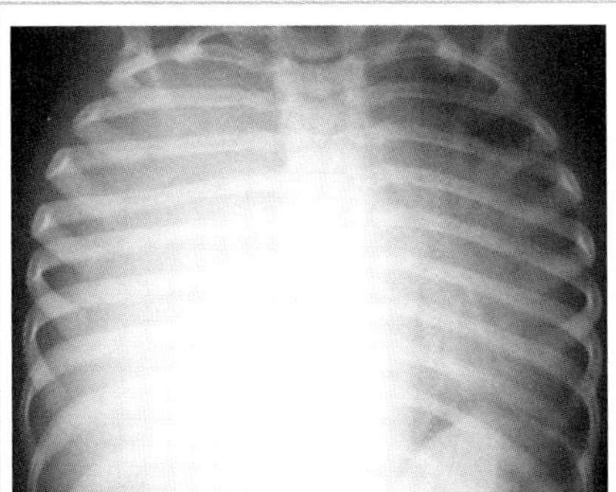 **Figure 3.2.18B:** Empyema right side *Photo Courtesy*: NC Gowrishankar, Chennai	• X-ray in a sick febrile child with respiratory distress (Fig. 3.2.18B) • Opaque right hemithorax • Absent bronchovascular markings • Mediastinal shift to opposite side	• Pleural tap—confirm pus • Intercostal drainage • IV antibiotics and supportive measures

Measles with Right-sided Empyema

Picture	Note	Management
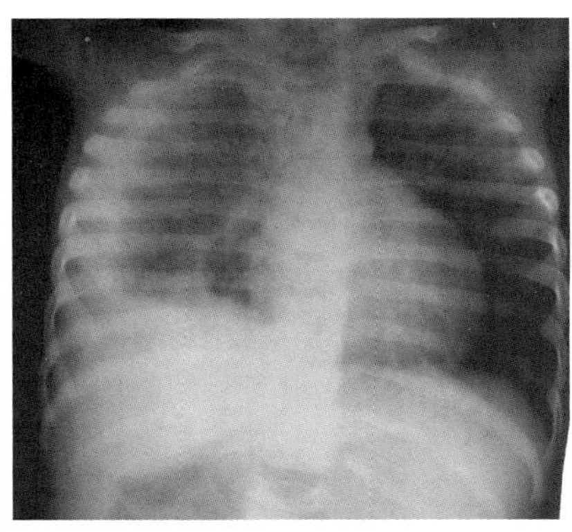 **Figure 3.2.19:** Measles with right-sided empyema *Photo Courtesy*: Devaraj Raichur, KB Shashikiran, Hubli	Opacification of peripheral right hemithorax with collapsed right lung (Fig. 3.2.19). Pleural tap yielded purulent material in this case of measles.	• Vitamin A and symptomatic therapy for measles • Management of empyema including antibiotics and surgical therapy (see above) Cover with antistaphylococcal antibiotic like cloxacillin or clindamycin in postmeasles lung pathology.

Pulmonary Tuberculosis

Picture	Note	Management
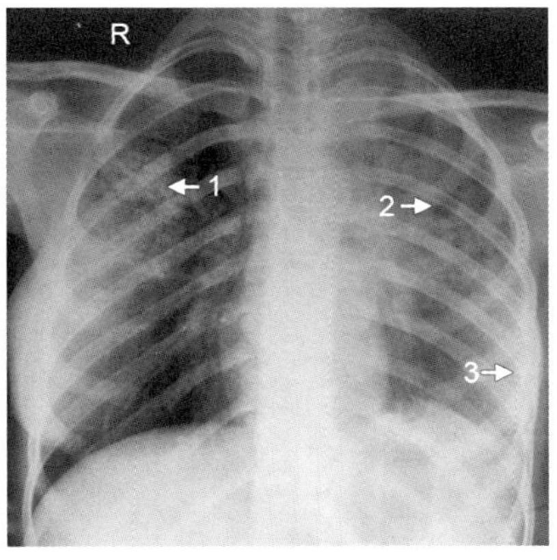 **Figure 3.2.20:** Pulmonary tuberculosis—(1) Extensive infiltrates with (2) Cavitations and (3) Pleural effusion *Photo Courtesy*: Vinod H Ratageri, Hubli	Extensive infiltrates (1) with cavity (2) and pleural effusion (3) are seen; the sputum was positive for AFB (Fig. 3.2.20).	Drug regimen for revised categories under Revised National Tuberculosis Control Program (RNTCP), 2011: • Cat I (New): 2HRZE3 + 4HR3 • Cat II (Previously treated): 2HRZES3 + 1HRZE3 + 5HRE3 Steroids—in bronchial obstruction, massive pleural effusion and miliary tuberculosis.

Picture	Note	Management

Cavitary Tuberculosis with Necrotizing Bronchopneumonia

Picture	Note	Management
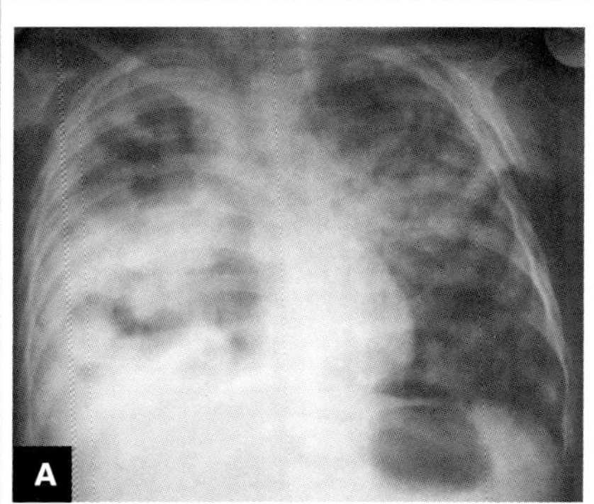	Cavities in both lungs and consolidation of the right lung and extensive infiltration of the left lung are evident (Fig. 3.2.21A). This child had acid fast bacilli in the sputum; he was not infected with HIV.	Drug regimen for revised categories under Revised National Tuberculosis Control Program (RNTCP), 2011: • Cat I (New): 2HRZE3 + 4HR3 • Cat II (Previously treated): 2HRZES3 + 1HRZE3 + 5HRE3 Steroids—in bronchial obstruction, massive pleural effusion and miliary tuberculosis.
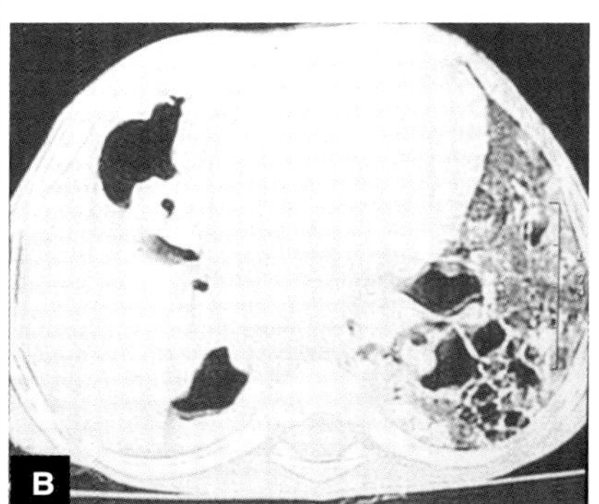 **Figures 3.2.21A and B:** (A) Cavitary tuberculosis with necrotizing bronchopneumonia—Chest X-ray; (B) Cavitary tuberculosis with necrotizing bronchopneumonia—CT scan *Photo Courtesy*: Devaraj Raichur, Hubli	Chest CT scan of the same child as above (Fig. 3.2.21B). Note extensive consolidation of right lung and bilateral pulmonary cavitation.	See above.

HIV with Tuberculosis

Picture	Note	Management
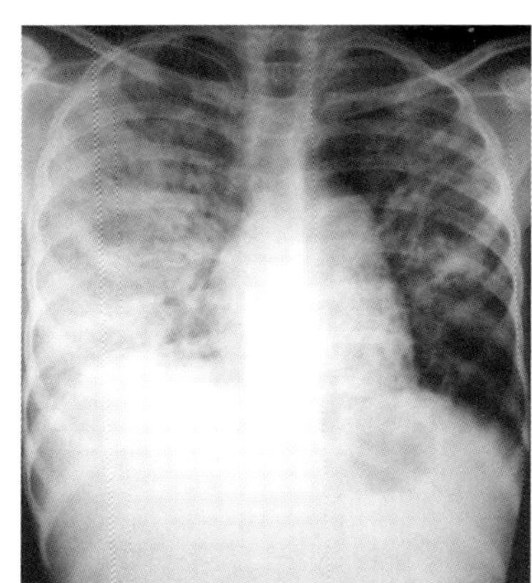 **Figure 3.2.22:** HIV with tuberculosis *Photo Courtesy*: TA Shepur, Bhavna Koppad, Hubli	Extensive pulmonary tuberculosis with consolidation, cavitation and bronchiectatic changes (Fig. 3.2.22). This child had HIV infection.	Treatment for tuberculosis should be started first. Total duration: At least 9 months. HIV infection is treated once there is improvement in the tuberculosis.

Picture	Note	Management

HIV with *Pneumocystis jiroveci (carinii)* Pneumonia—Early

Picture	Note	Management
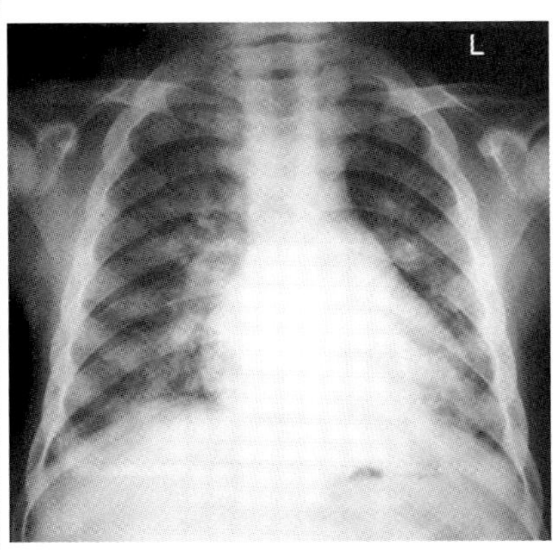 **Figure 3.2.23A:** HIV with *Pneumocystis jiroveci (carinii)* Pneumonia—Early *Photo Courtesy*: TA Shepur, Bhavna Koppad, Hubli	Bilateral almost symmetrical opacities are evident; this child had HIV infection (Fig. 3.2.23A).	• Trimethoprim-sulfamethoxazole [15–20 mg TMP/kg/day divided four times a day (qid)]. • Duration: 3 weeks in AIDS and 2 weeks for others. • Other drugs: Pentamidine is ethionate (4 mg/kg as a single daily dose IV). Atovaquone [750 mg twice a day (bid) with food, for age > 13 years]. Trimetrexate glucuronate or combinations of trimethoprim plus dapsone, or clindamycin plus primaquine • Prednisolone in moderate to severe cases.

HIV with *Pneumocystis jiroveci (carinii)* Pneumonia—Late

Picture	Note	Management
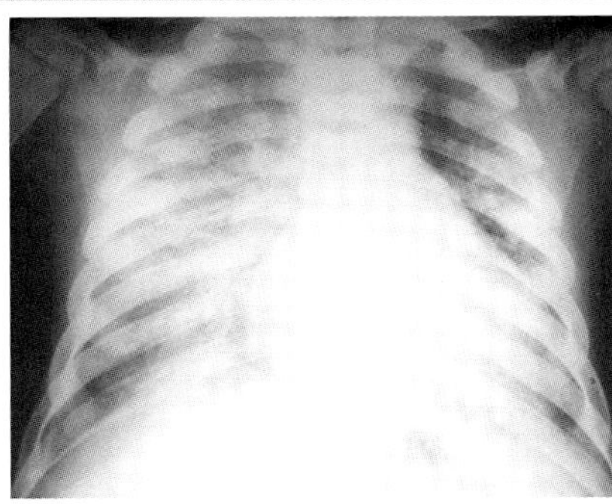 **Figure 3.2.23B:** HIV with *Pneumocystis jiroveci (carinii)* Pneumonia—Late *Photo Courtesy*: TA Shepur, Bhavna Koppad, Hubli	The same case as above. There is progression to ground-glass appearance of the opacities (Fig. 3.2.23B).	See above.

Lung Abscess with Bronchopneumonia

Picture	Note	Management
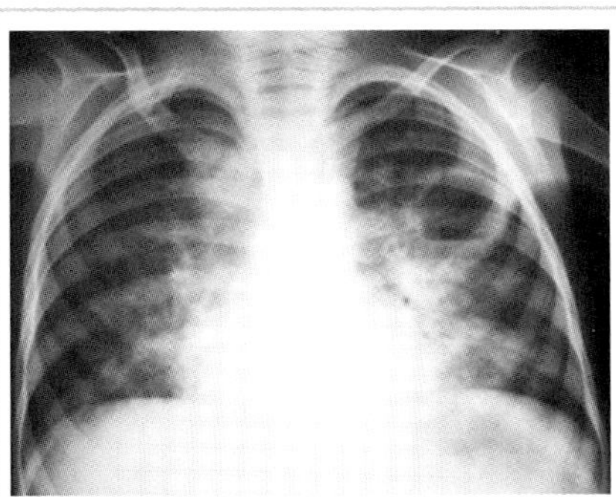 **Figure 3.2.24A:** Lung abscess with bronchopneumonia *Photo Courtesy*: Devaraj Raichur, Hubli	Note the air-fluid level in the cavity in left lung (Fig. 3.2.24A). Obliteration of both right and left borders of the heart indicates lesions in middle lobe of right lung and lingular segments of the left lung "cardiac silhouette sign". Pneumatoceles have thin-walled cavities and are usually multiple in staphylococcal infections.	• Antibiotics for 4–6 weeks, covering *S. aureus*, anaerobes and gram-negative bacteria. • If failed to improve in 7–10 days of antimicrobial therapy, surgical interventions like percutaneous aspiration techniques, and rarely thoracotomy with lobectomy and/or decortication may be necessary.

Picture	Note	Management

Lung Abscess with Right-Middle Lobe Consolidation

Picture	Note	Management
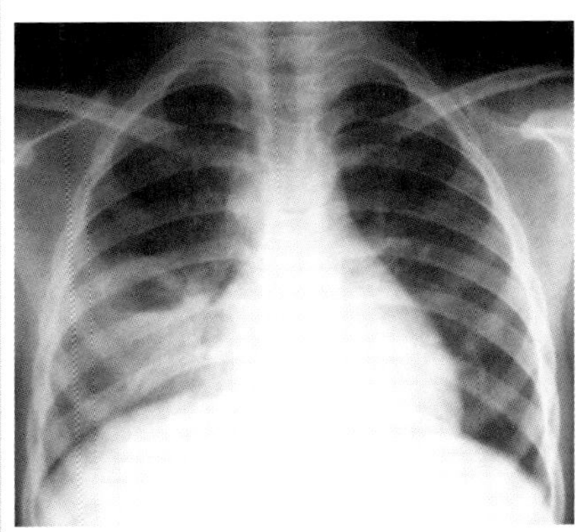 **Figure 3.2.24B:** Lung abscess with right-middle lobe consolidation *Photo Courtesy*: SR Fattepur, Hubli	Note the thick-walled cavity with air-fluid level below the horizontal fissure in the right lung (Fig. 3.2.24B). Blurring of the right-heart border indicates consolidation of the right middle lobe.	See above. History of measles, pyoderma, etc. is a pointer to staphylococcal infection.

Staphylococcal Pneumonia

Picture	Note	Management
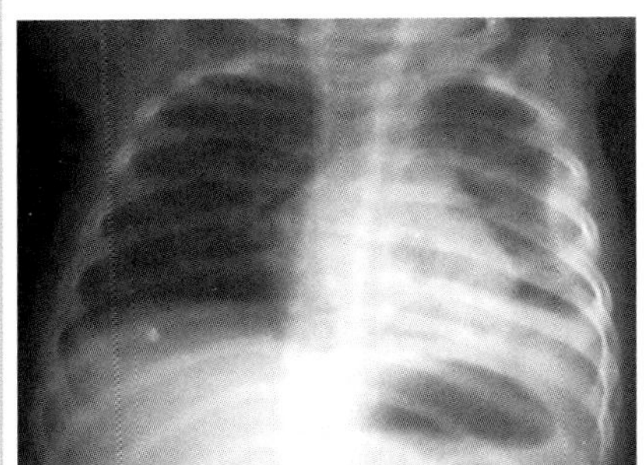 **Figure 3.2.25:** Staphylococcal pneumonia *Photo Courtesy*: Devaraj Raichur, Hubli	Note the cavities in left lower zone with formation of loculated pleural effusion/empyema along the rib cage. Staphylococcal pneumonia may be bronchopneumonia or lobar pneumonia and is characterized by rapid clinical progression and complications including formation of empyema, pyopneumothorax, bronchopleural fistula and pneumatoceles (Fig. 3.2.25).	• Cloxacillin or cefazolin in methicillin-susceptible *S. aureus* (MSSA). • Vancomycin in penicillin-allergy and suspected methicillin-resistant *S. aureus* (MRSA) (Alternatives: linezolid or teicoplanin). For MSSA cloxacillin is more efficacious than vancomycin.

Congenital Pneumonia

Picture	Note	Management
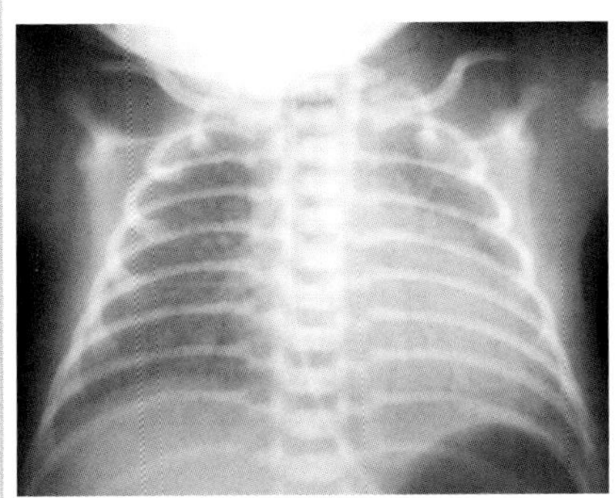 **Figure 3.2.26:** Congenital pneumonia *Photo Courtesy*: Devaraj Raichur, Hubli	Ground-glass appearance of the lungs with air-bronchogram is seen (Fig. 3.2.26). Other conditions producing air-bronchogram (which indicates alveolar lesion) are: Respiratory distress syndrome (RDS) and pulmonary edema. A history of risk factors for infection and a positive sepsis screen help in the diagnosis.	• Provide warmth • Maintain ABCs • Management of respiratory distress and shock, if present • Antibiotics (usually a betalactam + an aminoglycoside) covering mainly *K. pneumoniae*, *E. coli*, group B streptococci for 10–14 days.

Picture	Note	Management

Calcified Hilar Node—Tuberculosis

Picture	Note	Management
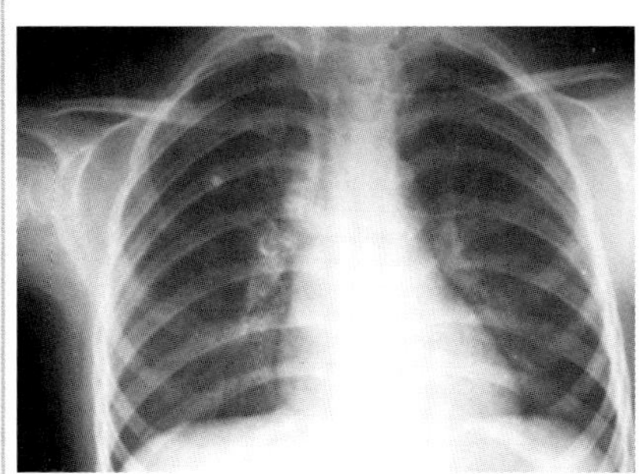 **Figure 3.2.27:** Calcified hilar node—tuberculosis *Photo Courtesy*: NC Gowrishankar, Chennai	X-ray chest shows bilateral calcified hilar nodes suggesting healed granulomatous disease like tuberculosis (Fig. 3.2.27)	Treatment for the calcified nodes alone is not necessary; if there is any evidence for active tuberculous disease, antitubercular treatment is indicated.

Multiple Cysts Left Side

Picture	Note	Management
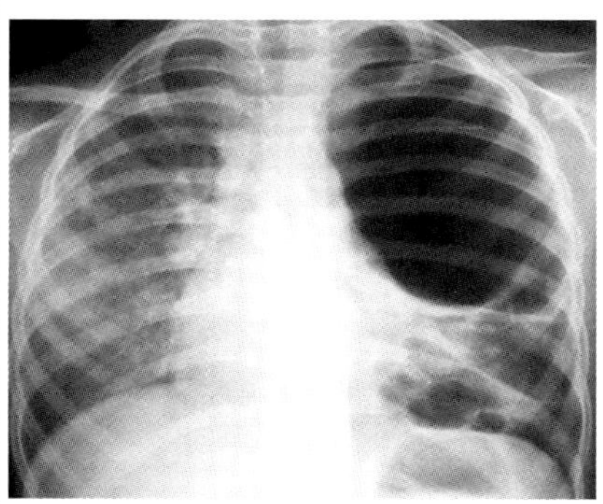 **Figure 3.2.28:** Multiple cysts left side *Photo Courtesy*: NC Gowrishankar, Chennai	Differential diagnosis: Staphylococcal cysts (pneumatoceles), congenital cystic adenomastoid malformation [CCAM (Fig. 3.2.28)].	Treatment depends on the cause, e.g. antibiotics for staphylococcal infection or surgery for CCAM.

Mass Lesion in Right Hemithorax

Picture	Note	Management
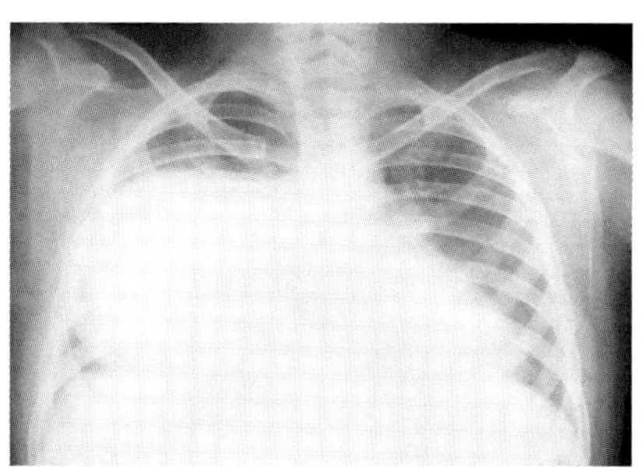 **Figure 3.2.29:** Mass lesion in right hemithorax *Photo Courtesy*: NC Gowrishankar, Chennai	Homogeneous opacity with smooth, round margins in right hemithorax, suggesting a mass lesion. It is unlikely to be the usual manifestation of an empyema as the costophrenic angle is free (Fig. 3.2.29).	Further imaging study with USG/CT scan is indicated to differentiate from other similar opacities like encysted empyema and to delineate the nature of the tumor. The child was found to have germ cell tumor.

Pneumonia both Lower Lobes

Picture	Note	Management
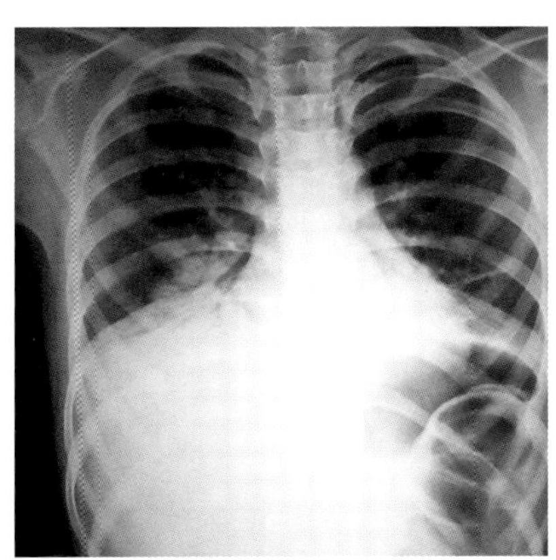 **Figure 3.2.30:** Pneumonia both lower lobes *Photo Courtesy:* NC Gowrishankar, Chennai	Non-homogeneous opacities in both lower zones with air-bronchograms are evident (Fig. 3.2.30).	Presentation like this should make one suspect aspiration into tracheobronchial tree. In older children, it can occur when child's sensorium is altered in any condition and if the secretions in the throat are not cleared properly. This child had status epilepticus following which pneumonia developed. This needs to be treated with antibiotics which cover gram-negative organisms and anerobes.

Pneumonia with Parapneumonic Effusion

Picture	Note	Management
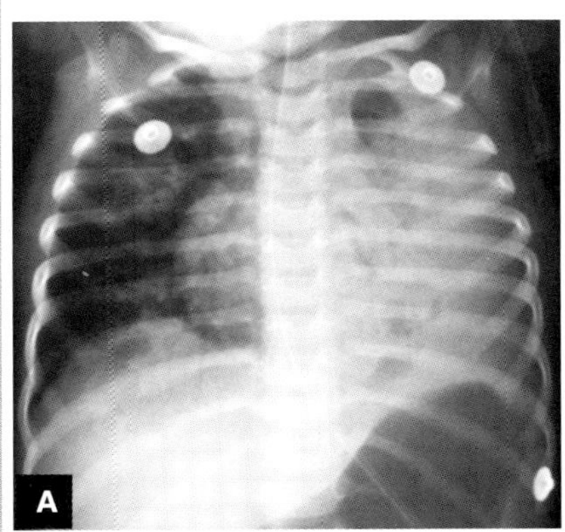 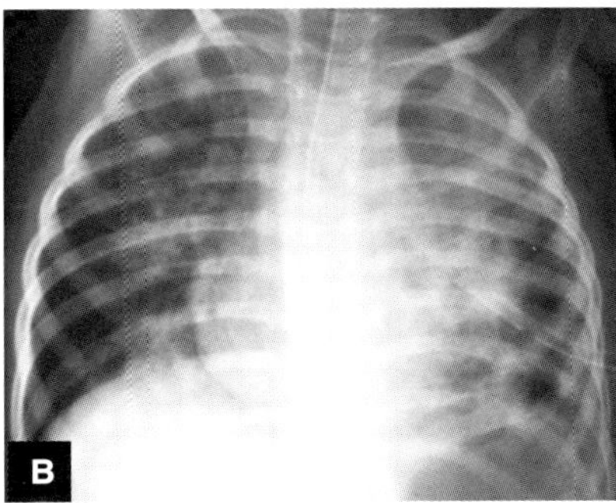 **Figures 3.2.31A and B:** Pneumonia with parapneumonic effusion *Photo Courtesy:* NC Gowrishankar, Chennai	Note the homogeneous opacity obliterating left costophrenic angle (Figs 3.2.31A and B); ICD was indicated for pleural fluid pH < 7.2, increasing respiratory distress even if pH > 7.2.	Treatment as for empyema.

Picture	Note	Management

Tension Pneumothorax with Pneumatoceles with Subcutaneous Emphysema

Picture	Note	Management
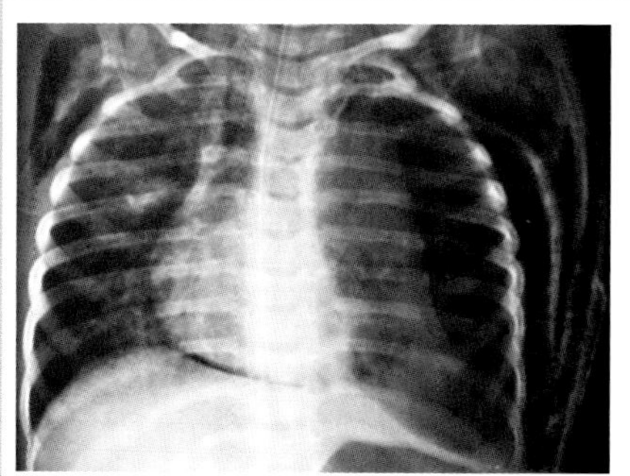 **Figure 3.2.32:** Tension pneumothorax with pneumatoceles with subcutaneous emphysema *Photo Courtesy*: NC Gowrishankar, Chennai	Left-sided tension pneumothorax is seen with mediastinal shift to right (Fig. 3.2.32). Subcutaneous emphysema with pneumomediastinum and pneumatoceles on left side are evident.	*Treatment*: ICD in the left side. For subcutaneous emphysema—observation. Antibiotics to cover *S. aureus*.

Postcardiac Repair State—Atelectasis both Lower Lobes Endobronchial Tuberculosis

Picture	Note	Management
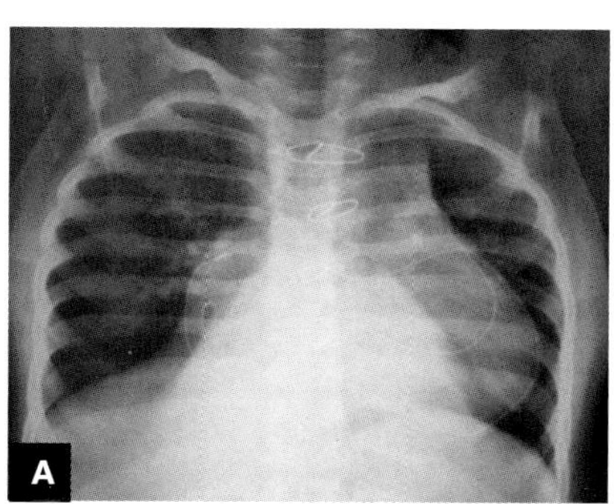 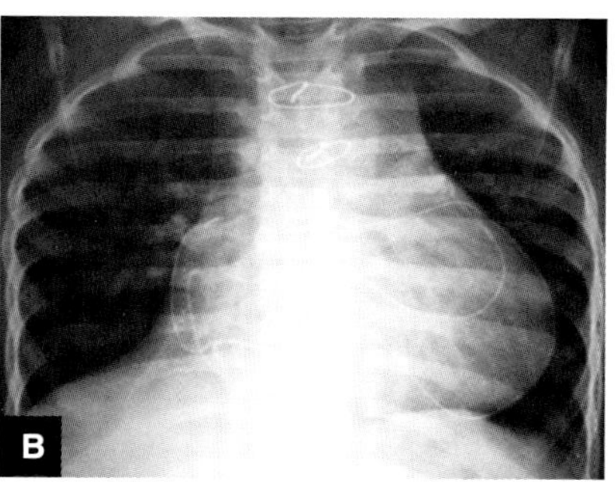 **Figures 3.2.33A and B:** Postcardiac repair state—atelectasis both lower lobes endobronchial tuberculosis *Photo Courtesy*: NC Gowrishankar, Chennai	On flexible bronchoscopy, bronchial stenosis on right side with endobronchial granulation on left side was seen (Figs 3.2.33A and B).	Post-ATT—Right segmental atelectasis and left atelectasis resolved.

Section 4

Gastrointestinal Infections

Section Editors

Neelam Mohan, Yogesh Waikar

Contributors

Neelam Mohan, Yogesh Waikar

Section Outline

4.1 Gastrointestinal Infections

- Ascariasis (Roundworms)
- Pseudomembranous Colitis
- Colitis
- Esophageal Candidiasis
- Abdominal Tuberculosis
- Appendicitis
- Necrotizing Enterocolitis

4.2 Hepatobiliary Infections

- Hydatid Cyst
- Amebic Liver Abscess
- Pyogenic Liver Abscess

Picture	Note	Management

4.1 GASTROINTESTINAL INFECTIONS

Ascariasis (Roundworms)

Picture	Note	Management
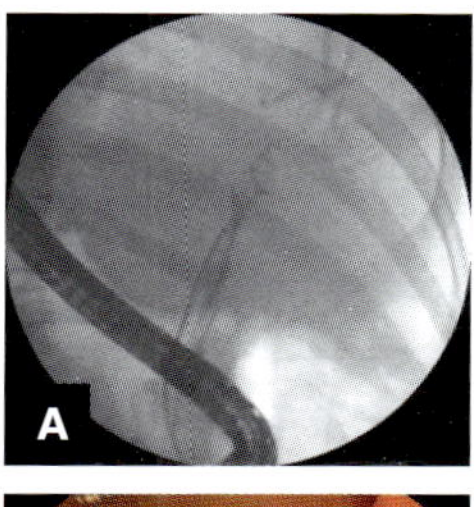 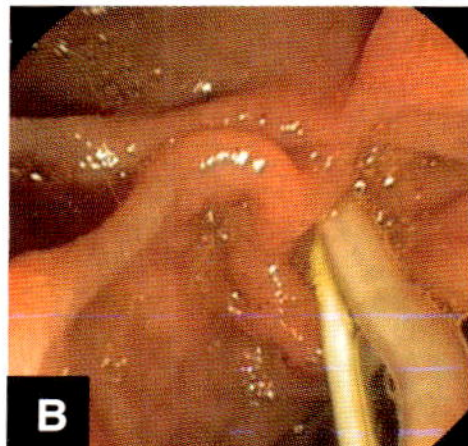 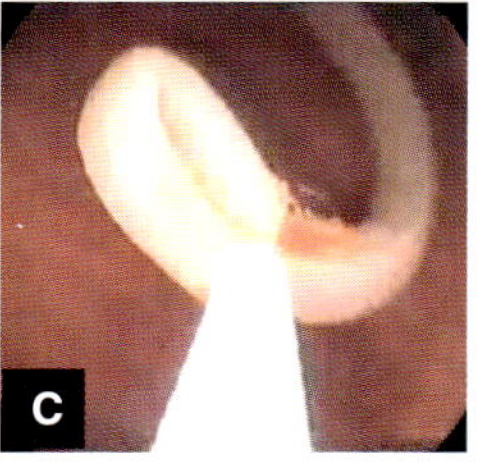 **Figures 4.1.1A to C:** Ascariasis (roundworm) *Photo Courtesy:* Neelam Mohan, Gurgaon	• *Ascaris lumbricoides*, which causes ascariasis, is the largest of the roundworms (nematodes), with females measuring 30 cm × 0.5 cm (Figs 4.1.1A to C). • Ascariasis is usually asymptomatic, but may be associated with anorexia, recurrent abdominal pain, nausea, vomiting and altered bowel habits. Heavy infestations can cause complications, including intestinal obstruction, appendicitis, bowel perforation, cholecystitis and pancreatitis. Worms can also cause obstruction of bile duct which can result into biliary colic and obstructive jaundice. Chronic cases can present with malabsorption and vitamin A deficiency. • On ultrasonography one may find the worms—may be single, multiple, in bundles and moving during the examination.	• Treatment includes single dose of albendazole. Mebendazole and pyrantel pamoate are other alternatives. • Prevention includes: Use of toilet facilities; safe excreta disposal; protection of food from dirt and soil; thorough washing of raw food products and hand washing.

Pseudomembranous Colitis

Picture	Note	Management
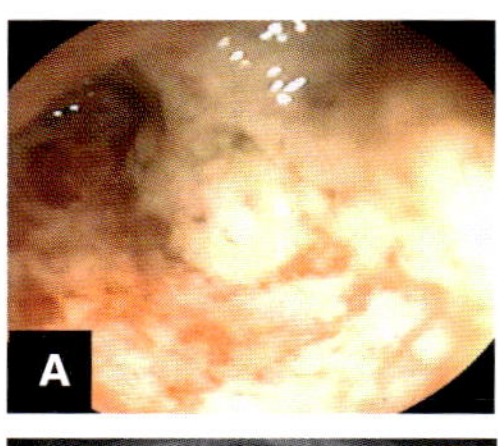 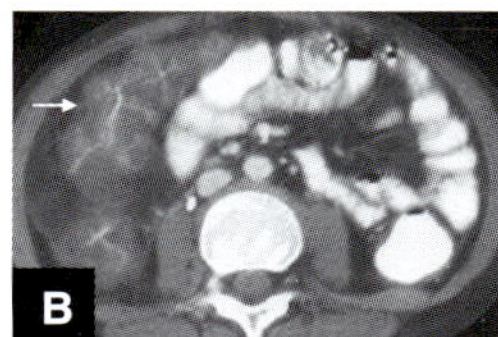 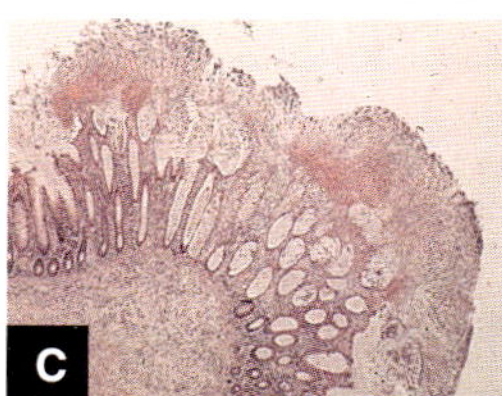 **Figures 4.1.2A to C:** Pseudomembranous colitis *Photo Courtesy:* Neelam Mohan, Gurgaon	• Pseudomembranous colitis is often, but not always, caused by the bacterium *Clostridium difficile* (Figs 4.1.2A to C). Prior use of antibiotic clinches the diagnosis. It is one of the commonest causes of antibiotic associated diarrhea. • The illness is characterized by offensive-smelling diarrhea, fever and abdominal pain. In severe cases, life-threatening complications can develop, such as toxic megacolon.	• The disease is treated either with oral vancomycin or with intravenous metronidazole.

Picture	Note	Management

Colitis

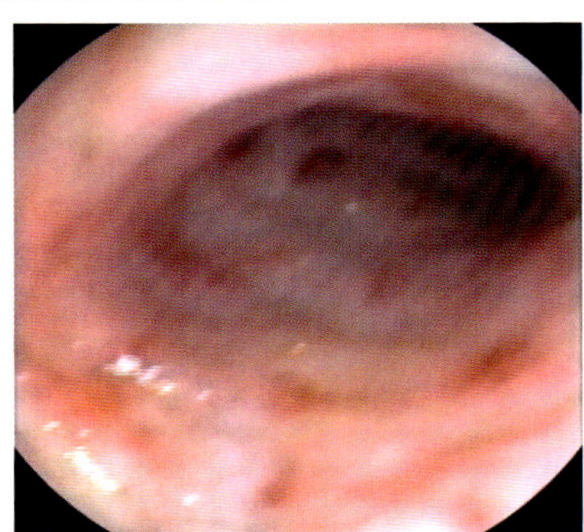 **Figure 4.1.3:** Colitis *Photo Courtesy:* Neelam Mohan, Gurgaon	• Infectious colitis is the most common cause of pediatric colitis, particularly beyond the first year of life (Fig. 4.1.3). • It can be caused by bacterial, viral and parasitic agents. • The most common bacterial causes of colitis in children are *Escherichia coli* (including both enterohemorrhagic *E. coli* [EHEC] and enteroinvasive *E. coli* [EIEC]) and species of *Shigella, Salmonella, Campylobacter,* and *Yersinia.* • The organism penetrates and proliferates in the cell, which leads to cell destruction, produces mucosal ulcerations, and causes bleeding.	• Oral rehydration solutions (ORS) and appropriate antibiotics are very important. Oral cefixime or quinolones are recommended for acute bloody diarrhea.

Esophageal Candidiasis

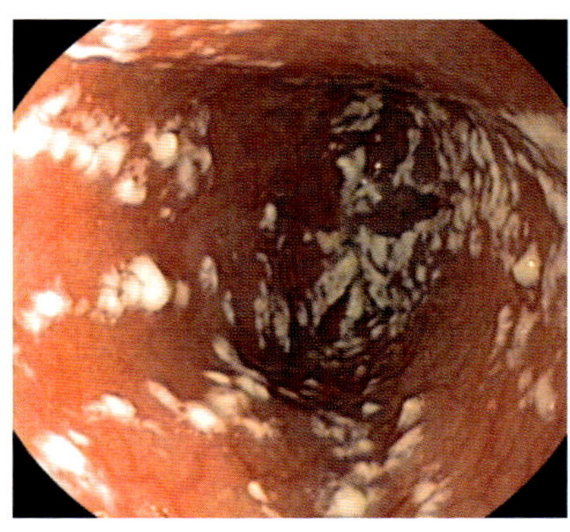 **Figure 4.1.4:** Esophageal candidiasis *Photo Courtesy:* Neelam Mohan, Gurgaon	• Esophageal candidiasis is an opportunistic infection of the esophagus by *Candida albicans* (Fig. 4.1.4). • The disease occurs in patients in immunocompromised states, including postchemotherapy and in acquired immunodeficiency syndrome (AIDS). • The patient complains of difficulty or pain with swallowing, or the sensation that food is "sticking" in the retrosternal chest along with nausea, vomiting weight loss. • Fever is not common with candidal esophagitis and if present, one should look for alternative cause. • Endoscopy often reveals classic diffuse raised plaques that characteristically can be removed from the mucosa by the endsocope. • Brushing or biopsy of the plaques shows yeast and pseudohyphae by histology that is characteristic of *Candida* species.	• Treatment includes oral fluconazole for 21 days or 14 days after the disappearance of symptoms. In refractory cases, caspofungin or amphotericin can also be used.

Picture	Note	Management

Abdominal Tuberculosis

Picture	Note	Management
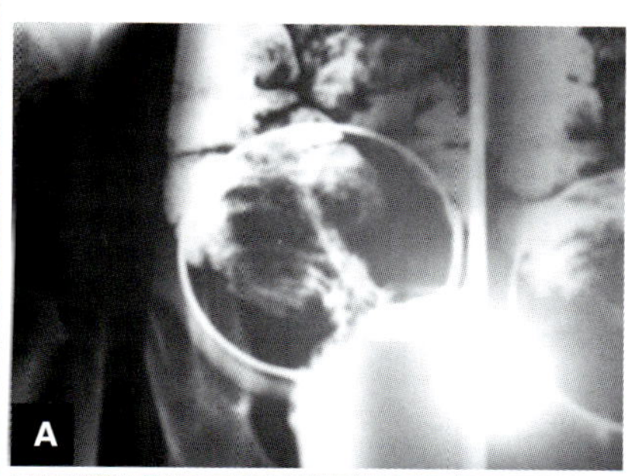 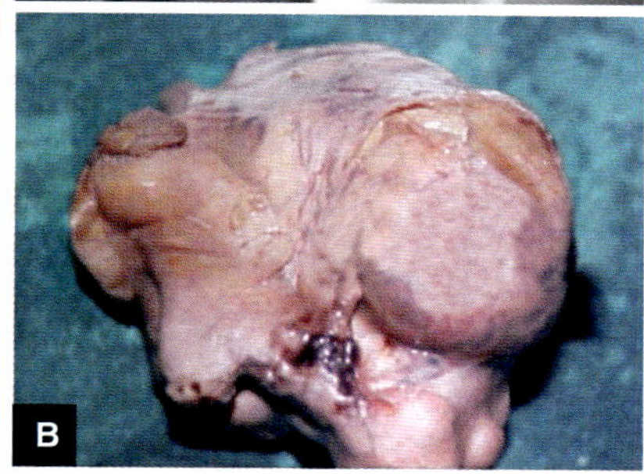 **Figures 4.1.5A and B:** Abdominal tuberculosis *Photo Courtesy:* Neelam Mohan, Gurgaon	• Tuberculosis (TB) can involve any part of the gastrointestinal tract and is the sixth most frequent site of extrapulmonary involvement. Out of all cases of abdominal TB, intestinal TB accounts for 65%, followed by peritoneal TB 30% and then lymph node TB only 5% (Figs 4.1.5A and B). • Both the incidence and severity of abdominal tuberculosis are expected to increase with increasing incidence of HIV infection. • Tuberculosis bacteria reach the gastrointestinal tract via hematogenous spread, ingestion of infected sputum, or direct spread from infected contiguous lymph nodes and fallopian tubes. • The gross pathology is characterized by transverse ulcers, fibrosis, thickening and stricturing of the bowel wall, enlarged and matted mesenteric lymph nodes, omental thickening and peritoneal tubercles. • Peritoneal tuberculosis occurs in three forms: (a) wet type with ascites, (b) dry type with adhesions, and (c) fibrotic type with omental thickening and loculated ascites. • The most common site of involvement of the gastrointestinal tuberculosis is the ileocecal region. Ileocecal and small bowel tuberculosis presents with a palpable mass in the right lower quadrant and/or complications of obstruction, perforation or malabsorption especially in the presence of stricture. Useful modalities for investigating a suspected case include small bowel barium meal, barium enema, ultrasonography, computed tomographic scan and colonoscopy.	• As per Revised National Tuberculosis Control Program (RNTCP), abdominal TB is considered category I. Regime includes 2 $H_3R_3Z_3E_3$ during intensive phase and 4 H_3R_3 during continuous phase.

Picture	Note	Management

Appendicitis

Picture	Note	Management
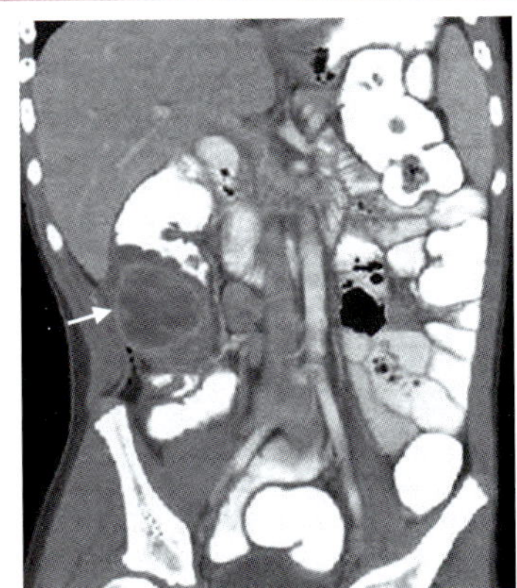 **Figure 4.1.6:** Appendicitis *Photo Courtesy:* Neelam Mohan, Gurgaon	• CT findings that suggest perforated appendicitis include periappendiceal or pericecal air, abscess, phlegmon and extensive free fluid (Fig. 4.1.6). • Because the disease is due to obstruction of the appendix and the inflammation occurs distal to the obstruction, extravasation of contrast or extensive free air is rarely seen. • If a patient is found to have free air throughout the abdomen or under the diaphragm, other diagnoses should be entertained. • CT scanning may be helpful in obese patients or those in whom a localized appendiceal abscess is clinically suspected. In patients with abscesses, CT scanning may also be helpful in the CT-guided drainage of the abscess.	• Acute appendicitis: Pediatric surgery referral and appendicetomy. • Recurrent acute appendicitis: In remission: Interval appendicetomy • Complicated appendicitis/perforation/abscess: Pediatric surgery referral.

Necrotizing Enterocolitis

Picture	Note	Management
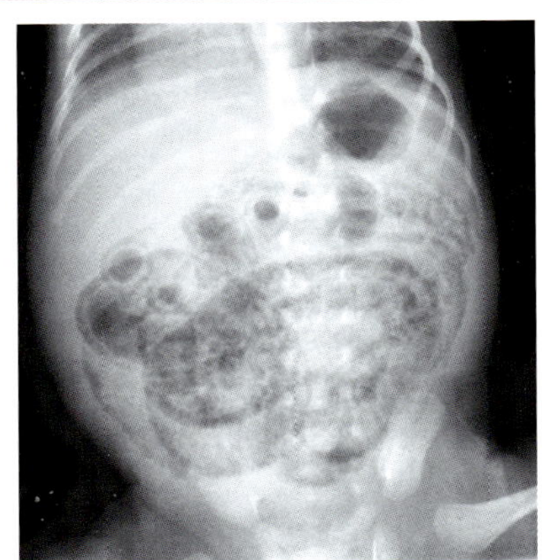 **Figure 4.1.7:** Necrotizing enterocolitis *Photo Courtesy:* Neelam Mohan, Gurgaon	The condition is typically seen in premature infants, and the timing of its onset is generally inversely proportional to the gestational age of the baby at birth, i.e. the earlier a baby is born, the later signs of *necrotizing enterocolitis* (NEC) are typically seen (Fig. 4.1.7). Initial symptoms include feeding intolerance, increased gastric residuals, abdominal distension and bloody stools. Symptoms may progress rapidly to abdominal discoloration with intestinal perforation and peritonitis and systemic hypotension requiring intensive medical support. The diagnosis is usually suspected clinically radiographic signs of NEC include dilated bowel loops, paucity of gas, a "fixed loop" (unaltered gas-filled loop of bowel), pneumatosis intestinalis, portal venous gas and pneumoperitoneum (extraluminal or "free air" outside the bowel within the abdomen). The pathognomic finding on plain films is pneumatosis intestinalis. Ultrasound may detect few of the positive findings.	Treatment consists primarily of supportive care including providing bowel rest by stopping enteral feeds, gastric decompression with intermittent suction, fluid repletion to correct electrolyte abnormalities and third space losses, support for blood pressure, parenteral nutrition, and prompt antibiotic therapy. Intestinal perforation may require surgical intervention.

4.2 HEPATOBILIARY INFECTIONS

Hydatid Cyst

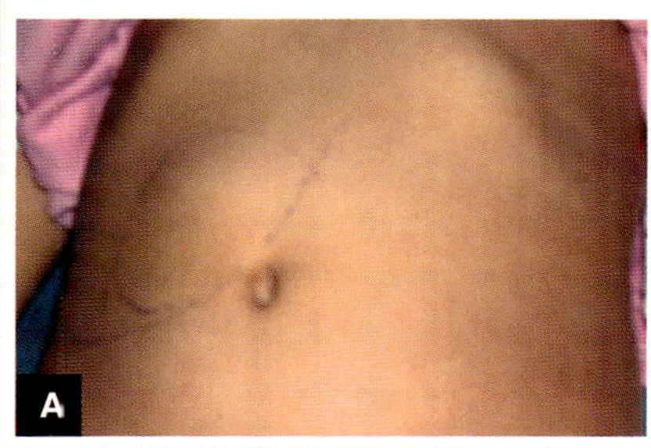

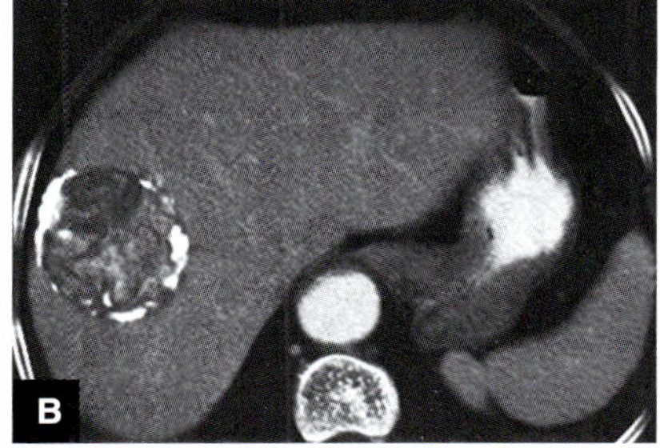

Figures 4.2.1A and B: Hydatid cyst
Photo Courtesy: Yogesh Waikar, Nagpur

- Hydatid disease (Figs 4.2.1A and B) is a parasitic infestation by a tapeworm of the genus *Echinococcus*.
- The right lobe is the most frequently involved portion of the liver.
- Imaging findings in hepatic hydatid disease depend on the stage of cyst growth, i.e. whether the cyst is unilocular, contains daughter vesicles, or daughter cysts, is partially calcified, or completely calcified (dead).
- Simple cysts do not demonstrate internal structures, although multiple echogenic foci due to hydatid sand may be seen within the lesion by repositioning the patient. The echogenic foci quickly fall to the most dependent portion of the cavity without forming visible strata. This finding has been referred to as the "snowstorm sign".
- Complete detachment of the membranes inside the cyst has been referred to as the "US water lily sign". Ultrasound is the most sensitive modality for the detection of membranes, septa and hydatid sand within the cyst.
- CT scan has an accuracy of 98% and the sensitivity to demonstrate the daughter cysts.
- A hydatid cyst typically demonstrates a high-attenuation wall at unenhanced CT even without calcification. Daughter vesicles manifest as round structures located peripherally within the mother cyst.

- For simple cases of cystic echinococcosis, the most common form of treatment is surgical removal of the cysts combined with chemotherapy using albendazole and/or mebendazole before and after surgery. However, if there are cysts in multiple organs or tissues, or the cysts are in risky locations, surgery becomes impractical. For such inoperable cases, chemotherapy and/or puncture-aspiration-injection-reaspiration (PAIR) become alternative options of treatment.
- Dose of albendazole—adult dosage of 400 mg orally, twice a day for 1–5 months and a pediatric dosage of 15 mg/kg/day (maximum of 800 mg) for 1–6 months. An alternative to albendazole is mebendazole at a dosage of 40–50 mg/kg/day for at least 3–6 months.

Picture	Note	Management

Amebic Liver Abscess

Picture	Note	Management
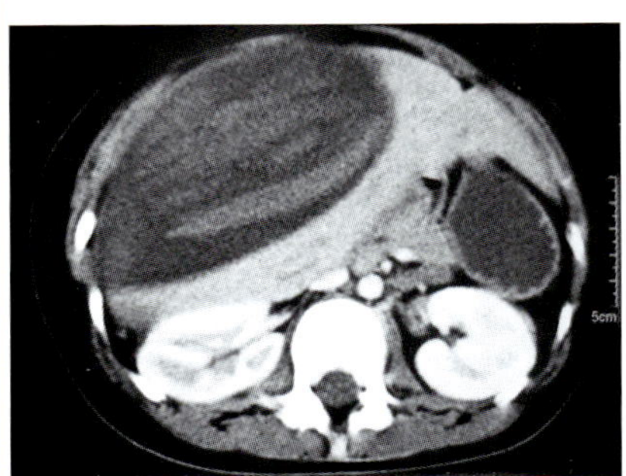 **Figure 4.2.2:** Amebic liver abscess *Photo Courtesy:* Neelam Mohan, Gurgaon	• Approximately two-thirds of liver abscess occur in the right lobe of the liver and majorities are solitary (Fig. 4.2.2). • Appearances of an abscess may be a rounded or an oval lesion which is usually hypoechoeic but may have heterogeneous echotexture. • The abscess cavity takes many months to finally resolve and lags behind clinical resolution by months.	• Therapy includes ultrasound-guided aspiration, culture and sensitivity and microbial study of aspirate. • *Antiamebic agents*: The treatment of invasive amebiasis should be directed to all sites where *E. histolytica* may be present. Hence the ideal amebicide should be able to act within the intestinal lumen, in the intestinal wall, and systemically, particularly in the liver. Systemic amebicidal drugs include emetine, dehydroemetine, chloroquine diphosphate, metronidazole and tinidazole. Metronidazole is safe and effective and widely used.

Pyogenic Liver Abscess

Picture	Note	Management
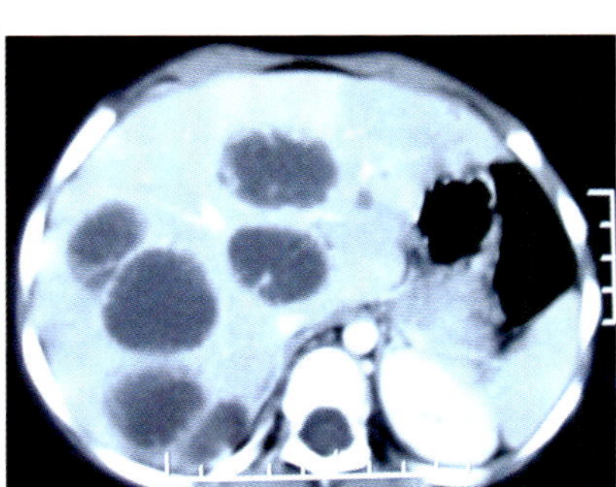 **Figure 4.2.3:** Pyogenic liver abscess *Photo Courtesy:* Neelam Mohan, Gurgaon	• Pyogenic liver abscess is a type of liver abscess caused by bacteria (Fig. 4.2.3). • Abscess can be caused by either ascending infection from the biliary tract, hematogenous spread of infection or direct traumatic introduction of infection. • Pyogenic abscess can be multiple or single and usually presents with fever, pain abdomen especially in the right upper quadrant with enlarged and tender liver. • Usual causes include *Streptococcus milleri, E. coli, Streptococcus fecalis, Klebsiella pneumoniae, Proteus vulgaris* and *Bacteroides*.	• Treatment includes broad spectrum antibiotics and if required percutaneous drainage of abscess cavity. Culture and sensitivity of aspirated material is a must.

Section 5

Urinary Tract Infections

Section Editors

Brigadier Madhuri Kanitkar, Pankaj V Deshpande

Contributors

Brigadier Madhuri Kanitkar, Pankaj V Deshpande

Section Outline

Picture	Note	Management

5.1 CLINICAL FEATURES AND PROCEDURES

PU Valves Presenting Late

Picture	Note	Management
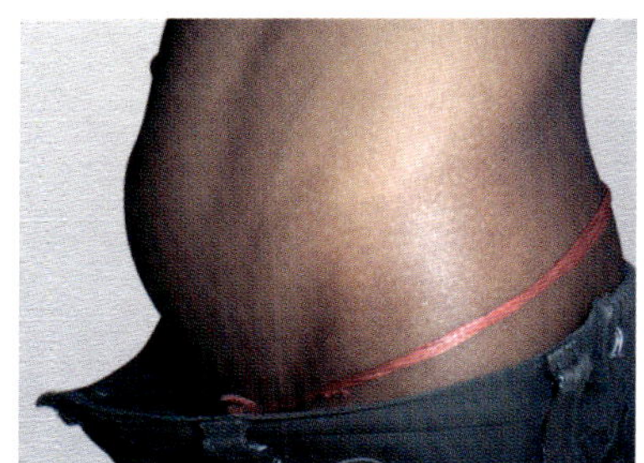 **Figure 5.1.1:** Well-developed abdominal muscles with suprapubic fullness in a boy with deranged renal function and short stature *Photo Courtesy:* Madhuri Kanitkar, New Delhi	Clinical examination of the abdomen and bladder can be very informative in any child presenting with deranged renal functions (Fig. 5.1.1). This boy had past history of recurrent episodes of high-grade fever requiring antibiotics but was never evaluated. He was found to have posterior urethral valves with obstructive nephropathy.	Besides surgery for the urethral valves, these children need long-term follow up for progression of chronic kidney disease. In spite of relieving the obstruction these children develop a 'Valve Bladder' characterized by poor emptying and recurrent urinary tract infection (UTI) resulting in progression of the chronic kidney disease (CKD).

Voiding Disorder—Underactive Bladder

Picture	Note	Management
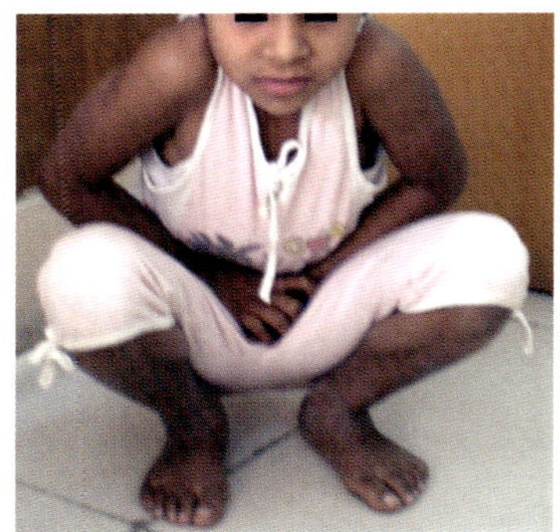 **Figure 5.1.2:** A six-year-old girl squatting and using pressure with both hands to help empty the bladder *Photo Courtesy:* Madhuri Kanitkar, New Delhi	Children presenting with recurrent UTI are more likely to have a functional voiding disorder. This young girl presented with recurrent UTI and had a lazy bladder on evaluation. Functional voiding disorders are abnormal voiding patterns in the presence of an anatomically normal bladder with intact neuronal control. Children presenting with recurrent UTI are more likely to have a dysfunctional voiding resulting from bladder sphincter dyssynergia or a lazy bladder (Fig. 5.1.2).	These children need bladder retraining consisting of timely relaxed voiding and may need biofeedback to help and relax the pelvic floor muscles during voiding. Antibiotic prophylaxis may be given for 3–6 months. Constipation needs to be treated adequately and child advised to increase the fluid intake.

Voiding Disorder—Overactive Bladder

Picture	Note	Management
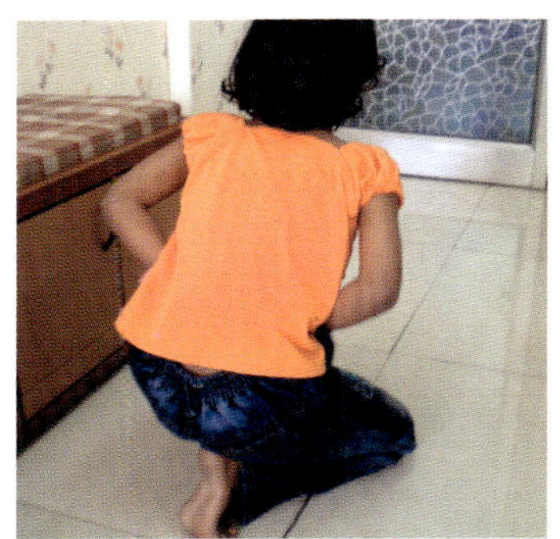 **Figure 5.1.3:** A five-year-old girl demonstrating the Vincent's Curtsy and using her heel for perineal pressure *Photo Courtesy:* Madhuri Kanitkar, New Delhi	Children presenting with UTI or daytime incontinence need to be specifically asked for a history of holding manoeuvres or squatting to be able to diagnose an underlying functional voiding disorder. Frequent small quantity voiding with negligent postvoid residue and squatting are predictive of an overactive bladder (Fig. 5.1.3).	These children need to be advised adequate fluid intake, relief of constipation, timely voiding and judicious use of anticholinergic medications.

Bladder Catheterization

Picture	Note	Management
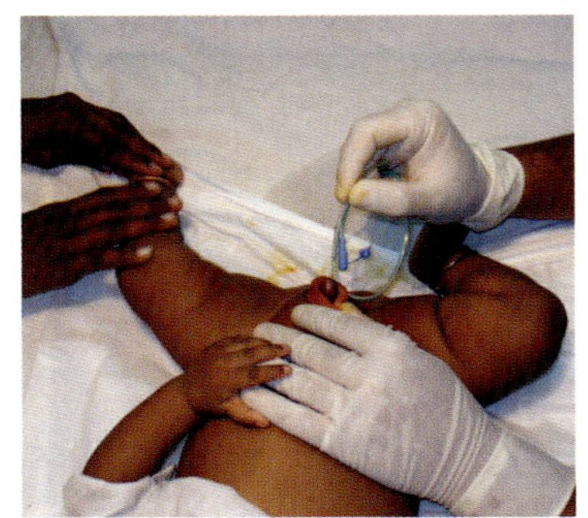 Figure 5.1.4: An infant being catheterized for an MCUG *Photo Courtesy:* Madhuri Kanitkar, New Delhi	A child needs to be catheterized whenever an MCUG is to be undertaken (Fig. 5.1.4). This needs to be performed under strict aseptic conditions.	It is advisable to provide antibiotic prophylaxis prior to catheterization. Injection amikacin 15 mg/kg may be administered 30 minutes prior to the procedure to prevent an UTI.

Urine Sample Collection using Urine Bag

Picture	Note	Management
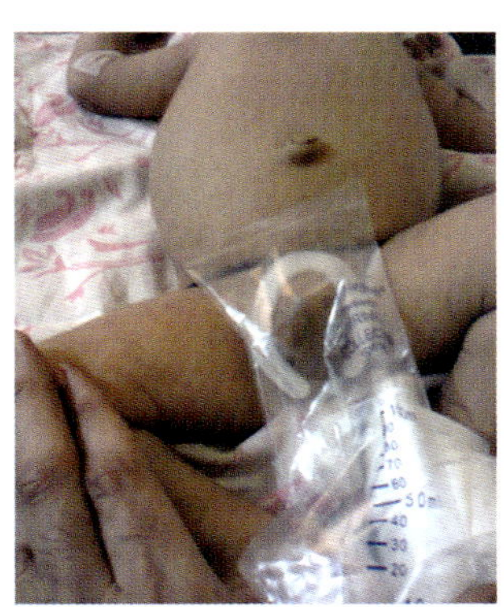 Figure 5.1.5: Urine bag being used for collecting a urine sample *Photo Courtesy:* Pankaj V Deshpande, Mumbai	Collection of urine is always the most difficult challenge in the diagnosis of urinary tract infection (UTI). Urine bag is one of the common methods of urine collection used for diagnosis of UTI (Fig. 5.1.5). Note that the infant is lying down. Proper precautions need to be taken while using a urine bag to minimize the contamination rate.	When a urine bag is used, proper care has to be taken to ensure the following precautions. The genital area needs to be cleaned with normal soap and water and then dried. The urine bag should be attached to the genital area. The infant should be upright till urine is passed to minimize the contamination occurring once the urine comes in contact with skin. As soon as urine is passed, the bag has to be taken off and the urine poured into the collection bottle. Remember, the first part of the urine is also collected in the urine bag and so is not a mid-stream sample. Despite the best efforts and precautions, urine bag carries a contamination rate of about 10%.

Picture	Note	Management

Urine Collection by Suprapubic Aspiration

Picture	Note	Management
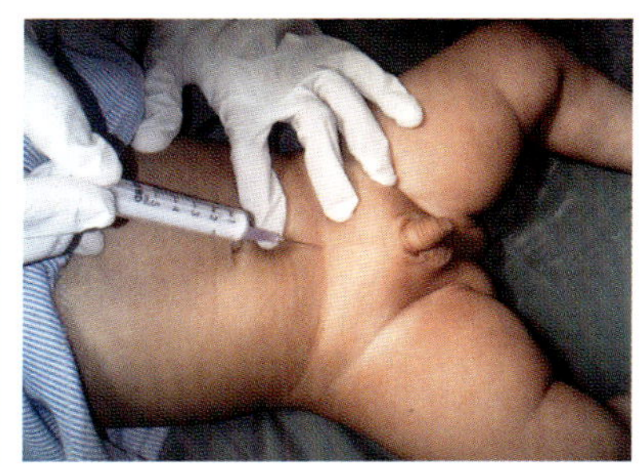 **Figure 5.1.6:** Suprapubic aspiration to collect urine sample *Photo Courtesy:* Pankaj V Deshpande, Mumbai	This method of urine collection is extremely important in the diagnosis of UTIs. Improperly collected samples are the bane of clinical practice and lead to unnecessary embarkation on treatment and multiple investigations. One of the main problems is contamination of the urine sample, especially if the sample is not mid-stream, the genital area is not cleaned or there is a delay in transporting the sample. In such cases, suprapubic aspiration is the ideal route to collect urine (Fig. 5.1.6).	The urinary bladder is an abdominal organ in children till about 5 years of age. To avoid contamination in the urine sample, it can be accessed by suprapubic aspiration to collect the urine sample. The timing is very important. Ensure the infant has not voided for at least half to 1 hour. Clean the suprapubic area with usual cleaning solution. Using a 2 or 5 mL syringe with a 23-gauge needle, aspirate as you enter just a centimeter or so above the pubic symphysis. Once urine is obtained, it is transferred to a container. The procedure carries virtually no risk and remember, any growth seen in the suprapubic aspirate is significant and indicates a UTI.

5.2 ABNORMALITIES ON US SCAN

USG showing Dilated Ureter

Picture	Note	Management
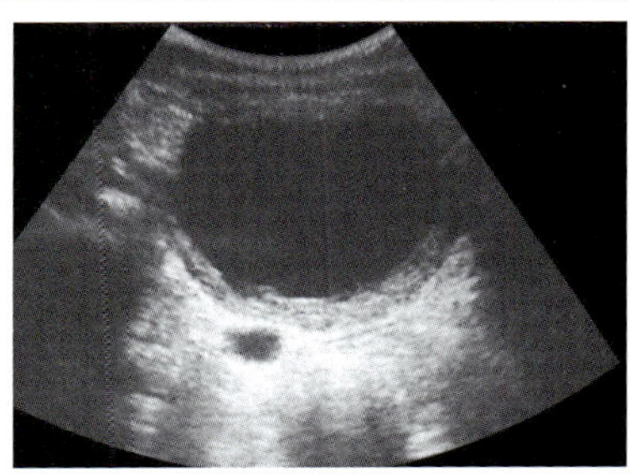 **Figure 5.2.1A:** Ultrasound scan in an infant showing the urinary bladder and dilated right ureter (seen as a golf-hole below the bladder) *Photo Courtesy:* Pankaj V Deshpande, Mumbai	Ultrasound scans are recommended in every child who has suffered from a UTI (Fig. 5.2.1A). Here the ureteric dilatation is seen on the right side along with thickened bladder wall. Note that comments on bladder thickness should be made only when the bladder is full.	Ultrasound scans should be done soon after a UTI in children. They are useful to show several abnormalities. The kidney sizes and shapes can be determined as well as the presence of ureteric and pelvis dilatation. Thickness of bladder wall and presence of urinary stones can be diagnosed. Dilatation needs to be investigated with further imaging.
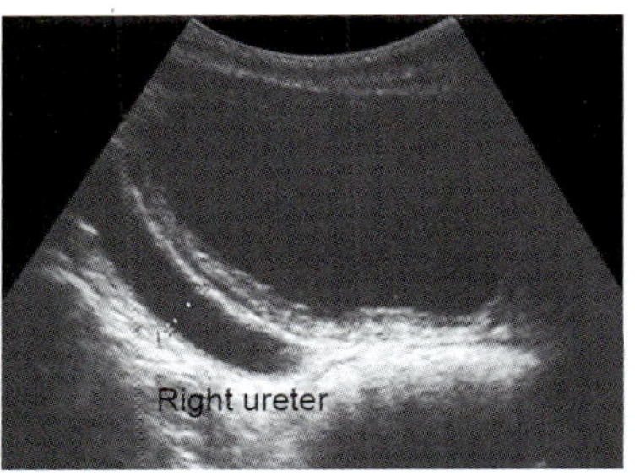 **Figure 5.2.1B:** Ultrasound scan in same patient tracing the ureteric dilatation on the right *Photo Courtesy:* Pankaj V Deshpande, Mumbai	Once dilatation is detected on ultrasound scan, further imaging is required depending on the site and degree of dilatation (Fig. 5.2.1B).	Ureteric dilatation is suggestive of vesico-ureteric reflux and will need a micturiting cystourethrogram (MCUG). Please remember to do the test under antibiotic cover. However, congenital megaureter and vesicoureteric obstruction also need to be kept in mind when ureteric dilatation is seen.

Picture	Note	Management

Hydronephrosis due to PUJ Obstruction

Picture	Note	Management
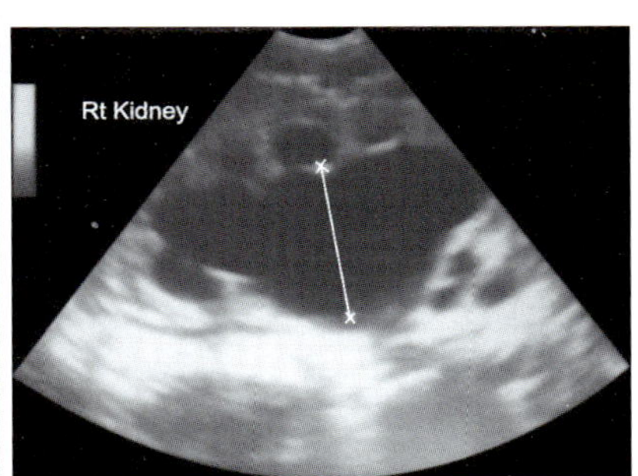 **Figure 5.2.2:** Renal ultrasonography showing gross hydronephrosis with pelvicalyceal dilatation. This is termed the "Mickey Mouse" appearance and is noted in pelviureteric junction (PUJ) obstruction *Photo Courtesy:* Madhuri Kanitkar, New Delhi	This is the postnatal ultrasonography (USG) of a three-day-old neonate detected to have antenatal hydronephrosis (Fig. 5.2.2). The "mickey mouse" appearance results from the proximal large cystic lesion of the obstructed pelvis and the dilated distal calyces giving the appearance of a face with the two ears. This helps to differentiate a multicystic dysplastic kidney which has multiple cysts of different sizes both proximal and distal often not communicating with each other.	A child with suspected PUJ obstruction needs to have a DTPA scan. In case the split function on the affected side is less than 30% or the child has recurrent UTI, the child requires surgical management. However most children have a resolution of the obstruction and conservative care and follow up is all that is required.

USG showing Ureterocele

Picture	Note	Management
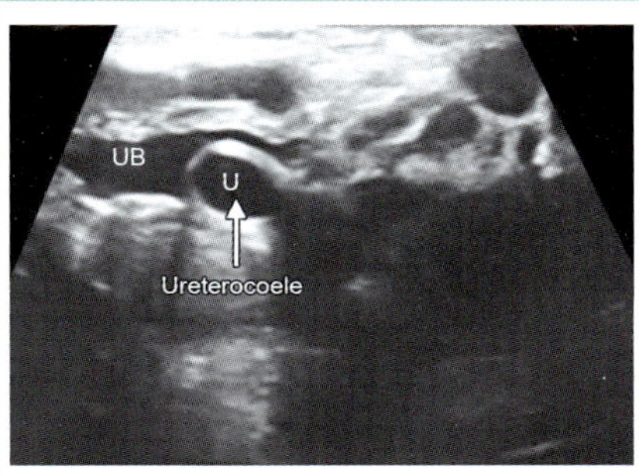 **Figure 5.2.3:** USG scan showing the presence of a ureterocele *Photo Courtesy:* Pankaj V Deshpande, Mumbai	This 2-month-old-baby girl presented with a UTI. Antenatal scans had shown dilatation unilaterally and MCUG, done under antibiotic cover had shown presence of vesicoureteric reflux on the other side (Fig. 5.2.3).	Ureterocele that is small and causes no symptoms or problems may not need intervention. However, if they cause obstruction, there will be urinary stasis and they will need puncturing to ensure good drainage. This should not be missed in an infant with a UTI.

Picture	Note	Management

5.3 ABNORMALITIES ON DMSA SCAN

DMSA Abnormalities 6–8 Weeks After UTI

Picture	Note	Management
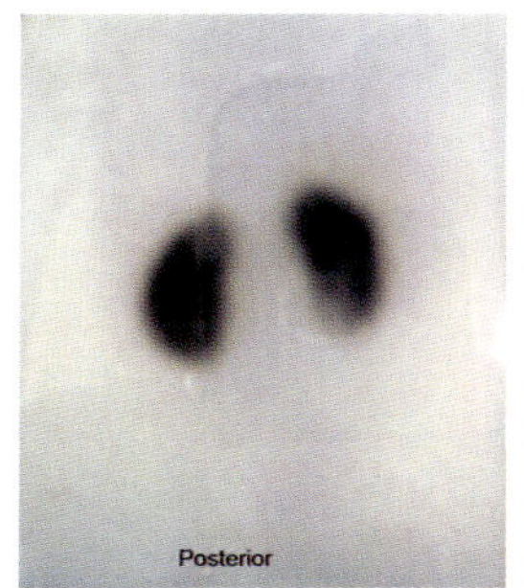 **Figure 5.3.1:** Dimercaptosuccinic acid (DMSA) scan in a 4-year-old girl *Photo Courtesy:* Pankaj V Deshpande, Mumbai	This girl developed a confirmed UTI with a positive urine culture. After the treatment was completed, she had a DMSA scan about 6–8 weeks after the UTI episode. As can be seen, reduced uptake was seen in both kidneys (Fig. 5.3.1).	This scan was interpreted as showing bilateral scarring. Normally both the kidneys appear uniformly dark. As areas of reduced uptake can be seen in both kidneys, it was labeled as scarring.

DMSA Abnormalities 6 Months After UTI

Picture	Note	Management
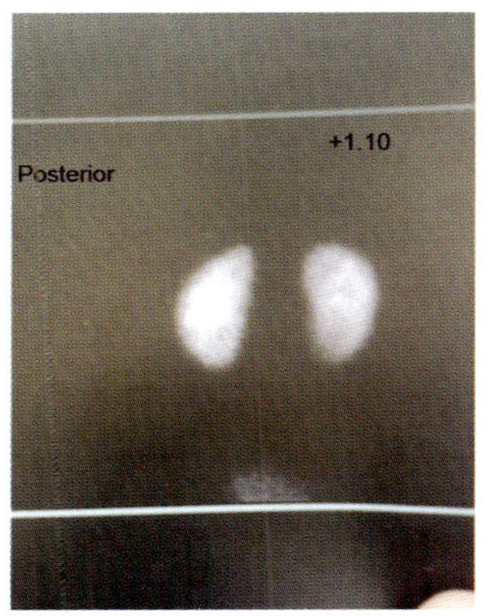 **Figure 5.3.2:** Dimercaptosuccinic acid (DMSA) scan in the same girl, repeated after 6 months *Photo Courtesy:* Pankaj V Deshpande, Mumbai	Dimercaptosuccinic acid (DMSA) scan was repeated in the same girl mentioned above 6 months after the UTI (Fig. 5.3.2). This showed normal kidneys with no evidence of reduced uptake in either of the kidneys. Clearly, no evidence of scarring.	The changes seen on a DMSA scan can be present only in the acute phase of a UTI. Consequently, DMSA scan should be done at least 4–6 months after an episode of UTI to look for scarring or long-term changes. Also remember that the DMSA scan can only show areas of reduced uptake. The interpretation of the picture has to be done by the clinician. It can represent dysplasia, acute changes due to UTI or even in some cases, nephritis. Also, the combined function of both the kidneys is always shown as 100%. This does not mean that the renal function is 100%. It shows you the differential function in each kidney of whatever the total kidney function is.

DMSA Scan showing Scarred Ectopic Kidney

Picture	Note	Management
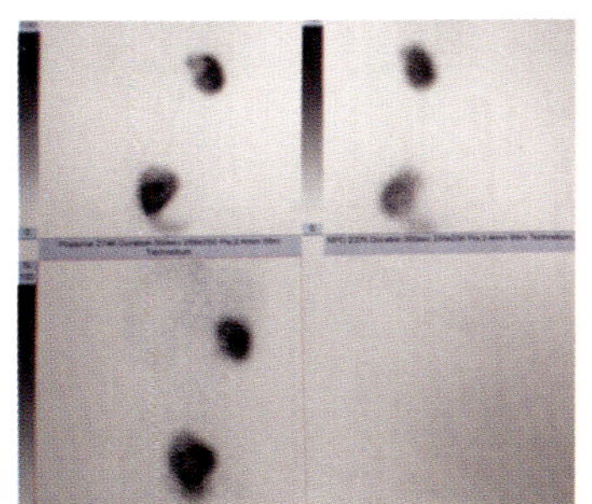 **Figure 5.3.3:** DMSA scan showing an ectopic scarred kidney *Photo Courtesy:* Madhuri Kanitkar, New Delhi	This is a DMSA scan of a 9-year-old girl who presented with UTI (Fig. 5.3.3). The USG revealed a single kidney. The DMSA scan confirmed the presence of an ectopic second kidney which was scarred.	A child with a renal scar needs follow up with annual check up for growth, blood pressure record, renal growth as determined by an ultrasound, serum creatinine and microalbuminuria.

Picture	Note	Management

5.4 ABNORMALITIES ON MCUG

PUV with Trabeculated Bladder and Grade V Reflux

Picture	Note	Management
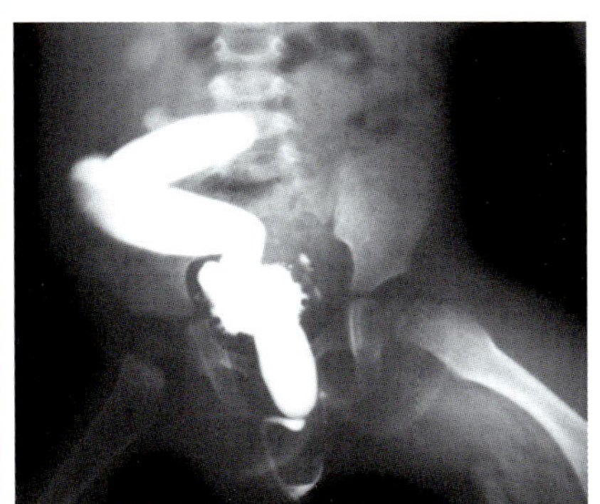 **Figure 5.4.1:** A micturating cystourethrogram showing trabeculated bladder with a grossly dilated posterior urethra and a high-grade reflux *Photo Courtesy:* Madhuri Kanitkar, New Delhi	A poorly developed noncompliant bladder results in worsening and progression of CKD in spite of fulguration (Fig. 5.4.1).	Children with valve bladders require detailed evaluation with urodynamic studies, judicious use of anticholinergic medications and complete emptying of the bladder to prevent recurrent UTI and progression of CKD. In spite of conservative measures if the postvoid residues are large (> 20 mL), the child requires clean intermittent catheterization to protect the kidneys.

Spinning Top Bladder

Picture	Note	Management
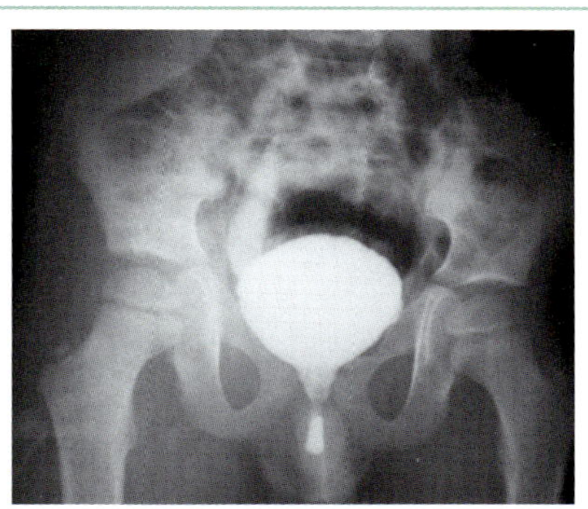 **Figure 5.4.2:** Micturiting cystourethrogram showing a spinning top configuration of the bladder *Photo Courtesy:* Madhuri Kanitkar, New Delhi	All infants with the first UTI, children from 1–5 years having a UTI and noted to have an abnormality on the ultrasonography or technetium ^{99m}Tc-dimercaptosuccinic acid (DMSA) scan or beyond 5 years with an abnormality in both the USG and the DMSA scan need to undergo a micturiting cystourethrogram (MCUG). It is also recommended in children with recurrent UTI. A spinning top configuration suggests an underlying functional voiding disorder (Fig. 5.4.2).	The management of a voiding disorder entails ruling out an anatomical or neurogenic anomaly, treatment of constipation, adequate fluid intake and bladder retraining.

Picture	Notes	Management

Christmas Tree Bladder

Picture	Notes	Management
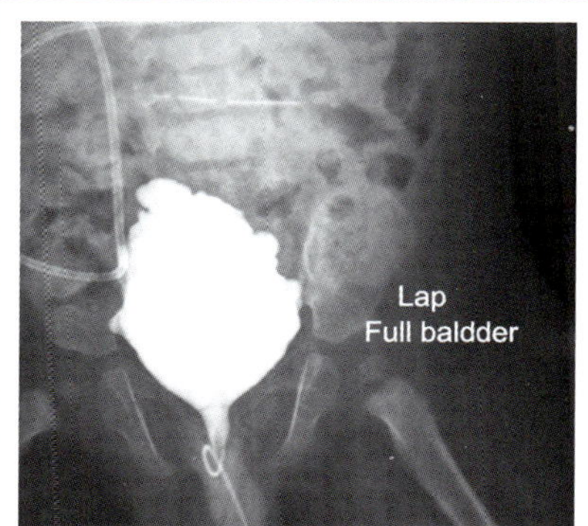 **Figure 5.4.3:** Micturiting cystourethrogram showing a Christmas-tree pattern of a trabeculated bladder *Photo Courtesy:* Madhuri Kanitkar, New Delhi	When a child undergoes the procedure of the MCUG, it is important to look at the bladder configuration besides the reflux if any and the bladder outlet obstruction. A Christmas tree bladder depicts a neurogenic bladder (Fig. 5.4.3).	A neurogenic bladder needs long term follow up to reduce bladder pressures and manage incontinence.

MCUG showing Vesico-colic Fistula

Picture	Notes	Management
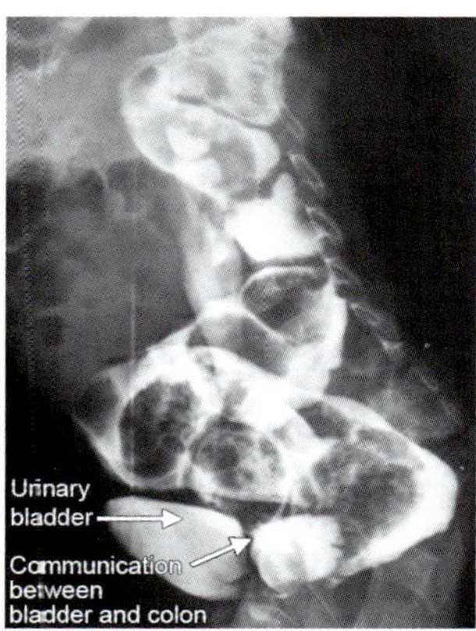 **Figure 5.4.4:** Micturating cystourethrogram (MCUG) showing communication between the urinary bladder and colon: complication of surgical intervention *Photo Courtesy:* Pankaj V Deshpande, Mumbai	This 3-year-old boy presented in an extremely ill state with severe persistent diarrhea for more than 6–9 months. He looked extremely cachectic and had severe electrolyte abnormalities that included severe hypokalemia, acidosis, hyperchloremia and a raised serum creatinine. He had had only 1–2 episodes of UTI and investigations had shown presence of bilateral vesico-ureteric reflux. He had undergone surgery for reimplantation of the ureters and "bladder surgery". These problems had driven the parents to despair (Fig. 5.4.4).	While surgical intervention for vesico-ureteric reflux has definite indications, it is important to remember that long-term studies have shown that medical management of reflux has a similar outcome to the surgical intervention. This boy actually has bilateral renal dysplasia that gets interpreted as scarring on DMSA and forces the hand into surgery. The fistula between the bladder and colon developed subsequently leading to persistent diarrhea and acidosis. The management was very difficult. Once he was metabolically stable, the fistula was excised and the boy's condition improved dramatically. He is now well with no diarrhea, growing well and needs monitoring of his renal function. Unfortunately, the bladder volume is low and hence that will need attention as well later.

MCUG showing Severe VUR

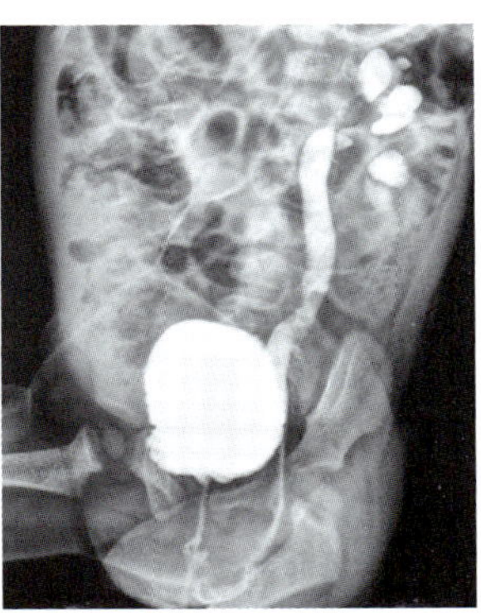

Figure 5.4.5A: Micturating cystourethrogram (MCUG) showing severe vesicoureteric reflux (VUR) on the left in an 18-month-old girl with an interesting history
Photo Courtesy: Pankaj V Deshpande, Mumbai

Table 5.4.5A: Interpretation of urine culture

Sample type	*Colony count*	*Probability of infection*
Suprapubic	Urinary pathogen in any number	99%
Catheterization	>50,000/mL	95%
Mid-stream clean catch	>100,000/mL	90-95%

This 18-month-old girl had been operated for an anorectal malformation at 3 months of age (Fig. 5.4.5A). Thereafter, she had developed confirmed UTIs every 2 weeks with turbid urine, high-grade fever, plenty of pus cells and a positive urine culture. She had undergone reimplantation of the ureters in the 5th month but the UTIs continued. She was advised to do clean intermittent catheterization and was even left with a continuous urinary catheter to improve bladder drainage (Table 5.4.5A). This also failed to stop the UTIs (continued in next picture).

Every UTI is in a class of its own. One can not make the illness fit into our knowledge. Reflux is not the whole and "soul" in terms of UTIs. Fixing reflux may not stop UTIs or renal deterioration. In this case, even bladder drainage seemed to be of little help. As she was having an enema every day, constipation was not a major concern.

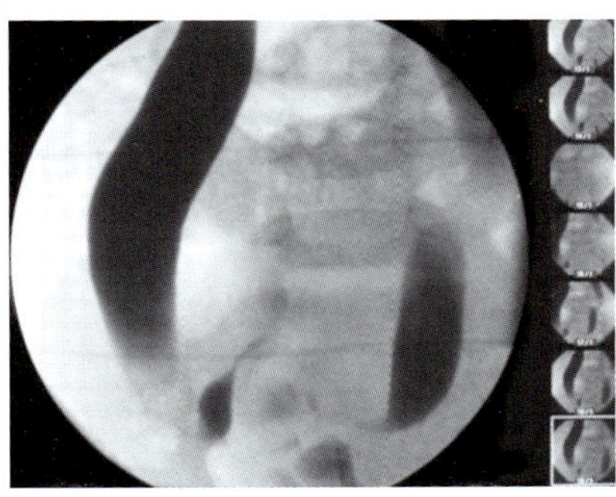

Figure 5.4.5B: Retrograde pyelogram showing right vesicoureteric junction narrowing and dilated left ureter
Photo Courtesy: Pankaj V Deshpande, Mumbai

The same girl above had an MCUG that showed persistent left VUR. However, it also showed that the drainage in the right system was poor as the VUJ was narrow after the reflux surgery (Fig. 5.4.5B). In any case, despite all measures the UTIs continued every 2 weeks. She was given prophylaxis with co-trimoxazole, nitrofurantoin and many other agents and even gentamicin bladder washes with no effect.

As can be understood, fixing reflux was of no help here and probably might have even worsened things. This child had an abnormal DMSA done 1 month after the first UTI that showed diffuse poor uptake though it was labeled as scarring. She also had proteinuria confirming dysplastic kidneys. Unfortunately, the whole system was dysplastic and the dysplastic ureters could not drain the urine effectively into the bladder. Hence, she would get better on IV antibiotics and get another UTI as soon as organisms multiplied in the ureters. She underwent bilateral ureterostomies and the UTIs stopped completely. Note that unilateral ureterostomy stopped UTIs in that kidney but the other side continued having UTIs. Be careful in blaming everything on reflux.

Picture	Note	Management

MCUG showing Bilateral VUR Grade 3

Picture	Note	Management
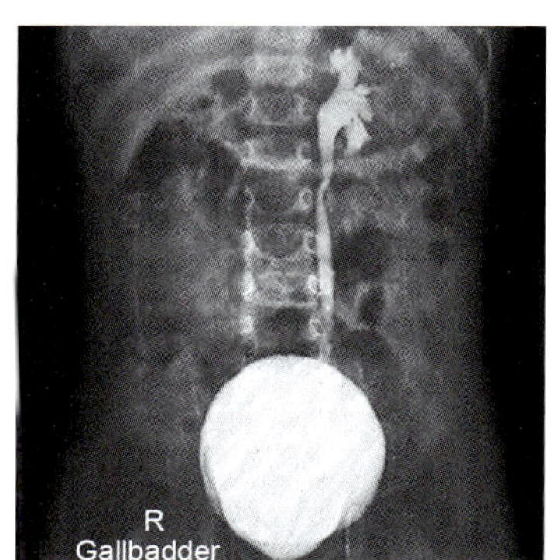 **Figure 5.4.6A:** MCUG in a 3-year-old girl showing bilateral vesicoureteric reflux, Grade 3 *Photo Courtesy:* Pankaj V Deshpande, Mumbai	This girl had presented with recurrent culture proven UTIs. She underwent an MCUG that showed bilateral Grade 3 VUR. Her US scan had shown normal kidneys with no dilatation (Figs 5.4.6A and B).	After appropriate management, the girl stopped having repeated UTIs. That management did not consist of surgical intervention. More important than presence of VUR is the presence of local factors that increase the propensity to develop UTIs. The MCUG shows not only VUR but also presence of constipation. This girl was severely constipated and as that had not been addressed; she had kept on developing UTIs. Once she had proper long-term management of constipation, the UTIs disappeared. Other important factors to consider are the amount of fluid intake by the child, the number of times the child voids urine, whether she empties her bladder (postmicturition residue) and whether she develops local inflammation or vulvovaginitis recurrently.
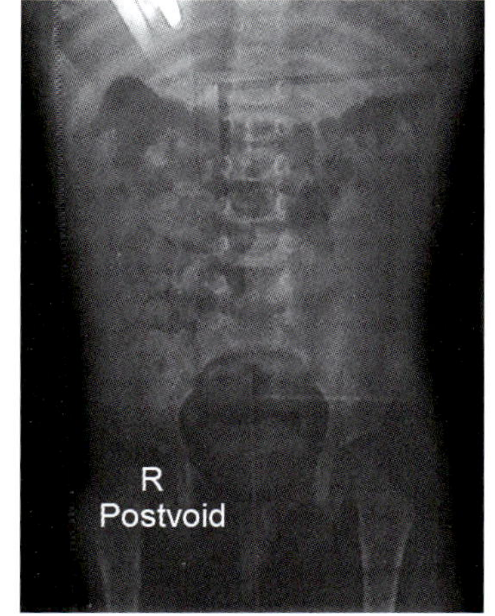 **Figure 5.4.6B:** X-ray of the same girl mentioned above showing severe constipation *Photo Courtesy:* Pankaj V Deshpande, Mumbai	Same as above.	Same as above.

5.5 OTHER STUDIES

Picture	Note	Management

X-ray showing Renal Calculus

Picture	Note	Management
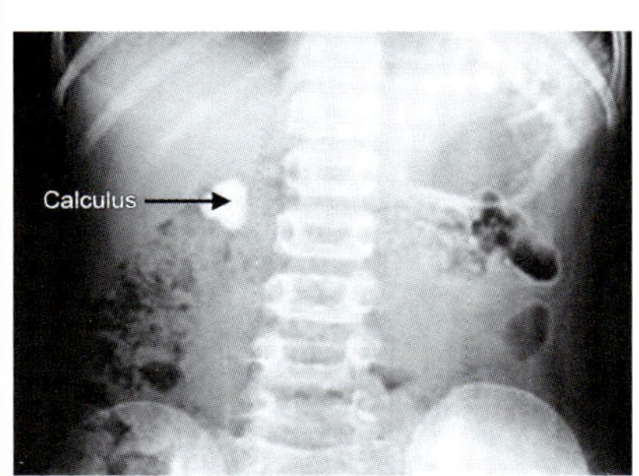 **Figure 5.5.1A:** Plain X-ray showing a large renal calculus in the right kidney *Photo Courtesy:* Pankaj V Deshpande, Mumbai	This little boy presented with recurrent UTIs, proven on culture. US scan shows presence of urolithiasis (Figs 5.5.1A and B).	Small urinary stones may be managed conservatively. However if they cause recurrent UTIs, recurrent pain, etc. they will need to be removed. Larger calculi clearly need to be removed as they will lead to the earlier mentioned problems. Remember the metabolic work-up to diagnose conditions like hypercalciuria, hypocitraturia, hyperoxaluria, etc. If not done and treatment initiated, the calculi recur. The treatments are very simple for prevention.
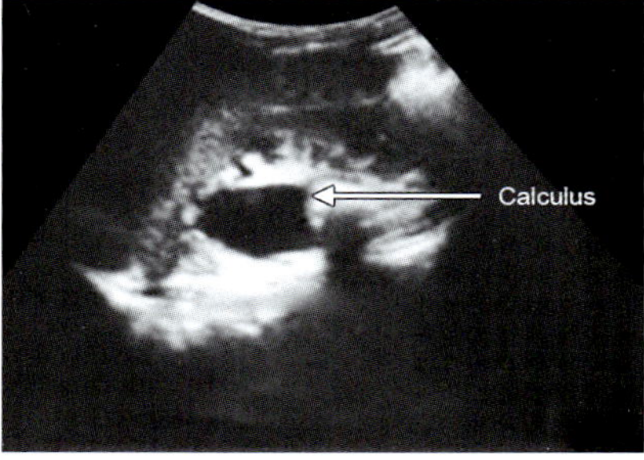 **Figure 5.5.1B:** US scan showing large calculus in pelvis causing dilatation and UTI *Photo Courtesy:* Pankaj V Deshpande, Mumbai	Same as above.	Same as above.

Picture	Note	Management

Nephrostogram in an Infant

Picture	Note	Management
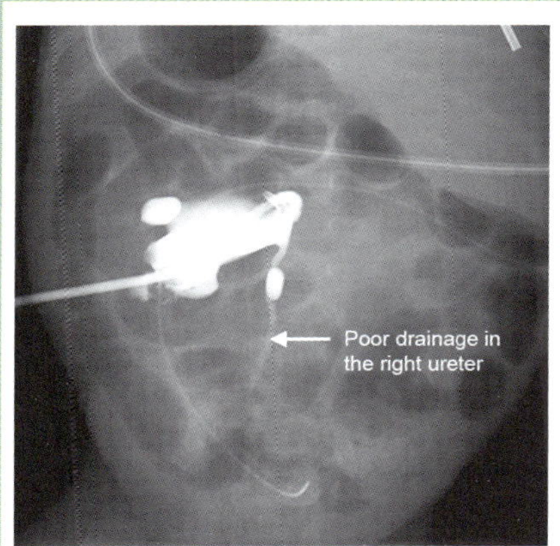 **Figure 5.5.2A:** Nephrostogram showing poor drainage of the dye into the right ureter with multiple filling defects *Photo Courtesy:* Pankaj V Deshpande, Mumbai	This interesting case is important to be remembered by everyone dealing with little babies. This preterm boy presented at about 4 months of age. He had been in NICU for about 3 months after birth. He was at home after discharge for about 2–3 weeks when he developed mild fever and URTI and received symptomatic treatment for a couple of days. Parents then noticed that he became completely anuric. Subsequent investigations showed a raised creatinine, blood urea nitrogen (BUN), hyperkalemia and ultrasound showed mild bilateral dilatation with increased echogenicity in the kidneys and pelvis. Urine and blood culture showed growth of *Candida* (Fig. 5.5.2A).	He underwent peritoneal dialysis and was given antifungal therapy with fluconazole and amphotericin as the urine and blood culture showed *Candida* sensitive to both. In a week, he started good diuresis and dialysis could be stopped. But within 48 hours, he became anuric again.
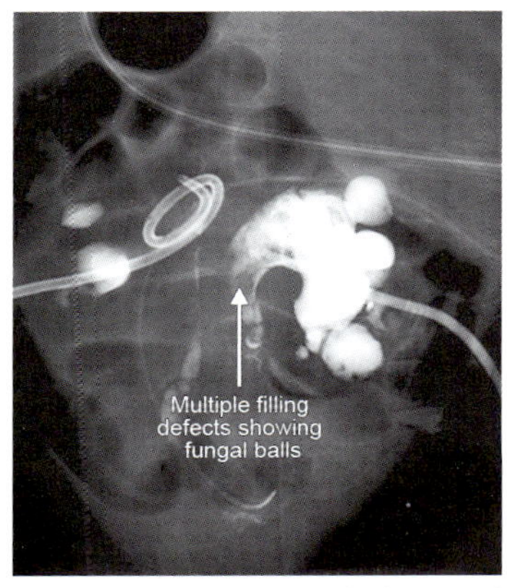 **Figure 5.5.2B:** Nephrostogram in the same baby showing poor drainage in the left ureter and multiple filling defects denoting fungal balls *Photo Courtesy:* Pankaj V Deshpande, Mumbai	In this second episode of renal shutdown, the ultrasound showed similar picture to earlier. He underwent a kidney biopsy that showed tubulointerstitial nephritis and a follow-up ultrasound scan a few days later showed massive enlargement of the pelvicalyceal systems suggesting obstruction by fungal balls. He underwent nephrostograms that are shown above depicting the degree of blockage and the fungal balls clearly delineated (Fig. 5.5.2B).	Bilateral nephrostomies were done and irrigation with amphotericin was done through the nephrostomies. After 7–10 days, methylene blue was also used to irrigate the nephrostomies and ureters. Subsequent nephrostograms showed good drainage and clearance of the ureters. Nephrostomies were closed. At follow-up 3 months later, the ultrasound scan showed no evidence of dilatation or obstruction. At 1 and 2 years follow-up, the child remains well with no further infective episodes. It is important to remember fungal infections, especially UTIs in neonates who are in NICU for a long time and receive multiple antibiotics. They may not have high-grade fever and signs of infection may be subtle.

Picture	Note	Management

DRCG showing VUR

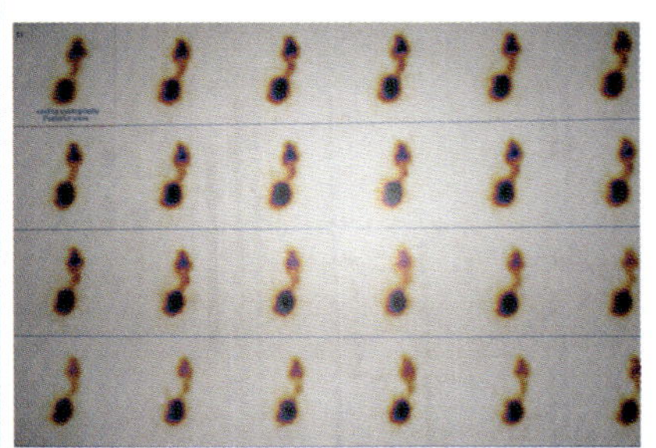 **Figure 5.5.3:** A direct radionuclide cystogram (DRCG) scan showing high-grade reflux on the right *Photo Courtesy:* Madhuri Kanitkar, New Delhi	A DRCG scan may be preferred to the MCUG for follow up scan as it causes less radiation and may be performed without bladder catheterization. However, it cannot be used for imaging the urinary tract for the first time as it does not characterize the urethra and cannot grade the severity of reflux accurately (Fig. 5.5.3).	Vesicoureteric reflux (VUR) is best managed conservatively with antibiotic prophylaxis. Surgery may be considered for a child with persisting bilateral high-grade reflux or when the child has recurrent breakthrough UTI while on prophylaxis.

Section 6

Infections in Central Nervous System

Section Editors

Ritesh C Shah, Shekhar Patil

Contributors

Shekhar Patil, Ritesh C Shah,
Vrajesh Udani, Ananda Kesavan

Section Outline

6.1 Viral CNS Infections

- Japanese B Encephalitis
- Herpes Simplex Virus Encephalitis
- Acute Disseminated Encephalomyelitis
- Subacute Sclerosing Panencephalitis
- Viral Encephalitis
- Minimal Encephalopathy with Reversible Splenial Lesion
- Intrauterine Infection—Cytomegalovirus Illness
- Postherpes Zoster Facial Palsy
- Human Immunodeficiency Virus Encephalopathy
- Postinfectious Transverse Myelitis

6.2 Bacterial CNS Infections

- Brain Abscess
- Ventriculitis
- Recurrent Meningitis
- Subdural Empyema
- Tuberculous Meningitis
- Tuberculoma with Hydrocephalus

6.3 Parasitic CNS Infections

- Neurocysticercosis
- Multiple Neurocysticercosis
- Hydatid Cyst
- Toxoplasmosis

Picture	Note	Management

6.1 VIRAL CNS INFECTIONS

Japanese B Encephalitis

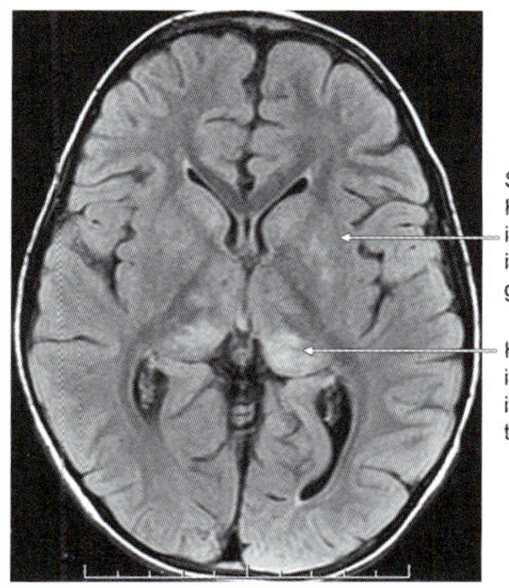

Figure 6.1.1: Japanese B encephalitis
Photo Courtesy: Vrajesh Udani, Mumbai

Bilateral near symmetric hyperintensities in axial FLAIR image involving both thalami with subtle hyperintensities in bilateral basal ganglia region (Fig. 6.1.1). MRI may have characteristic "panda" sign.

- Most common form of epidemic encephalitis in India, mainly during monsoon.
- Japanese B encephalitis (JE) usually presents as high-grade fever followed by signs and symptoms of cranial nerve palsies, raised intracranial pressure, extrapyramidal symptoms and seizures.
- Immunoglobulin M (IgM) antibody in cerebrospinal fluid (CSF) and/or serum is specific diagnostic test. MRI shows typical thalamic involvement (giant panda sign).
- Treatment is supportive. Severe encephalitis carries mortality around 20–40% and remaining have neurological sequelae.
- Mosquito protective measures and JE vaccination are important preventive tools.

Herpes Simplex Virus Encephalitis

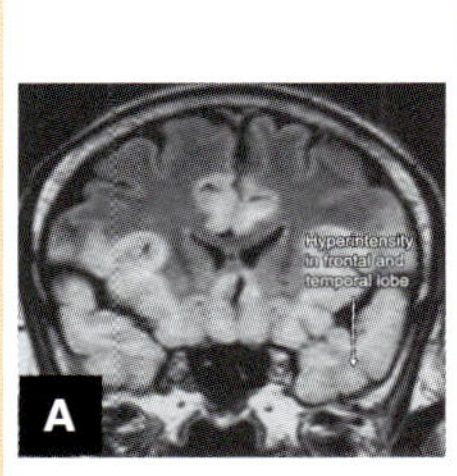

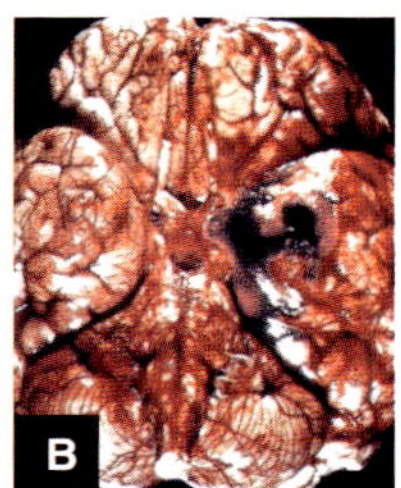

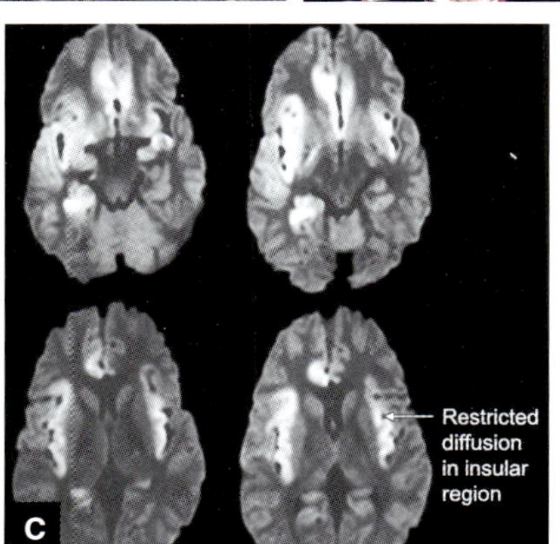

Figures 6.1.2A to C: Herpes simplex virus (HSV) encephalitis
Photo Courtesy: Vrajesh Udani, Mumbai

Coronal FLAIR image: Bilateral symmetric cortico-subcortical hyperintensities in frontotemporal, opercular, insular and cingulated gyrus region.

- Axial diffusion weighted image of same patient showing hypersignals (diffusion restriction) in the same areas suggest herpes encephalitis.
- Postmortem specimen of brain showing necrosis in temporal lobe on right side (Figs 6.1.2A to C).

- Herpes simplex encephalitis (HSE) usually presents as acute illness with fever, irritability, malaise for 1–7 days followed by progressive neurological symptoms like refractory status epilepticus and leads to coma and death within next 3–7 days. HSE has predilection for temporal lobe involvement.
- Cerebrospinal fluid demonstrates pleocytosis with raised protein and decrease sugar. RBCs due to hemorrhagic necrosis are highly suggestive.
- Polymerase chain reaction (PCR) for HSV DNA is very specific and sensitive test (> 90% sensitivity and specificity).
- Electroencephalography (EEG) shows periodic lateralized epileptiform discharges (PLEDs).
- MRI shows frontal (orbitofrontal) and temporal lobe involvement.
- IV acyclovir 10 mg/kg/dose 8 hourly for 14 days is the drug of choice. If untreated mortality is around 75%.

Acute Disseminated Encephalomyelitis

Picture	Note	Management
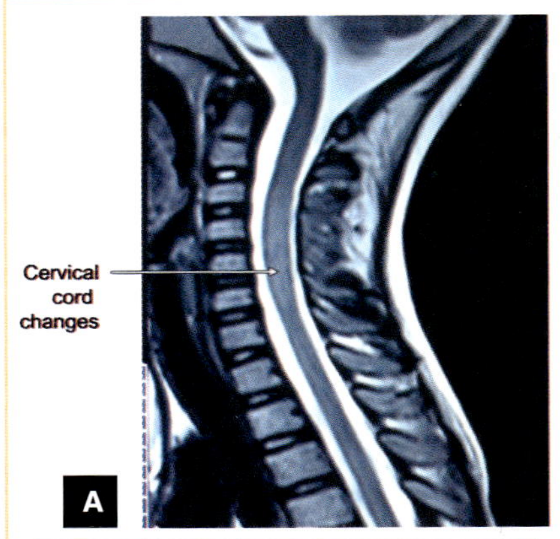 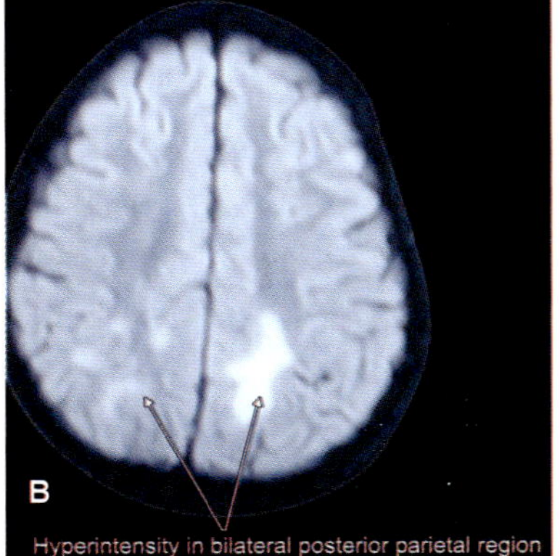 **Figures 6.1.3A and B:** Acute disseminated encephalomyelitis (ADEM) *Photo Courtesy*: Ritesh C Shah, Surat	Sagittal T2W image showing ill-defined intramedullary and short segment hyperintensity in cervical cord (Fig. 6.1.3A). Axial FLAIR image showing subcortical hyperintensity in bilateral posterior parietal region consistent with vasogenic edema of demyelination (Fig. 6.1.3B).	• ADEM is acute immune mediated perivenous, demyelinating disorder. It presents as acute onset of signs and symptoms like altered sensorium, seizures, hemi/paraparesis, cranial nerve palsy, optic neuritis, bowel/bladder disturbance and fever. Usually occurs after viral illness or immunization. • Often difficult to differentiate from encephalitis. MRI shows multiple T2 hyperintensity in white matter and also in basal ganglia and gray matter. • Cerebrospinal fluid may show mild lymphocytic pleocytosis (100–200 cell/cm^3) and mildly raised protein. • Treatment is high dose steroids (methylprednisolone 30 mg/kg/day or dexamethasone 5 mg/kg/day) for 7 days. Outcome is usually good without sequelae. • Intravenous immunoglobulin (IVIg) is also helpful.

Subacute Sclerosing Panencephalitis

Picture	Note	Management
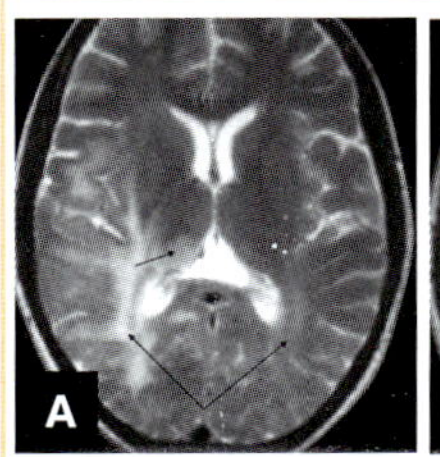 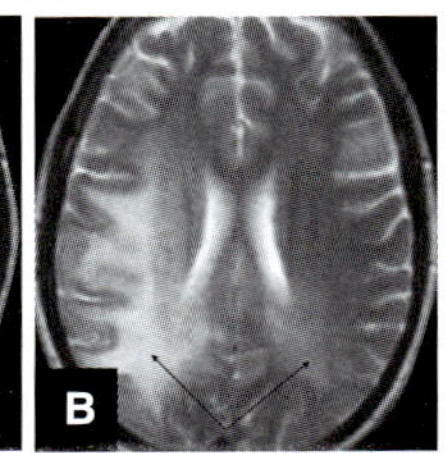 **Figures 6.1.4A and B:** Subacute sclerosing panencephalitis (SSPE) *Photo Courtesy*: Ritesh C Shah, Surat	Axial T2W images show asymmetric hyperintensity in bilateral (right > left) periventricular and subcortical white matter and altered signal in right thalamus and putamen (Figs 6.1.4A and B).	• SSPE is progressive neurological disease related to measles infection in past. It usually presents as seizures (periodic myoclonus typical), change in behavior and cognitive decline. Worsening school performance and intellectual deterioration in otherwise previously normal child with past history of measles is most common presentation. EEG is often characteristic. It is universally fatal disease and person usually dies 1–2 years after diagnosis but some may survive longer.

Picture	Note	Management

Viral Encephalitis

Picture	Note	Management
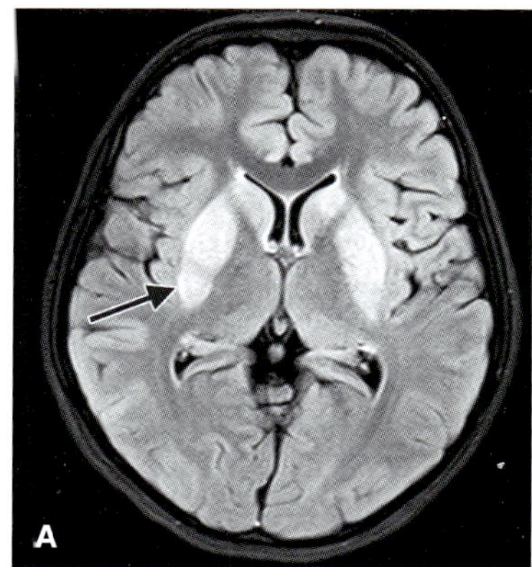 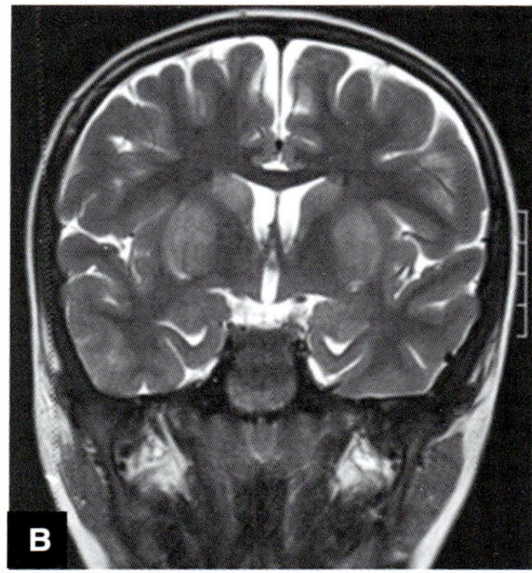 **Figures 6.1.5A and B:** Viral encephalitis *Photo Courtesy*: Shekhar Patil, Mumbai	FLAIR Images (A) and T2 weighted images (B) show hyperintense signal in the basal ganglia with swelling of the corpus striatum (Figs 6.1.5A and B). The diffusion-weighted images show restricted diffusion in the cortex as seen in Figures 6.1.5A and B. MR spectroscopy of the same sites reveals reduced N-acetyl-aspartate (NAA) peak and a lactate peak. The reduced NAA peak on the spectroscopy images suggests neuronal injury and heralds a poor outcome.	• Viral encephalitis presents as an acute illness with fever with catarrh, altered sensorium and convulsions and possibly viral exanthem. • Imaging shows a variable picture, e.g. HSV being classic for involvement of the limbic structures and Japanese B encephalitis for abnormality in the basal ganglia and thalami. • Most common imaging picture in presumed viral encephalitis is nonspecific signal abnormality in the cortex and basal ganglia. • The imaging features as seen in adjoining picture are quite reminiscent for Leigh's disease and needs to be considered in the differential diagnosis. • Investigations in the line of mitochondrial disease may help in separating the two entities. Treatment is usually supportive supplemented by care of the unconscious child, management of seizures/status epilepticus. In such a setting, the outcome is extremely guarded with long-term sequelae in the cognitive, visual and motor domain and possibly refractory epilepsy.

Minimal Encephalopathy with Reversible Splenial Lesion

Picture	Note	Management
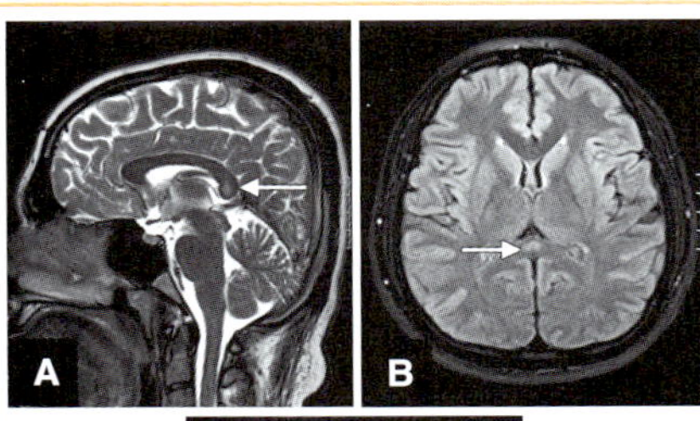 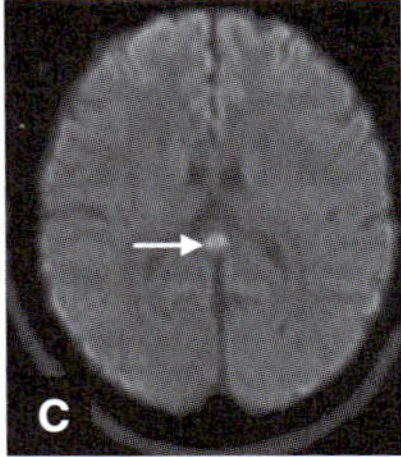 **Figures 6.1.6A to C:** Minimal encephalopathy with reversible splenial lesion *Photo Courtesy*: Shekhar Patil, Mumbai	T2W sagittal image (A) and FLAIR (B) axial show hyperintense signal in the splenium of corpus callosum. The diffusion image (C) shows an area of restricted diffusion corresponding to the hyperintense signal (Figs 6.1.6A to C).	• Commonly seen in Asian population. Presents with acute and occasionally severe encephalopathy at the onset with prompt and complete recovery. Investigations reveal minimal to absent CSF pleocytosis and characteristic reversible hyperintense lesion in the splenium of corpus callosum. Additionally, there may be involvement of the frontoparietal white matter and the cerebellum, which is reversible. • Influenza, Epstein-Barr virus (EBV), human herpesvirus 6 (HHV-6) are said to be associated with this condition. • Treatment with supportive care is associated with prompt and complete recovery. Repeat MRI scan which shows complete resolution of the splenial lesion.

Intrauterine Infection—Cytomegalovirus Illness

Picture	Note	Management
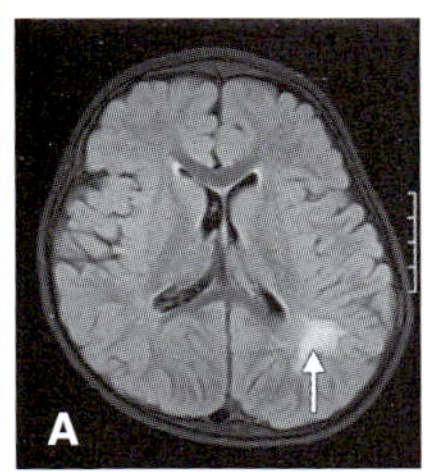 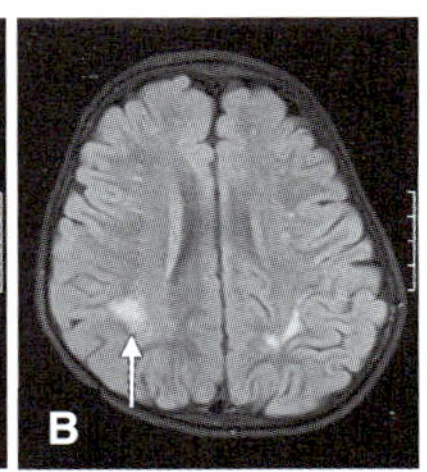 **Figures 6.1.7A and B:** Intrauterine infection—Cytomegalovirus (CMV) illness *Photo Courtesy*: Shekhar Patil, Mumbai	The FLAIR axial images show hyperintense signal in the parieto-occiptal white matter. This is one of the features of CMV disease and may additionally show more widespread white matter involvement, neuronal migration abnormalities and anterior temporal cysts (Figs 6.1.7A and B).	Cytomegalovirus illness may be diagnosed at birth or during childhood, typically like this patient who underwent an MRI scan for a cochlear implant program. These patients present with developmental delay, infrequent seizures, sensorineural hearing deficit and microcephaly. Neonatal presentation is quite different to that of later presentation.

Postherpes Zoster Facial Palsy

Picture	Note	Management
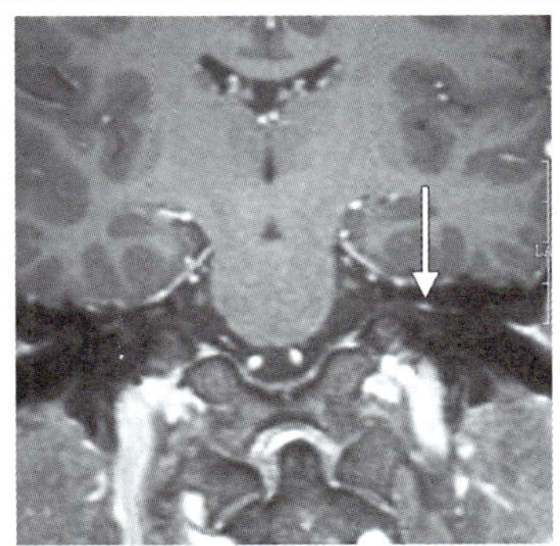 **Figure 6.1.8:** Postherpes zoster facial palsy *Photo Courtesy*: Shekhar Patil, Mumbai	Postcontrast T1W image shows enhancement of the facial nerve of the left side (Fig. 6.1.8).	• This is a complication of pediatric herpes zoster. Facial weakness is seen as a part of herpes zoster oticus or isolated facial nerve involvement. • Facial palsy may be seen as a part of acute illness or during reactivation phase seen during diminished cellular immunity. • Treatment includes antivirals such as oral acyclovir, valacyclovir and corticosteroids. Postherpetic neuralgia is quite uncommon in children.

Picture	Note	Management

Human Immunodeficiency Virus Encephalopathy

Picture	Note	Management
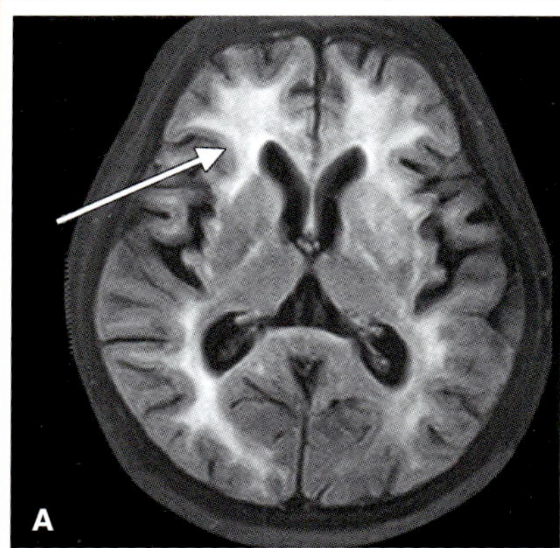 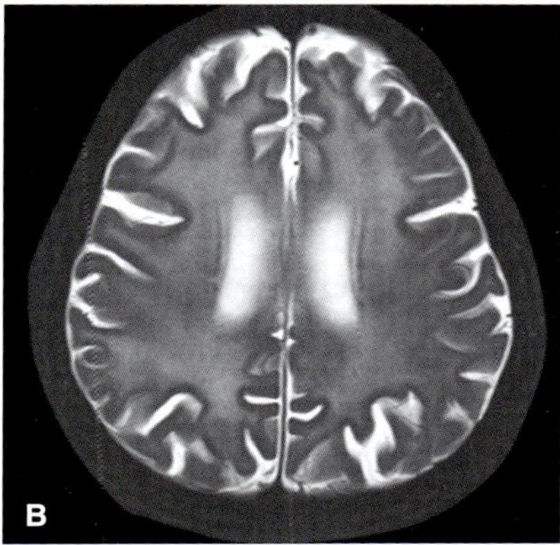 **Figures 6.1.9A and B:** Human immunodeficiency virus encephalopathy *Photo Courtesy*: Shekhar Patil, Mumbai	FLAIR and T2W images show abnormal white matter signal, cortical atrophy and mild ventricular enlargement (Figs 6.1.9A and B).	• Progressive encephalopathy in the setting of human immunodeficiency virus (HIV) infection was quite common in the pre-highly active antiretroviral therapy (HAART) era and this has reduced to 5–10% in the HAART era. Progressive encephalopathy in HIV is quite similar to progressive white matter disease. Perinatally acquired HIV can manifest symptoms of HIV encephalopathy as early as 2 months after birth to as late as 5 years after birth. • Human immunodeficiency virus encephalopathy usually manifests with microcephaly, progressive bilateral pyramidal signs, developmental delay and loss of milestones or developmental stagnation. Adolescents may manifest as HIV dementia similar to adults. Focal signs are rarely seen in HIV encephalopathy. • Cerebrospinal fluid study shows nonspecific changes and the diagnosis is based on clinical impression and radiological features with MRI being preferred modality. MRI brain shows cortical atrophy, ventricular dilatation, white matter signal abnormality beginning in the periventricular area and then spreading towards the cortex and basal ganglia calcification. • Treatment includes the same antiretroviral agents as used to treat symptomatic HIV disease with similar goal of reducing the viral load and reversing the immune suppression.

Picture	Note	Management

Postinfectious Transverse Myelitis

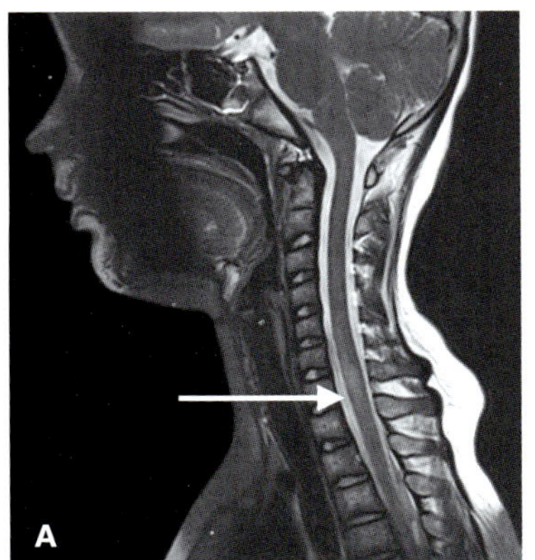 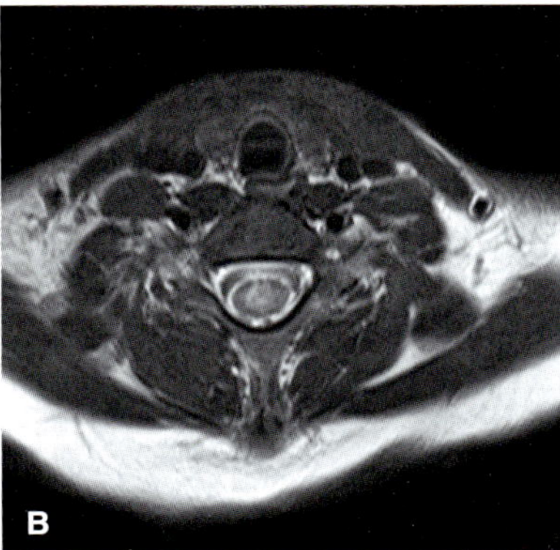 **Figures 6.1.10A and B:** Postinfectious transverse myelitis *Photo Courtesy*: Shekhar Patil, Mumbai	The sagittal T2W (A) image shows a long-segment hyperintense signal in the cervical cord (white arrow) and the T2W axial (B) image at the same level shows the hyperintensity in the central gray matter and the surrounding white matter (Figs 6.1.10A and B).	• The clinical syndrome of postinfective transverse myelitis is seen in patients 2–15 days after a febrile illness usually of viral origin. • Acute transverse myelitis presents with cord symptoms such as paraparesis or quadriparesis, backache, sphincter disturbances and sensory phenomena. The symptoms usually occur as rapid as within a span of 4 hours or slow progression over 10–15 days. The 4 hours period is so defined to separate postinfectious/inflammatory cause from vascular causes. • Cerebrospinal fluid and neuroimaging are required for diagnosis. The CSF shows pleocytosis and the MRI images show a long segment and central gray matter signal abnormality extending over a number of cord segments. Serological tests and other appropriate tests need to be carried out to exclude vasculitides. Tests to exclude neuromyelitis optica (NMO) and multiple sclerosis. • Treatment includes high dose corticosteroids and in majority of cases results in good clinical recovery. Supportive care for sphincter disturbance and medication such as gabapentin, amitryptiline for sensory phenomena is advised.

6.2 BACTERIAL CNS INFECTIONS

Brain Abscess

Picture	Note	Management
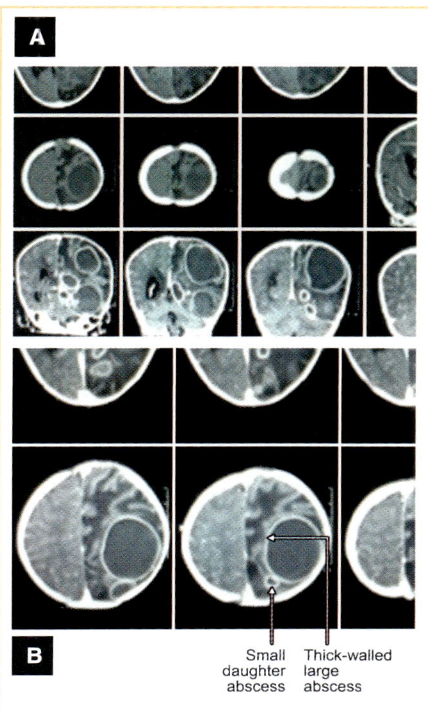 **Figures 6.2.1A and B:** Brain abscess *Photo Courtesy*: Ritesh C Shah, Surat	Postcontrast axial and coronal CT images showing large peripherally enhancing thick-walled abscess in left high frontoparietal region with diffuse edema. Also note the multiple small daughter abscesses adjacent to main abscess (Figs 6.2.1A and B).	• Brain abscess presents as fever (40–80%), headache, vomiting, focal neurological signs (25–50%) and irritability, drowsiness and stuporous state (40–50%). • Absence of fever does not rule out brain abscess. • Underlying cyanotic congenital heart disease (CHD) and acute otitis media may be there. • Cerebrospinal fluid is not helpful and should not be done. Contrast enhanced CT or MRI is the most useful investigation. • Antibiotics should be selected based on polymicrobial etiology and specific organism suspected on basis of predisposing condition and should be given for 4–6 weeks. Surgical treatment is indicated in some selected patients with large and accessible abscess, impeding herniation and impending rupture of abscess.

Ventriculitis

Picture	Note	Management
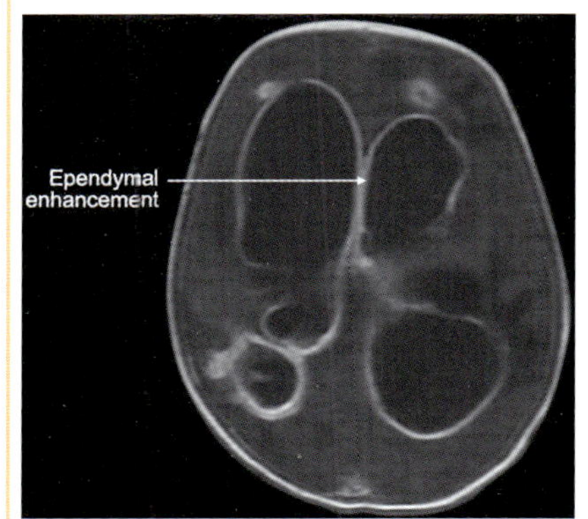 **Figure 6.2.2:** Ventriculitis *Photo Courtesy*: Ritesh C Shah, Surat	Postcontrast T1W axial image showing enhancement of ependymal margin of both the lateral ventricle and few nodular enhancing areas in periventricular region (Fig. 6.2.2).	Ventriculitis is a common complication of neonatal pyogenic meningitis. It must be suspected on the basis of failure to respond clinically and bacteriologically to appropriate antimicrobial therapy and increasing head size. Use of intraventricular antibiotics should be avoided as it increases mortality as compared to intravenous antibiotics (given for 4–6 weeks).

Picture	Note	Management

Recurrent Meningitis

Picture	Note	Management
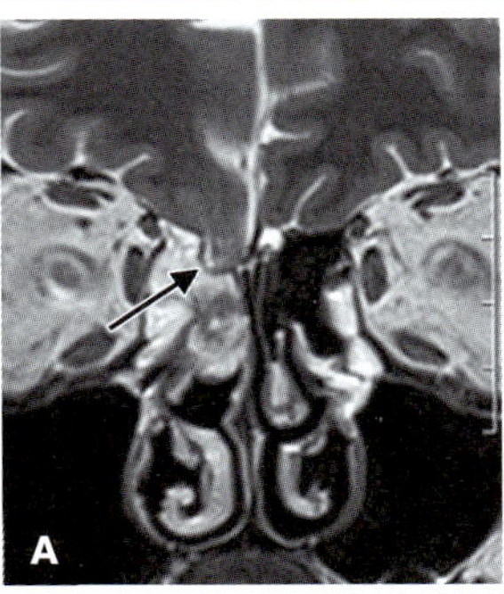 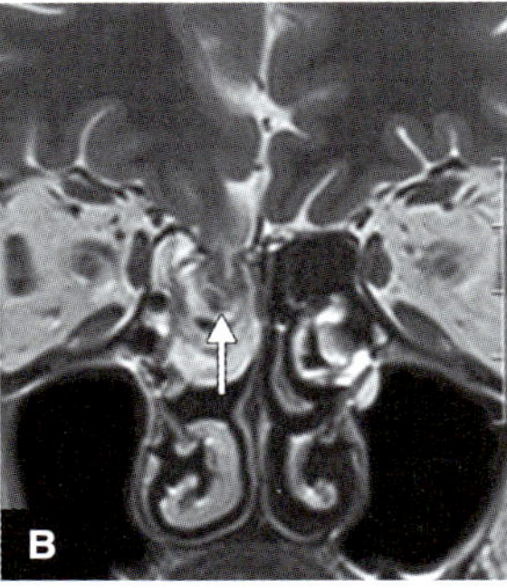 **Figures 6.2.3A and B:** Recurrent meningitis *Photo Courtesy:* Shekhar Patil, Mumbai	The T2W coronal images show a defect in the cribriform plate with a small encephalocele (Figs 6.2.3A and B).	Recurrent meningitis may be recurrent aseptic meningitis (Mollaret's meningitis), or due to structural causes like fracture/defect of the cribriform plate, Mondini type dysplasia, skull base defects, and dermal sinus tracts and rarely due to immunodeficiency states. Recurrent meningitis is of two types, bacterial and nonpurulent. These patients manifest with typical features of meningitis such as fever, altered sensorium, seizures, meningism and possibly CSF otorrhea or rhinorrhea. Treatment includes medical management with antibiotics and detailed investigations to look for structural defects, blood tests to screen for immunodeficiency states, detailed ENT evaluation. Closure of the structural defect that may be primary or post-traumatic usually results in complete cure. Appropriate treatment for immunodeficiency states under expert guidance.

Subdural Empyema

Picture	Note	Management
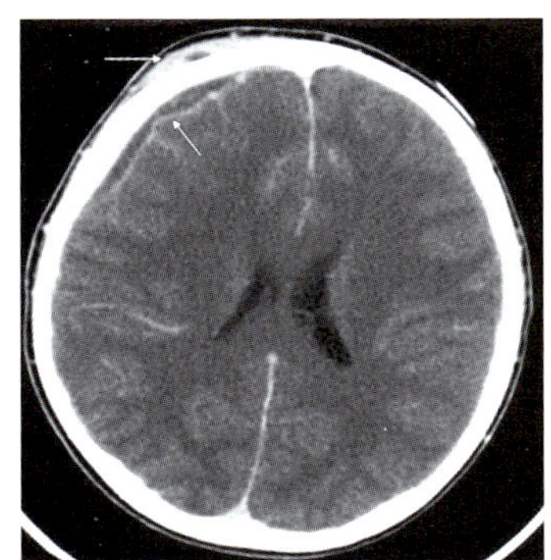 **Figure 6.2.4:** Subdural empyema *Photo Courtesy*: Ritesh C Shah, Surat	Postcontrast axial CT showing thin subdural collection with enhancing dural consistent with subdural empyema in right anterior frontal region (Fig. 6.2.4). Also note the small enhancing abscess in subgaleal region of right frontal scalp tissue which may indicate spread of infection through emissary veins.	Subdural empyema is suspected in cases of pyogenic meningitis when there is recrudescence of fever, increasing head size and CT/MRI show enhancing margin of effusion. Subdural tap confirms the diagnosis. It needs drainage. Deterioration of otherwise responsive child of acute bacterial meningitis (ABM) is an indication for subdural tapping. Confirmation by CT is a must.

Picture	Note	Management

Tuberculous Meningitis

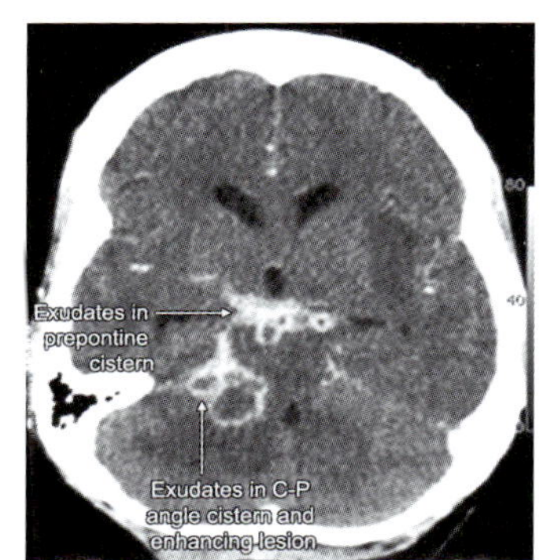 **Figure 6.2.5:** Tuberculous meningitis (TBM) *Photo Courtesy*: Ritesh C Shah, Surat	Postcontrast CT shows multiple conglomerated peripherally enhancing nodular lesions and exudates in prepontine cistern, left sylvian fissure and left C-P angle cistern consistent with TBME (Fig. 6.2.5).	• Tuberculous meningitis is the most important cause of chronic meningitis and can have acute or insidious onset. Most common between 6–24 months of age. Conventionally, it is divided in three stages based on clinical features (I: prodromal stage, II: meningitis, III: coma). • Cerebrospinal fluid is the most useful investigation and CT scan demonstrates some abnormality in majority of patients like basal exudates, calcification, infarcts, tuberculoma and hydrocephalus. The triad of basal exudates, thalamic infarcts and hydrocephalus is typical of TBM. • Recommended treatment is 2 HRZE/S +10 HRE. Dexamethasone is recommended for 6 weeks.

Tuberculoma with Hydrocephalus

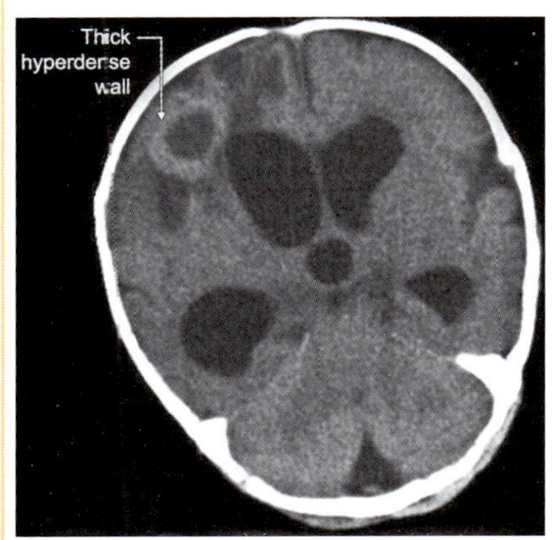 **Figure 6.2.6:** Tuberculoma with hydrocephalus *Photo Courtesy*: Ritesh C Shah, Surat	Coronal Plain CT shows fluid hypodense lesion with thick hyperdense wall in right high frontal region with perilesional edema. Moderate dilatation of both the lateral and third ventricle is also noted (Fig. 6.2.6).	• Tuberculoma sometimes presents only as seizures and creates confusion with neurocysticercosis. It must be differentiated from NCC. In tuberculoma, the lesions are larger in size with greater perilesional edema. • Features of raised intracranial tension like headache, vomiting, altered sensorium is more commonly associated with tuberculoma. Shunt is required for hydrocephalus apart from treatment for tuberculous meningitis.

6.3 PARASITIC CNS INFECTIONS

Neurocysticercosis

Picture	Note	Management
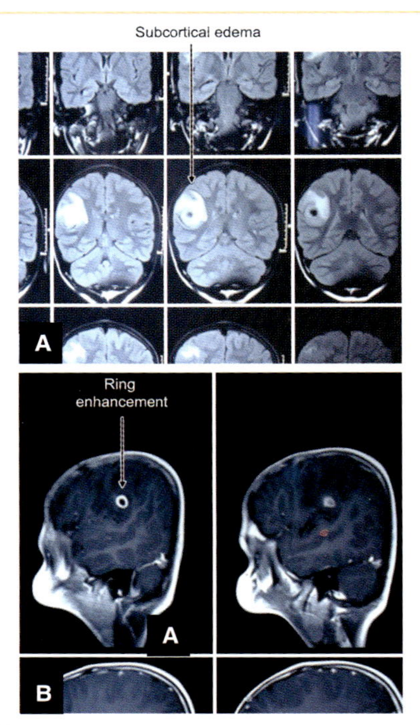 **Figures 6.3.1A and B:** Neurocysticercosis *Photo Courtesy*: Ritesh C Shah, Surat	Coronal Fluid attenuated inversion recovery (FLAIR) images (Figs 6.3.1.A and B) showing diffuse subcortical edema with central hypointense area suggestive of single ring enhancing lesion of neurocysticercosis. The same lesion on postcontrast sagittal study shows well-defined ring enhancement. Tuberculoma is an important differential diagnosis. Magnetic resonance spectroscopy (MRS) is useful, where in TB we will get lipid and lactate peaks.	• Neurocysticercosis usually presents as focal seizures either simple or complex depending on location of cyst. Treatments consist of "corticosteroids (dexamethasone or prednisolone), anticysticercal therapy (albendazole or praziquantel) and anticonvulsants (usually for 3–9 months, not for long time like in epilepsy)". • Albendazole is more effective than praziquantel. • Dose of albendazole is 15 mg/kg/day in two divided doses for 28 days. • Cysticidal therapy should be preceded by steroid therapy to prevent severe raised intracranial pressure (ICP) and precipitation of seizures.

Multiple Neurocysticercosis

Picture	Note	Management
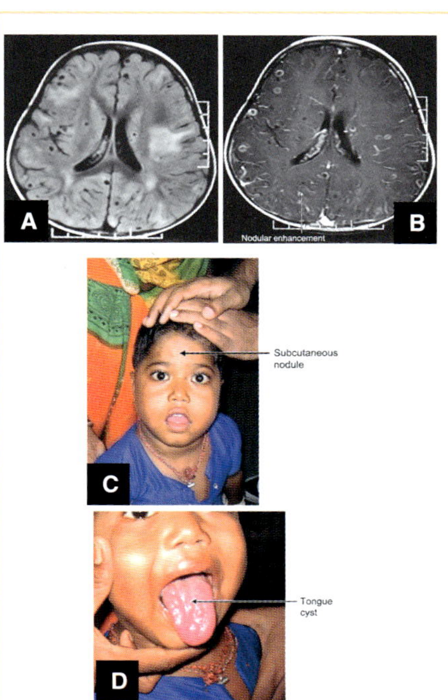 **Figures 6.3.2A to D:** Multiple neurocysticercosis *Photo Courtesy*: Ritesh C Shah, Surat; Vrajesh Udani, Mumbai	Axial FLAIR image (Fig. 6.3.2A) showing multiple tiny scattered fluid intensity areas in cortico-subcortical and periventricular region with mild brain edema. Axial postcontrast T1W image of same patient (Fig. 6.3.2B) showing peripheral regular ring enhancement. Some of the lesions in right occipital region also shows nodular enhancement. Subcutaneous nodule and tongue cyst in the same patient (Figs 6.3.2C and D).	• Disseminated neurocysticercosis presents as seizures and other manifestations like raised ICP, neurological deficit, ocular cyst and subcutaneous nodules. • Before starting anticysticidal therapy look for ocular cyst, ventricular cyst, spinal cysts and hydrocephalous and if they are there cysticidal therapy is contraindicated. • There is high possibility of precipitating raised ICP when cysticidal drugs are used in presence of multiple lesions. So if MRI "shows starry night appearance" on contrast, give only steroids.

Picture	Note	Management

Hydatid Cyst

Picture	Note	Management
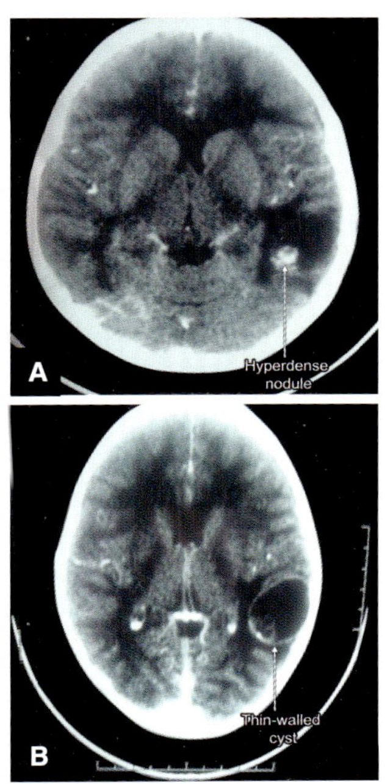 **Figures 6.3.3A and B:** Hydatid cyst *Photo Courtesy:* Ananda Kesavan, Thrissur	Axial postcontrast CT shows well-defined fluid density cyst with thin wall and hyperdense nodular area in the dependent portion of the cyst consistent with hydatid cyst (Figs 6.3.3A and B). (Usually hydatid cyst in brain does not show enhancing nodule or scolex as in liver hydatid cyst).	• Intracranial hydatid cysts are commonly solitary. Multiple intracranial cysts are rare. The patients with intracranial hydatid cysts usually present with focal neurological signs and features of raised intracranial pressure and few patients with seizures. • The treatment of hydatid cyst is surgical and the aim of surgery is to excise the cyst in toto without rupture of the cyst to prevent recurrence and anaphylactic reaction. • Studies have shown complete disappearance of multiple intracranial hydatid cysts with albendazole therapy in a daily dose of 10 mg/kg, three times a day for 4 months. Better effectiveness of the drug therapy is more effective in recurrent cases and in cases with rupture during surgery.

Toxoplasmosis

Picture	Note	Management
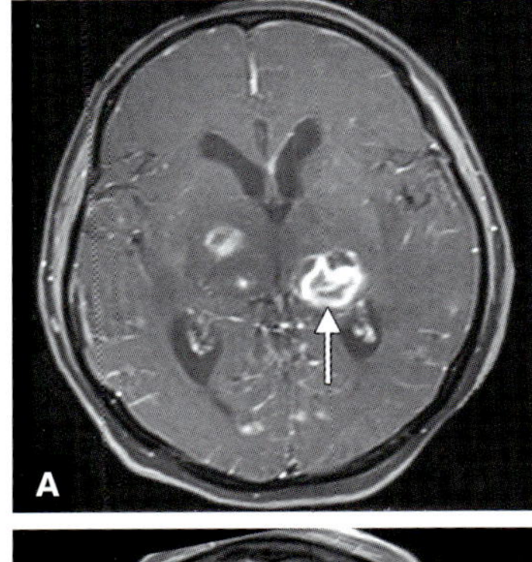 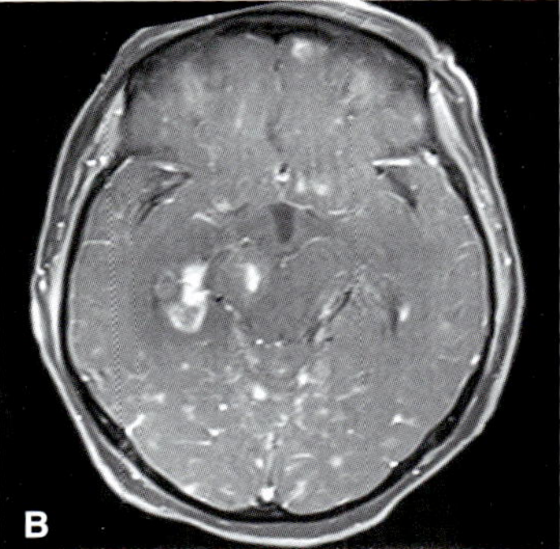 **Figures 6.3.4A and B:** Toxoplasmosis *Photo Courtesy:* Shekhar Patil, Mumbai	Postcontrast T1W images show multiple ring enhancing lesions with shaggy margins, the largest located in the thalamus (Figs 6.3.4A and B).	• Toxoplasmosis in children is congenital or acquired and in the acquired setting this manifests as an acute condition with seizures, headaches, vomiting and focal neurological deficit. Central nervous system (CNS) toxoplasmosis is usually due to reactivation of latent infection and seen in context of low CD4 counts. Serologic testing is sensitive but not specific for diagnosis. Treatment is usually empiric with periodic reassessment to ascertain clinical and radiological recovery. The only definitive diagnosis is biopsy of the intracranial lesion. • Standard regime includes combination of pyrimethamine, sulfadiazine and folinic acid. Alternative regimes with single drug trimethoprim-sulfamethoxazole and for patients allergic to sulpha drugs clindamycin is a good option. In appropriate setting antiretroviral therapy is indicated.

Section 7

Skin and Soft Tissue Infections

Section Editor

C Vijayabhaskar Chandran

Contributors

C Vijayabhaskar Chandran, V Anandan, R Madhu, V Suganthy, R Akila

Section Outline

7.1 Viral Skin Infections

- Hand-Foot-and-Mouth Disease
- Herpes Zoster in a One-and-Half-Year-Old Boy
- Herpes Zoster in a 2-Year-Old Child
- Molluscum Contagiosum
- Giant Molluscum Contagiosum in an HIV Child
- Herpes Simplex

7.2 Bacterial Skin Infections

- Furunculosis
- Impetigo
- Impetigo with Staphylococcal-Scalded Skin Syndrome
- Cutaneous Tuberculosis – Lupus Vulgaris
- Impetigo-Cellulitis
- Necrotizing Fasciitis

7.3 Fungal Skin Infections

- Pityriasis Versicolor
- Pityriasis Versicolor on Forehead
- Tinea Capitis
- Kerion – A Type of Tinea Capitis

7.4 Parasitic Skin Infections

- Scabies
- Cutaneous Larva Migrans

7.5 Miscellaneous

- Acne Vulgaris

Picture	Note	Management

7.1 VIRAL SKIN INFECTIONS

Hand-Foot-and-Mouth Disease

Picture	Note	Management
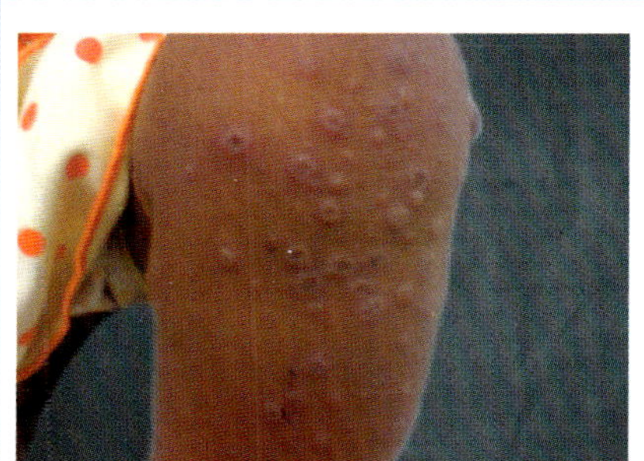 **Figure 7.1.1:** Hand, foot and mouth disease involving the knee and leg *Photo Courtesy*: C Vijayabhaskar Chandran, Chennai	• Hand, foot and mouth disease. • Multiple vesicles and papules are seen with central umbilication seen over the leg and knee (Fig. 7.1.1). • Caused by coxsackie virus Type A and B and enterovirus.	• Reassurance. • Symptomatic management. • Soothening lotions like calamine lotion and oral antihistamines like cetrizine hydrochloride if itching present.

Herpes Zoster in a One-and-Half-Year-Old Boy

Picture	Note	Management
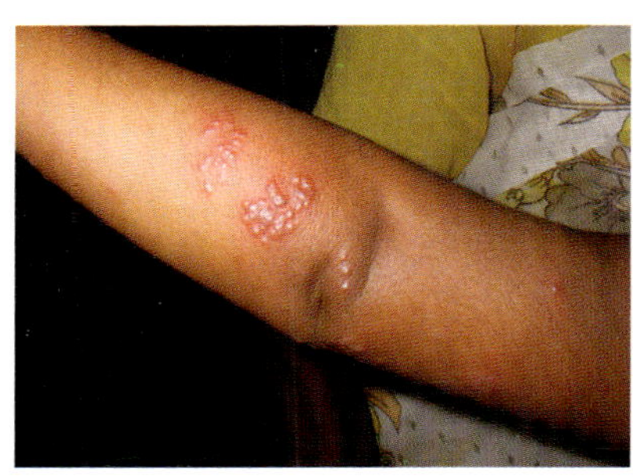 **Figure 7.1.2:** Herpes zoster involving the left arm and forearm in a one-and-half-year-old child with history of mother with chickenpox in the second trimester of pregnancy *Photo Courtesy*: R Madhu, Chennai	• Herpes zoster in a one-and-half-year-old boy. Multiple vesicles seen over the erythematous base in a linear pattern over the back of arm and forearm involving one side of the body (Fig. 7.1.2). • Caused by HHV 3-Varicella zoster virus. Previous history of chickenpox is usually present. In this picture child with one-and-half-year-old had herpes zoster and there was no previous history of chickenpox. But mother had chickenpox in the second trimester of pregnancy infecting the baby *in utero*.	Topical antibiotics and acyclovir 20 mg/kg body weight given five times a day for 7 days. If pain occurs oral NSAIDs could be given.

Picture	Note	Management

Herpes Zoster in a 2-Year-Old Child

Picture	Note	Management
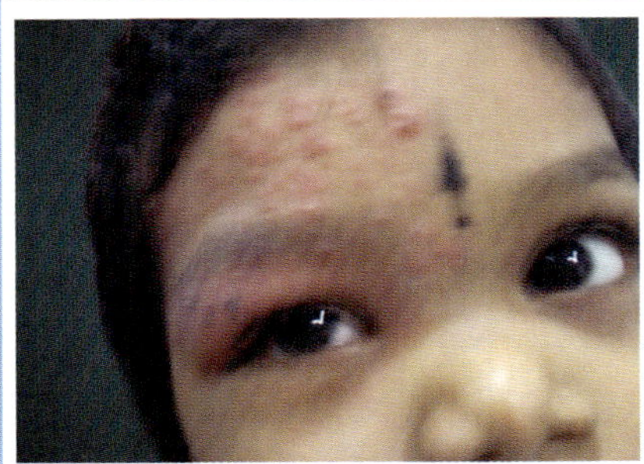 **Figure 7.1.3A:** Herpes zoster in a 2-year-old female child with history of mother with chickenpox during her second trimester of pregnancy *Photo Courtesy*: C Vijayabhaskar Chandran, Chennai	Herpes zoster in a 2-year-old child (Fig. 7.1.3A).	Same as above.
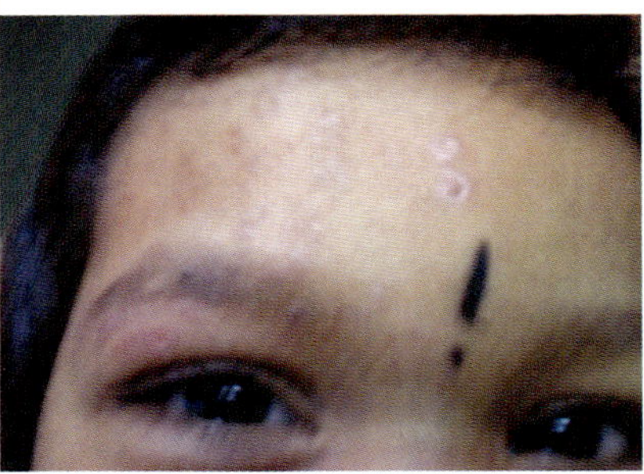 **Figure 7.1.3B:** Resolving herpes zoster in the previous child with treatment within 7 days *Photo Courtesy*: C Vijayabhaskar Chandran, Chennai	Same child as Figure 7.1.3A after treatment with acyclovir (Fig. 7.1.3B).	

Molluscum Contagiosum

Picture	Note	Management
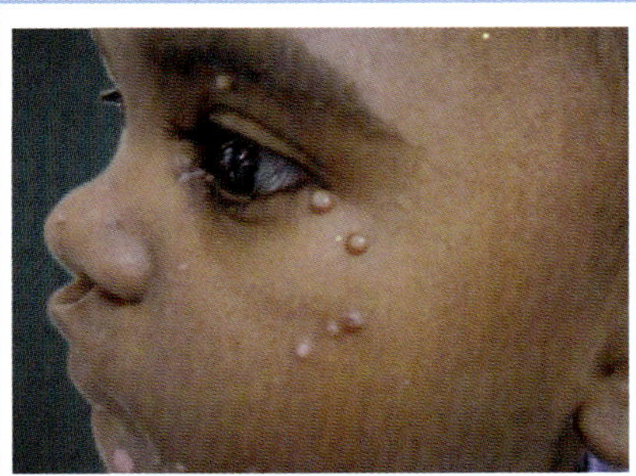 **Figure 7.1.4:** Molluscum contagiosum in a 3-year-old child *Photo Courtesy*: V Anandan, Chennai	• Molluscum contagiosum in a 3-year-old child. Multiple umblicated pearly translucent papules on the face (Fig. 7.1.4). • Caused by pox virus family—Molluscum contagiosum virus (MCV).	• Needling and removal. • 5% KOH twice daily could be applied topically for a week which causes irritant dermatitis and MC bodies are extruded out.

Picture	Note	Management

Giant Molluscum Contagiosum in an HIV Child

Picture	Note	Management
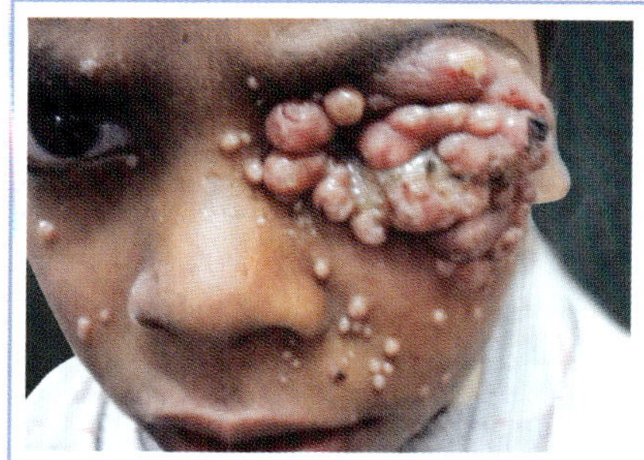 **Figures 7.1.5:** Molluscum contagiosum in an HIV child who is on antiretroviral therapy *Photo Courtesy*: C Vijayabhaskar Chandran, Chennai	Giant molluscum contagiosum over the eyelids and face in an HIV child of 10 years of age on antiretroviral therapy (Fig. 7.1.5).	• Needling and removal. • Liquid nitrogen therapy could be tried.

Herpes Simplex

Picture	Note	Management
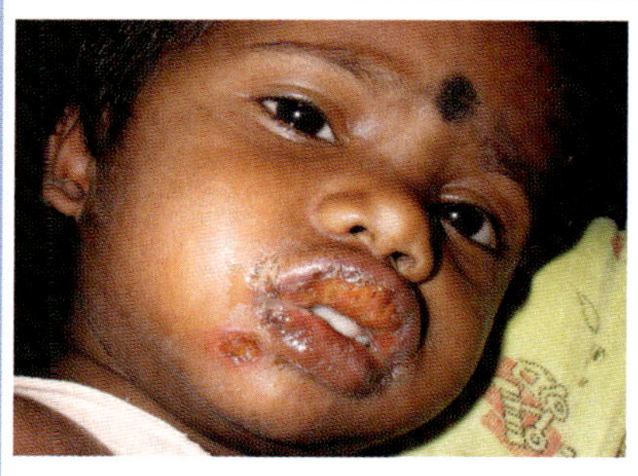 **Figure 7.1.6:** Herpes simplex *Photo Courtesy*: V Anandan, Chennai	• Erosions seen over the lips and chin area in a 1-year-old child with fever (Fig. 7.1.6). • Caused by herpes simplex virus Type 1.	Saline soaks and topical acyclovir may be given. In severe cases oral acyclovir 10 mg/kg body weight given five times a day for 1 week.

Picture	Note	Management

7.2 BACTERIAL SKIN INFECTIONS

Furunculosis

Picture	Note	Management
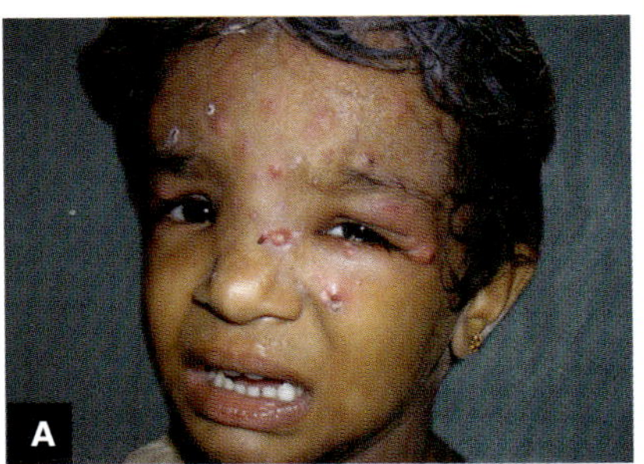 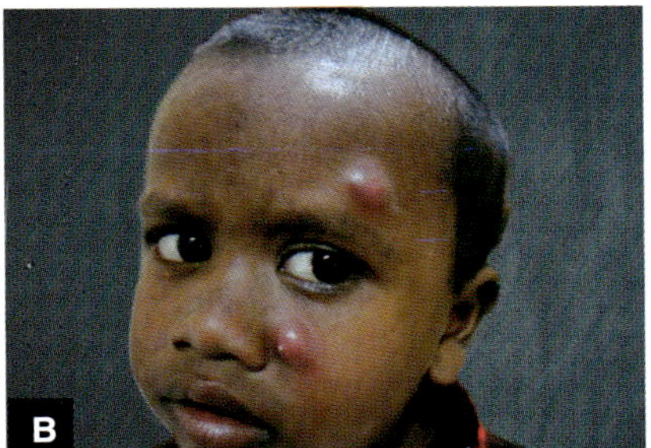 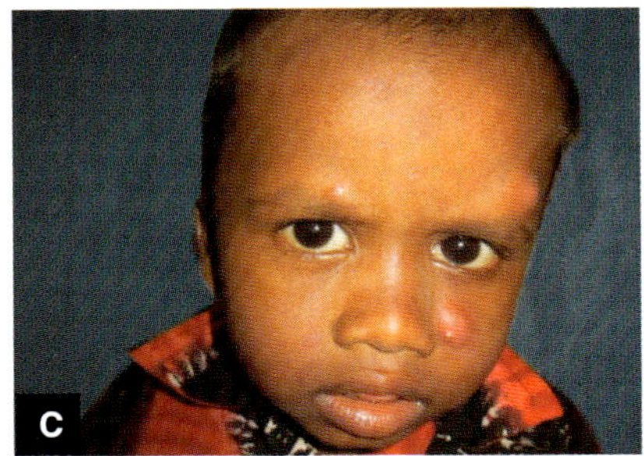 **Figures 7.2.1A to C:** Furunculosis *Photo Courtesy*: (A) C Vijayabhaskar Chandran, Chennai; (B) V Anandan, Chennai; (C) V Suganthy, Chennai	• Furunculosis—Multiple nodules seen over the face (Figs 7.2.1A to C). • Common during summer. Caused by *Staphylococcus* and *Streptococcus*.	Orally penicillin group of drugs cloxacillin/dicloxacillin, cephalexin or erythromycin.

Impetigo

Picture	Note	Management
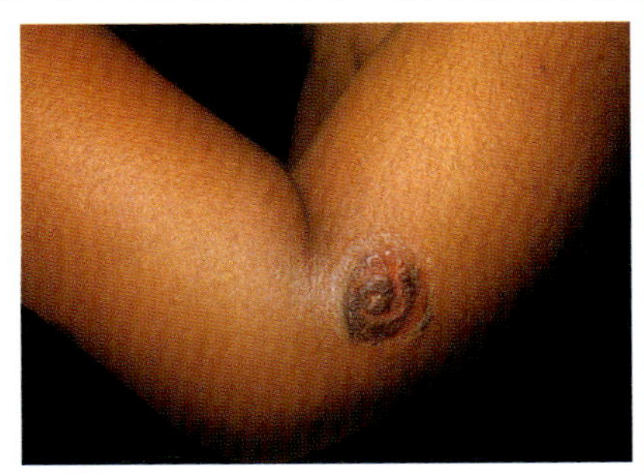 **Figure 7.2.2:** Impetigo *Photo Courtesy*: R Akila, Chennai	Impetigo—*Staphylococcus* and *Streptococcus* common cause (Fig. 7.2.2).	• A few lesions—Topical antibiotics are preferred. Mupirocin/Fusidic acid thrice daily for 10 days. • Severe lesions—Topical antibiotics and systematically penicillin group of antibiotics like cloxacillin/dicloxacillin, cephalexin or erythromycin.

Picture	Note	Management

Impetigo with Staphylococcal-Scalded Skin Syndrome

Picture	Note	Management
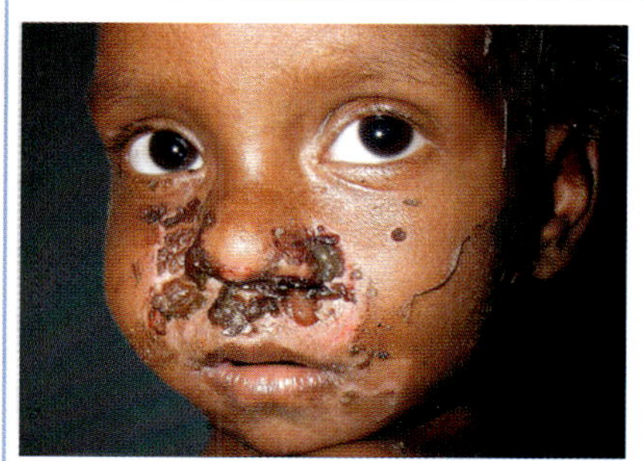 **Figure 7.2.3:** Impetigo with staphylococcal-scalded skin syndrome *Photo Courtesy*: V Anandan, Chennai	Impetigo with Staphylococcal-scalded skin syndrome. Impetigenous lesions seen over the paranasal area and peeling of skin perioral area and over the sides of the face (Fig. 7.2.3).	• Mild—Oral antibiotics preferably penicillin group. • Severe—Admit the child and start parenteral antibiotics like cloxacillin or clindamycin.

Cutaneous Tuberculosis—Lupus Vulgaris

Picture	Note	Management
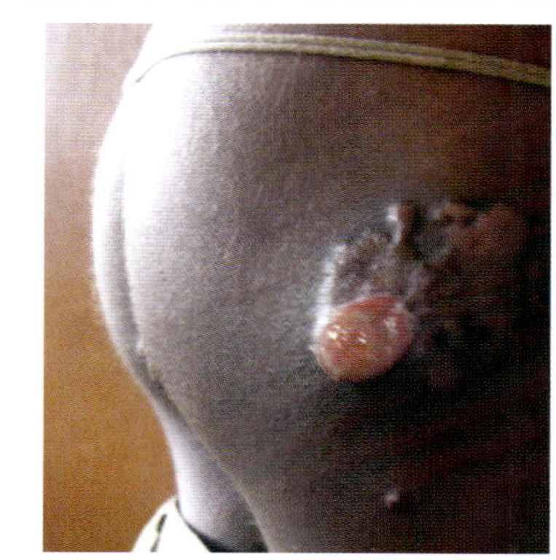 **Figure 7.2.4:** Cutaneous tuberculosis—Lupus vulgaris *Photo Courtesy*: V Anandan, Chennai	• Cutaneous tuberculosis—Lupus vulgaris—a large plaque with healing on one end and progression and ulceration at the other end seen (Fig. 7.2.4). • Caused by *Mycobacterium tuberculosis*.	Antituberculosis therapy (ATT) with isoniazid (INH), rifampicin, ethambutol and pyrazinamide daily for 2 months followed by INH and rifampicin daily for 4 months.

Impetigo-Cellulitis

Picture	Note	Management
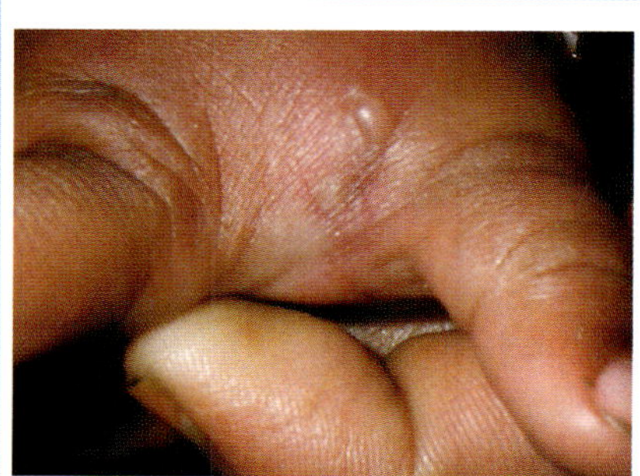 **Figure 7.2.5:** Impetigo-cellulitis *Photo Courtesy*: V Anandan, Chennai	• Bullous impetigo with swelling of the hand seen—cellulitis. • Impetigo occurs due to *Staphylococcus* and *Streptococcus* (Fig. 7.2.5).	Child needs oral antibiotics and if necessary intravenous antibiotics are required.

Picture	Note	Management

Necrotizing Fasciitis

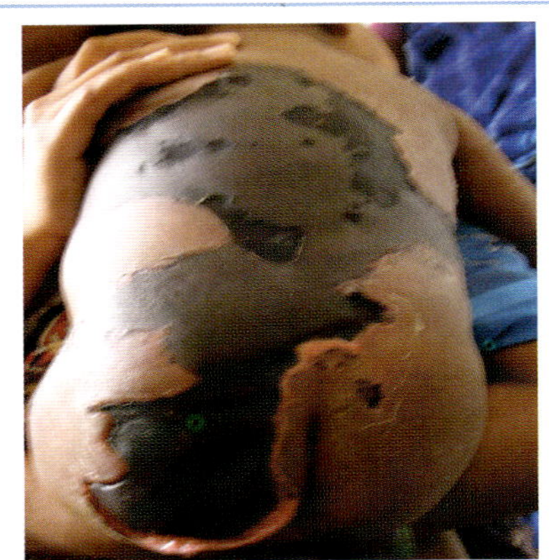 **Figure 7.2.6:** Necrotizing fasciitis *Photo Courtesy*: V Anandan, Chennai	• Large area of necrosis seen over the back of this sick child. • Necrotizing fasciitis—Flesh eating disease (Fig. 7.2.6). • Caused by *Staphylococcus, Streptococcus, Clostridium*, etc. More common in immunocompromised patients and may start on the site of trauma and can progress very fast.	Mortality is very high with this condition. As soon as diagnosed intravenous antibiotics like penicillin, vancomycin and clindamycin to be started and culture and sensitivity could be done meanwhile and antibiotics changed accordingly. Surgical debridement of wound is also required.

7.3 FUNGAL SKIN INFECTIONS

Pityriasis Versicolor

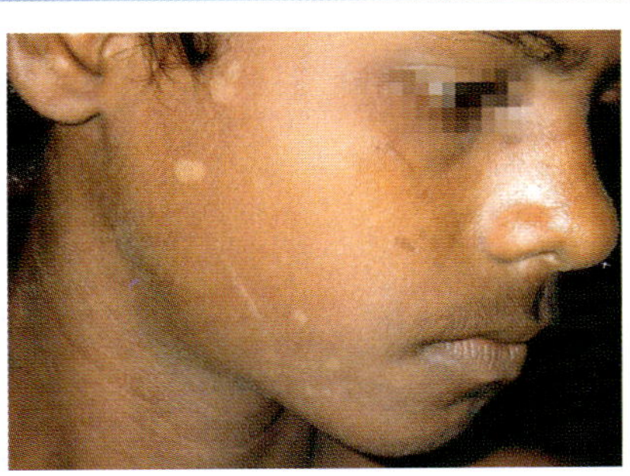 **Figure 7.3.1:** Pityriasis versicolor on the face *Photo Courtesy*: C Vijayabhaskar Chandran, Chennai	• Pityriasis versicolor—multiple hypopigmented patch with well-defined border with scales in it seen on the side of the face (Fig. 7.3.1). • Caused by dimorphic fungi *Malassezia furfur*.	• Topical azole group of drugs like clotrimalzole, Ketoconazole and miconazole twice daily for 6 weeks will help. • When extensive on the trunk topical selenium sulfide with clotrimazole combination could be used over the body 10 minutes before bath daily once for 2 weeks along with oral fluconazole 8–12 mg/kg body weight can be given as single dose and to repeat after 1 week.

Pityriasis Versicolor on Forehead

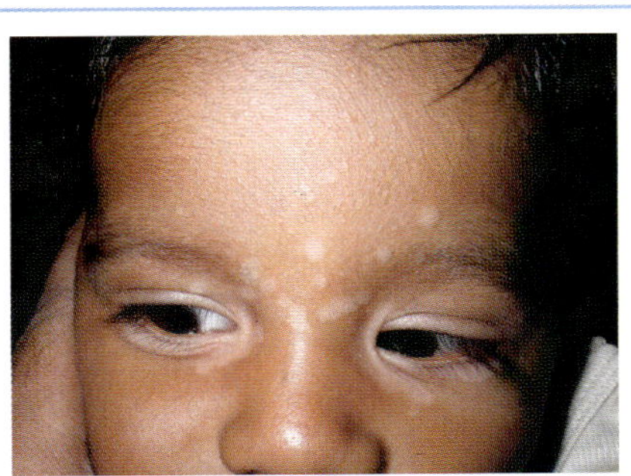 **Figure 7.3.2:** Pityriasis versicolor *Photo Courtesy*: V Anandan, Chennai	• Multiple scaly macules and patches seen over the forehead and also over the inner canthal region with well-defined border and scaling (Fig. 7.3.2). • Pityriasis versicolor caused by *Malassezia furfur*.	Topical azoles twice daily for a period of 6 weeks clear the lesion.

Picture	Note	Management

Tinea Capitis

Picture	Note	Management
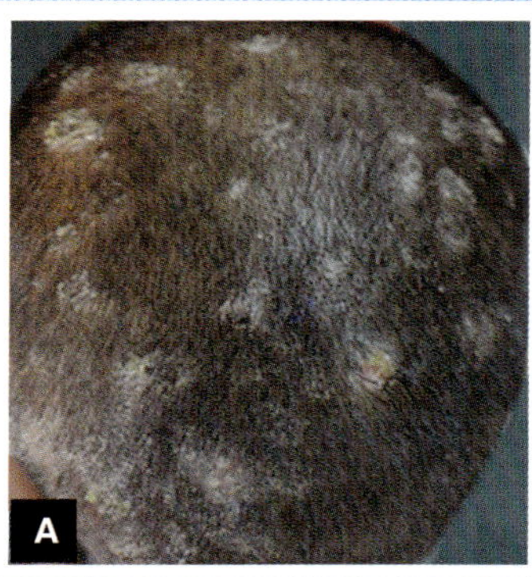	• Tinea capitis—multiple scaly patches seen over the scalp with areas of alopecia (Fig. 7.3.3A). • History of tonsuring may be positive in majority of the cases.	• In children topical ketoconazole based shampoos could be used. • Oral griseofulvin twice daily for 12 weeks along with food preferably fatty meal. • Terbinafine once daily for 4 weeks 10–20 kg—62.5 mg daily once a day. • More than 20 kg up to 40 kg—125 mg once a day. • More than 40 kg—250 mg once a day.
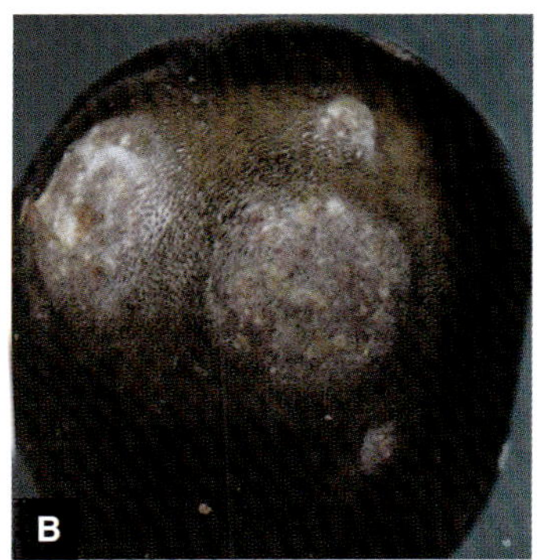	Tinea capitis—Large patches with alopecia seen over the scalp (Fig. 7.3.3B).	
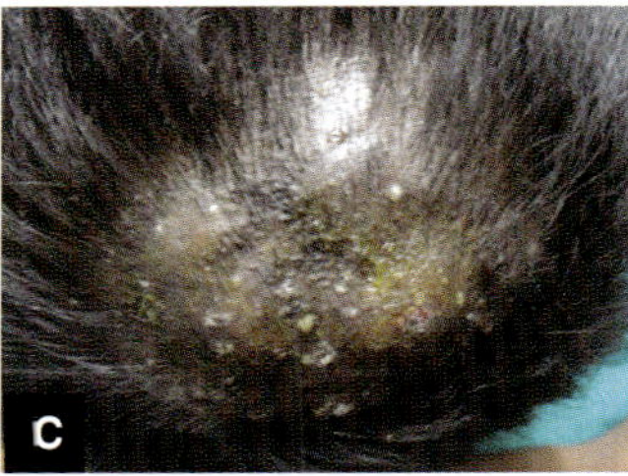 **Figures 7.3.3A to C:** Tinea capitis *Photo Courtesy*: R Madhu, Chennai	Tinea capitis—Large patch with pustules and alopecia seen (Fig. 7.3.3C).	

Kerion—A Type of Tinea Capitis

Picture	Note	Management
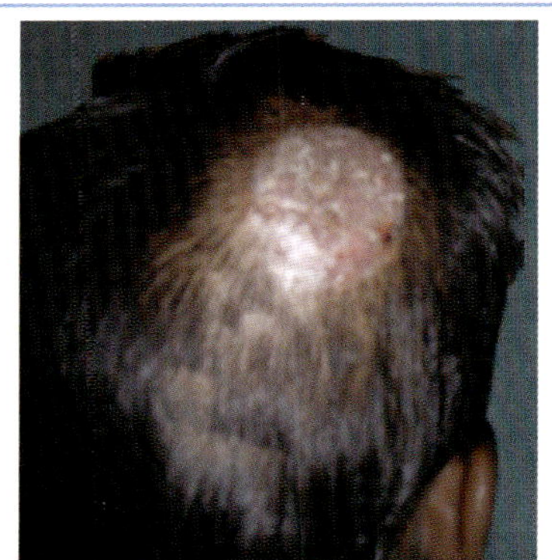 **Figure 7.3.4:** Kerion – A type of tinea capitis *Photo Courtesy*: R Madhu, Chennai	Boggy swelling seen over the scalp with alopecia in a child with history of tonsuring 2 months back (Fig. 7.3.4).	• Common in children and often mistaken for abscess. Scraping for fungus in 10% KOH will help in diagnosis. • Best treatment option is Tab griseofulvin 20–25 mg/kg body weight in two divided doses given for a period of 12 weeks will help. • Terbinafine could be tried as described earlier.

Picture	Note	Management

7.4 PARASITIC SKIN INFECTIONS

Scabies

Picture	Note	Management
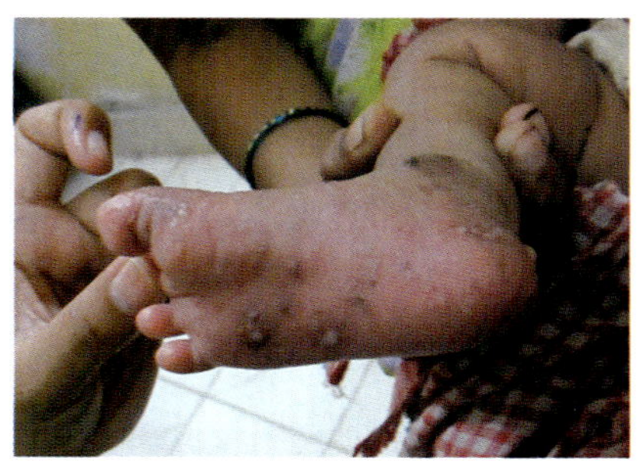 **Figure 7.4.1:** Scabies lesion involving the soles in an infant *Photo Courtesy*: C Vijayabhaskar Chandran, Chennai	• Scabies—both soles of a 2-month-old infant showing pustules and scaling of skin. • Face, palms and soles are commonly involved in infants (Fig. 7.4.1). • Caused by *Sarcoptes scabiei* variety *hominis*.	• Below 2 months of age—5% Sulfur ointment to be applied below the neck throughout the body daily for 3 days. • Above 2 months of age—5% Permethrin cream to be applied below the neck throughout the body and to give bath after 8–12 hours. • Above 5 years of age—Ivermectin orally 0.2 mg/kg body weight given two doses 1 week apart.

Cutaneous Larva Migrans

Picture	Note	Management
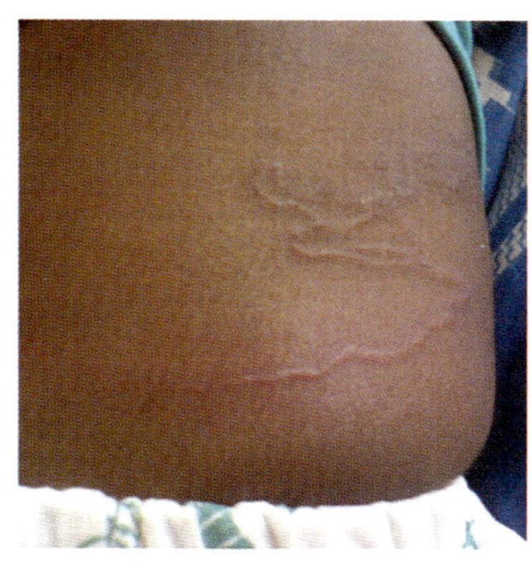 **Figure 7.4.2A:** Cutaneous larva migrans in a 4-month-old child *Photo Courtesy*: C Vijayabhaskar Chandran, Chennai	• Cutaneous larva migrans. A serpiginous migratory skin lesion over the back of a 4-month-old baby (Fig. 7.4.2A). • Caused by larval stages of hook-worms such as *Ancylostoma caninum* and *Ancylostoma braziliense*.	• Below 1 year of age—liquid nitrogen spray over the advancing end or ethyl chloride spray and freezes the advancing end. • Above 1 year—albendazole once daily for 3 days.
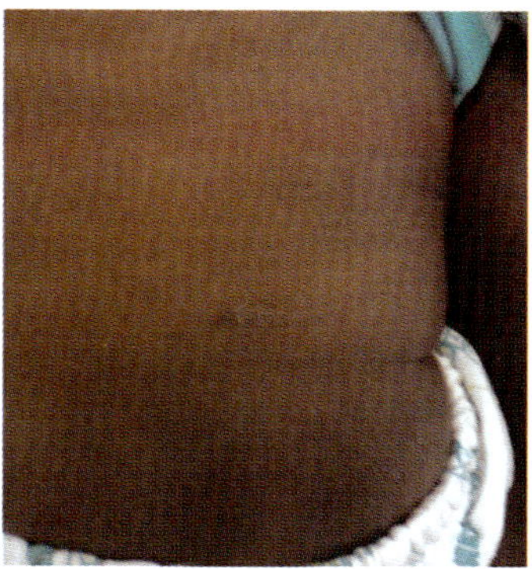 **Figure 7.4.2B:** Resolving cutaneous larva migrans after treatment *Photo Courtesy*: C Vijayabhaskar Chandran, Chennai	• Same child as above (Fig. 7.4.2A) with treatment. • Lesion has disappeared (Fig. 7.4.2B).	

Picture	Note	Management

7.5 MISCELLANEOUS

Acne Vulgaris

Picture	Note	Management
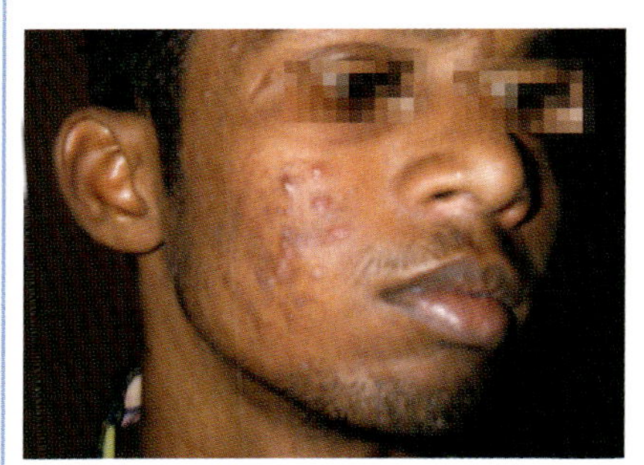 **Figure 7.5.1:** Acne vulgaris in adolescent male *Photo Courtesy*: V Anandan, Chennai	• Acne vulgaris in a 16-year-old male. • Multiple papules and pustules seen over the face with postinflammatory scars (Fig. 7.5.1).	• Frequent face wash. • Benzoyl peroxide 2.5% over the whole face in the morning and adapelene over the entire face in the night and if pustules seen doxycyline 100 mg once a day or azithromycin pulse therapy could be given.

Section 8

Ophthalmic Infections

Section Editor

Atul Seth

Contributors

Atul Seth, Hrishikesh A Tadwalkar, Mihir Kothari,
Parul M Deshpande, Vishram A Sangit, Mamta V Manglani

Section Outline

8.1 Lid and Orbital Infections
- Blepharitis
- Hordeolum Internum
- Preseptal Cellulitis
- Orbital Cellulitis
- Orbital Myocysticercosis
- Lid Abscess
- Tuberculous Lid Mass

8.2 Lacrimal Sac Infections
- Congenital Dacryocele
- Acute Dacryocystitis

8.3 Conjunctival Infections
- Viral Pseudomembranous Conjunctivitis

8.4 Corneal Infections
- Bacterial Corneal Ulcer
- Fungal Corneal Ulcer
- Herpes Simplex Keratitis
- Herpes Zoster Ophthalmicus

8.5 Retinal and Posterior Segment Infections
- Toxoplasma Retinitis
- Cytomegalovirus Retinitis

Picture	Note	Management

8.1 LID AND ORBITAL INFECTIONS

Blepharitis

Picture	Note	Management
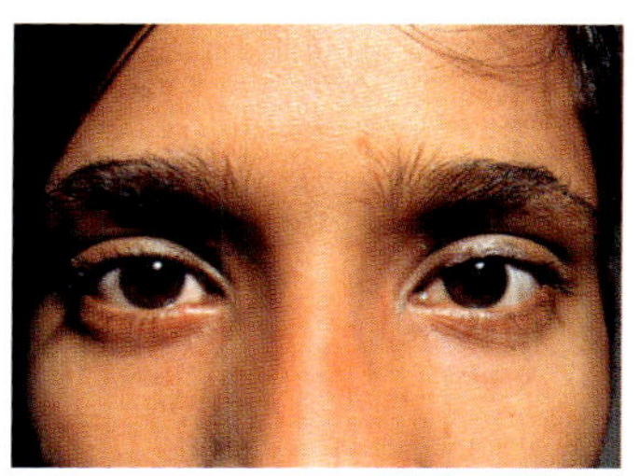 **Figure 8.1.1:** Left upper lid seborrheic blepharitis *Photo Courtesy*: Atul Seth, Navi Mumbai	Note the left upper lid margin appears red and irritated with scales that cling to the base of the eyelashes. Blepharitis may be seborrheic (as in Fig. 8.1.1) or staphylococcal.	• Warm, moist compresses. • Lid scrubs with baby shampoo. Topical antibiotic ointment (erythromycin or bacitracin).

Hordeolum Internum

Picture	Note	Management
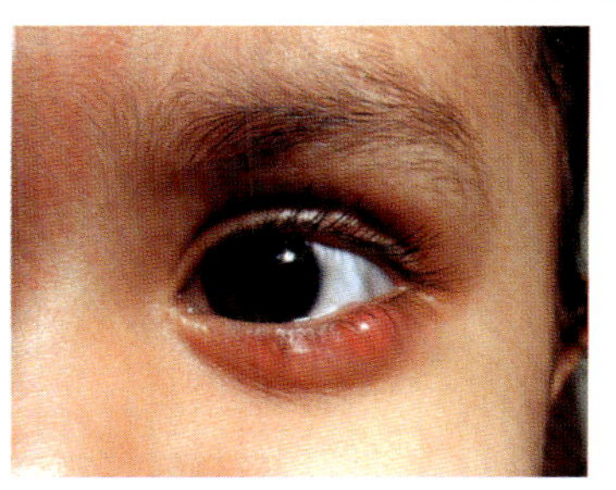 **Figure 8.1.2:** Left lower lid hordeolum internum *Photo Courtesy*: Atul Seth, Navi Mumbai	Note the localized and erythematous left lower lid swelling. It is a focal infection arising within the meibomian glands in the eyelid. Commonly caused by *Staphylococcus*. It needs to be differentiated from a *hordeolum externum* [Fig. 8.1.2 (stye: abscess of root of an eyelash)].	• Warm, moist compresses. • Topical antibiotic ointment to the lid margins. • Systemic antibiotic and NSAID therapy.

Preseptal Cellulitis

Picture	Note	Management
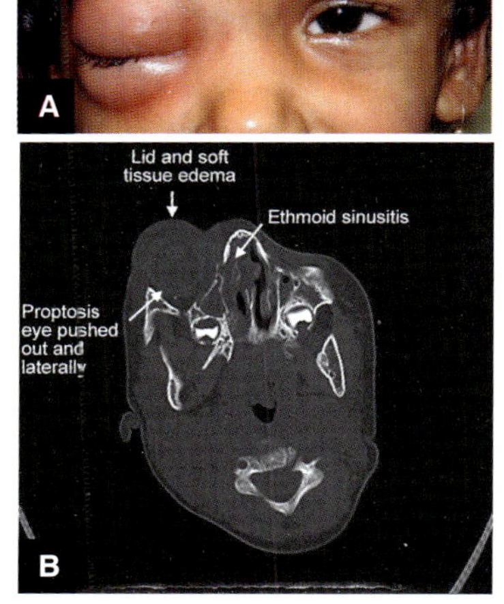 **Figures 8.1.3A and B:** (A) Preseptal cellulitis in a 2-year-old girl; (B) CT scan right orbit shows ethmoid sinus haziness and preseptal haze *Photo Courtesy*: Atul Seth, Navi Mumbai	• Note right eyelids swelling, erythema with conjunctival hyperemia (Figs 8.1.3A and B). • The absence of proptosis and presence of normal eye movements differentiated it from an orbital cellulitis. • CT scan showed ethmoid sinusitis (commonest cause of preseptal and orbital cellulitis in children). • Commonest organisms are staphylococci, streptococci and *H. influenzae*. • Preseptal cellulitis can spread into an orbital cellulitis especially in younger children.	• Oral or parenteral antibiotics with broad spectrum antibiotics (amoxicillin-clavulanate or cephalexin). • CT scan of orbit and sinuses indicated if symptoms worsen or fever present. • Concurrent management of the sinus pathology by ENT surgeon.

Picture	Note	Management
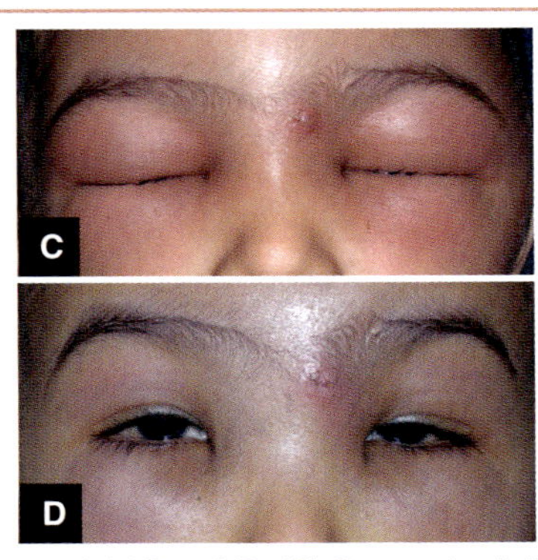 **Figures 8.1.3C and D:** (C) Preseptal cellulitis: Pretreatment; (D) Post-treatment *Photo Courtesy*: Mihir Kothari, Thane	Bilateral preseptal cellulitis resulting from a left forehead folliculitis (Fig. 8.1.3C) and resolution following systemic antibiotics in a 3-year-old male child (Fig. 8.1.3D). Staphylococcal folliculitis and other localized infective lid lesions can spread into a preseptal cellulitis.	Treatment of the infective lid lesion with topical antibiotic ointment and systemic antibiotic and nonsteroidal anti-inflammatory drug (NSAID) therapy.

Orbital Cellulitis

Picture	Note	Management
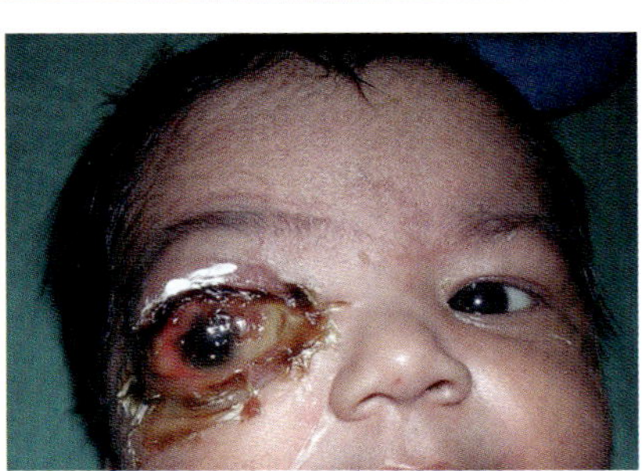 **Figure 8.1.4:** A 5-month-old child with orbital cellulitis and orbital abscess formation *Photo Courtesy*: Hrishikesh A Tadwalkar, Navi Mumbai	Note severe proptosis, conjunctival chemosis, loss of eye movements and corneal exposure (Fig. 8.1.4). Pupils were reacting briskly to light. • CT scan confirmed diagnosis of orbital cellulitis with orbital abscess. • Contiguous spread from adjacent sinuses (Gram-positive cocci) is the commonest cause. Other causes are spread from preseptal cellulitis or rarely a fungal etiology in immunocompromised patients.	• Urgent admission and CT scan orbit with paranasal sinuses. • Systemic antibiotics (ceftriaxone or vancomycin or other appropriate treatment). • Orbital abscess cavity if formed may need to be surgically drained. • In case of fever and neurological signs, consider cavernous sinus thrombosis.

Orbital Myocysticercosis

Picture	Note	Management
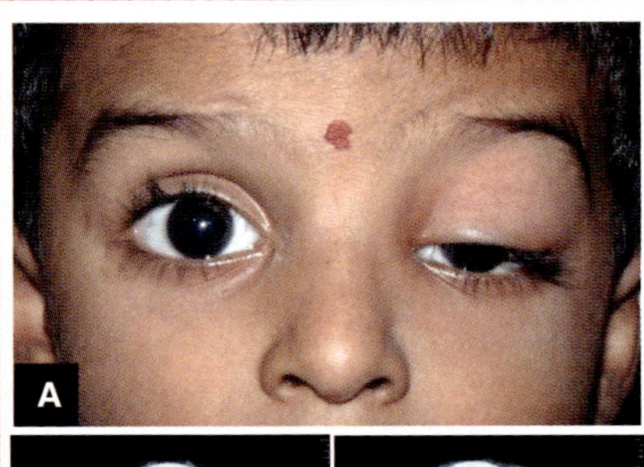 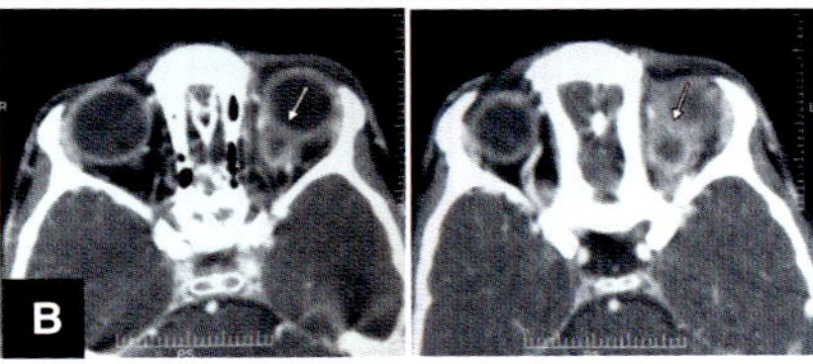 **Figures 8.1.5A and B:** Orbital myocysticercosis in a 3-year-old boy *Photo Courtesy*: Hrishikesh A Tadwalkar, Navi Mumbai	Chief complaint was ptosis since 15 days (Fig. 8.1.5A). • Axial CT scan (Fig. 8.1.5B) showed a ring-enhancing cystic lesion in the levator-superior rectus muscle complex. • Complete resolution of ptosis occurred with medical treatment.	• Diagnosis is confirmed by CT scan of orbit and brain. • Systemic anticysticercal therapy under cover of systemic steroids is given.

Picture	Note	Management

Lid Abscess

Picture	Note	Management
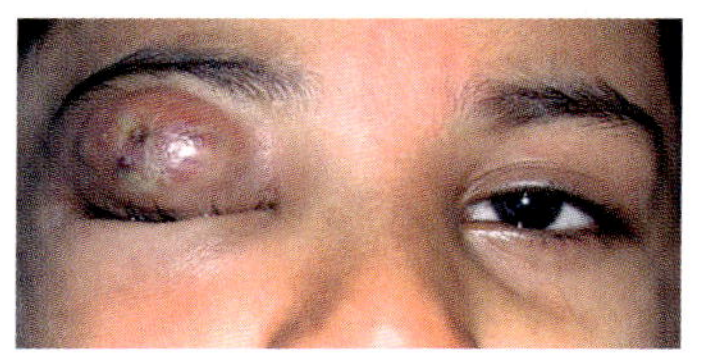 **Figure 8.1.6:** Lid abscess in a 10-year-old boy *Photo Courtesy*: Hrishikesh A Tadwalkar, Navi Mumbai	Note the pointing preseptal cellulitis with fluctuant feel indicating a lid abscess formation (Fig. 8.1.6). This abscess is limited to the space anterior to the orbital septum.	Surgical drainage necessary under cover of systemic antibiotics.

Tuberculous Lid Mass

Picture	Note	Management
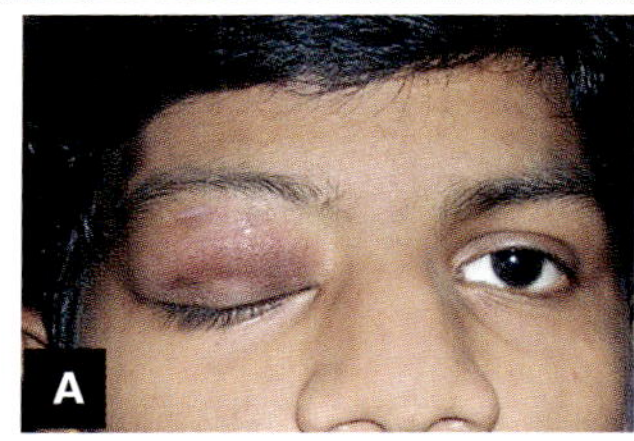 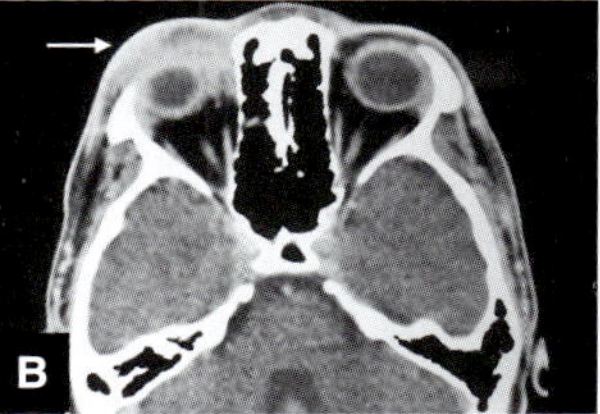 **Figures 8.1.7A and B:** Tuberculous lid mass in a 15-year-old boy *Photo Courtesy*: Hrishikesh A Tadwalkar, Navi Mumbai	Note right upper lid firm, indurated, immobile lid mass (Fig. 8.1.7A). Axial CT scan (Fig. 8.1.7B) shows diffuse swelling in the right preseptal space. Incisional biopsy showed a tuberculous involvement of the eyelid.	Excision of the mass followed by antituberculous therapy.

8.2 LACRIMAL SAC INFECTIONS

Congenital Dacryocele

Picture	Note	Management
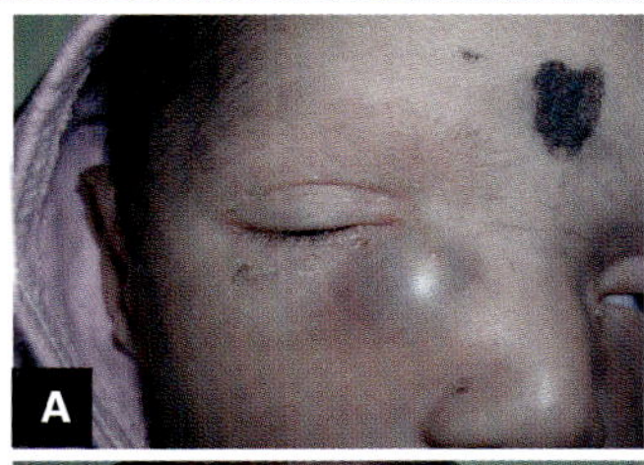 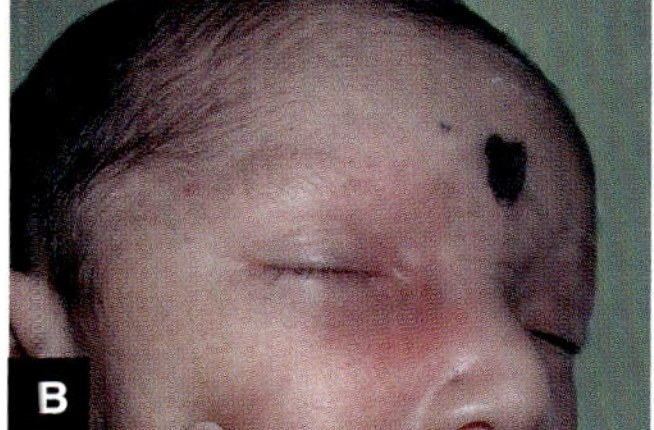 **Figures 8.2.1A and B:** Congenital dacryocele (Amniocele) in a 15-day-old child *Photo Courtesy*: Hrishikesh A Tadwalkar, Navi Mumbai	Note swelling and bluish or purplish discoloration of the soft tissues medial to the inner canthus present since birth. It is secondary to congenital blockage of nasolacrimal duct. Postprobing photograph shows resolution of the amniocele (Figs 8.2.1A and B).	Treatment consists of prompt nasolacrimal duct probing in the neonatal period, which can be done at this age without general anesthesia.

Picture	Note	Management

Acute Dacryocystitis

Picture	Note	Management
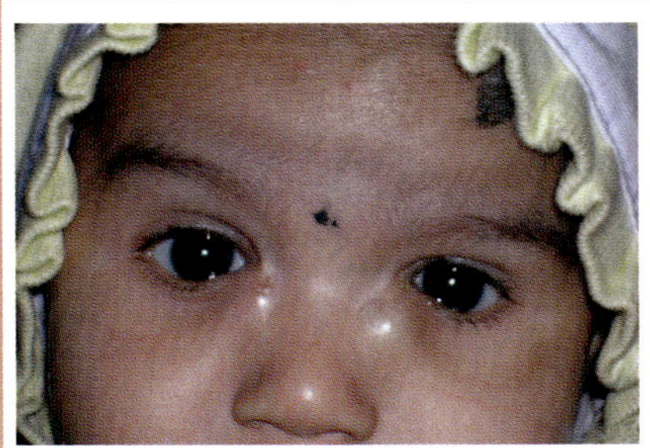 **Figure 8.2.2:** Acute dacryocystitis in a 4-month-old child *Photo Courtesy*: Mihir Kothari, Thane	An infection of both the lacrimal sacs resulting from blocked nasolacrimal ducts (Fig. 8.2.2). Both sides have formed a lacrimal abscess and the right side has burst open to form a lacrimal fistula. Ten percent neonates have a blocked nasolacrimal duct at birth which rarely may get infected.	• Acute stage treated with systemic antibiotics, warm moist compresses and topical antibiotic therapy. • A pointing lacrimal abscess needs to be drained surgically. • Definitive management to open the blocked nasolacrimal duct [Probing or a dacryocystorhinostomy (DCR) surgery] is done after resolution of acute phase.

8.3 CONJUNCTIVAL INFECTIONS

Viral Pseudomembranous Conjunctivitis

Picture	Note	Management
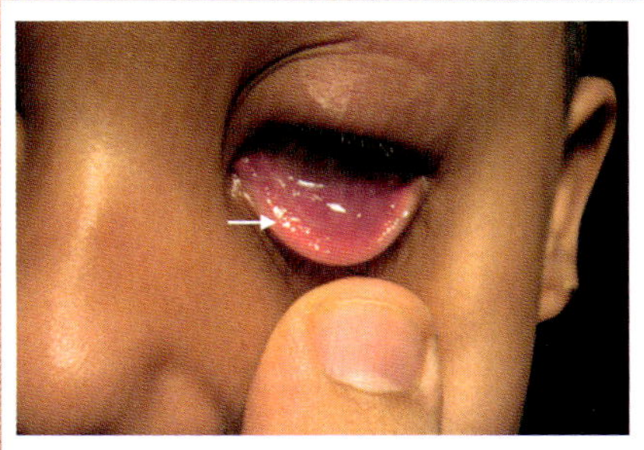 **Figure 8.3.1:** Left eye pseudomembranous conjunctivitis in a 10-year-old boy *Photo Courtesy*: Atul Seth, Navi Mumbai	Viral conjunctivitis with typical follicular reaction and whitish pseudomembrane formation [Fig. 8.3.1 (arrow)]. Often associated preauricular lymphadenopathy is present. This may lead to postviral subepithelial corneal infiltrates.	• Topical antibiotics and lubricant therapy given. • Thick pseudomembranes may need peeling with a sterile bud and supervised local steroid therapy.

8.4 CORNEAL INFECTIONS

Bacterial Corneal Ulcer

Picture	Note	Management
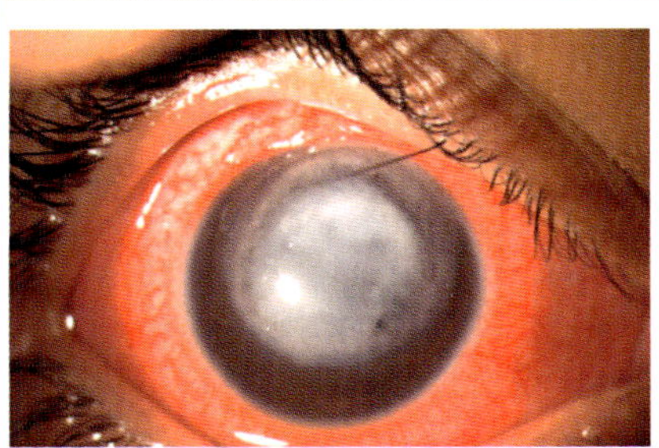 **Figure 8.4.1:** Slit-lamp image of bacterial (pseudomonas) corneal ulcer in an 8-year-old girl *Photo Courtesy*: Vishram A Sangit, Panvel	Note the large moist ulcer with severe corneal thinning (Fig. 8.4.1). Symptoms of redness, pain, photophobia and a white infiltrate on the cornea are characteristic of a bacterial keratitis.	• Microbiological diagnosis of corneal scrapings is ideal. • Intensive treatment with appropriate local antibiotics and cycloplegic eyedrops is essential. • Therapeutic keratoplasty is done in case of perforation of the ulcer.

Picture	Note	Management

Fungal Corneal Ulcer

Picture	Note	Management
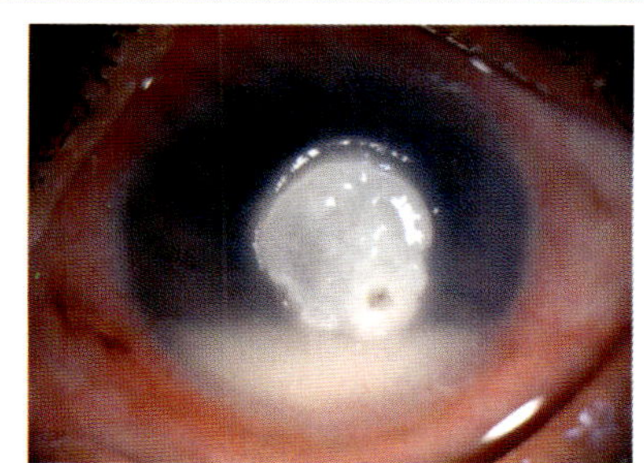 **Figure 8.4.2:** Slit-lamp image of fungal corneal ulcer in a 10-year-old boy *Photo Courtesy*: Vishram A Sangit, Panvel	Note left eye fungal corneal ulcer with a hypopyon following injury with tree branch. Note the dry plaque which looks like typical of a fungal ulcer (Fig. 8.4.2).	• Intensive treatment with antifungal eyedrops and cycloplegics after microbiological confirmation. • Perforation following thinning requires therapeutic keratoplasty.

Herpes Simplex Keratitis

Picture	Note	Management
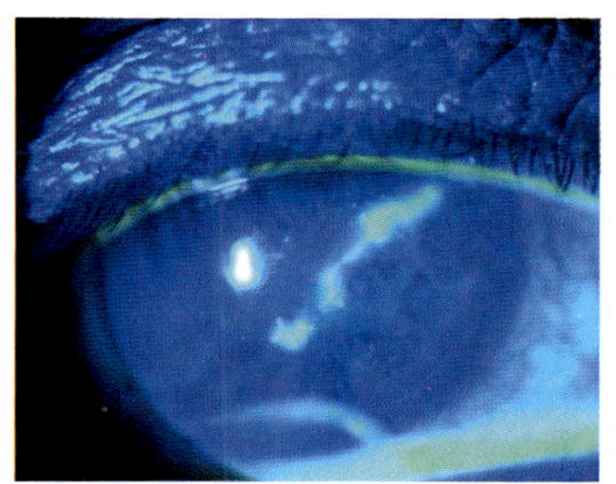 **Figure 8.4.3:** Slit-lamp image of herpes simplex keratitis in a 7-year-old girl *Photo Courtesy*: Vishram A Sangit, Panvel	Classical corneal dendritic (branching) pattern seen on slit-lamp examination with fluorescein staining (Fig. 8.4.3). Symptoms are watering, redness and photophobia. Corneal lesion is not easily seen on torch light examination.	Local acyclovir ointment five times a day for 2–3 weeks.

Herpes Zoster Ophthalmicus

Picture	Note	Management
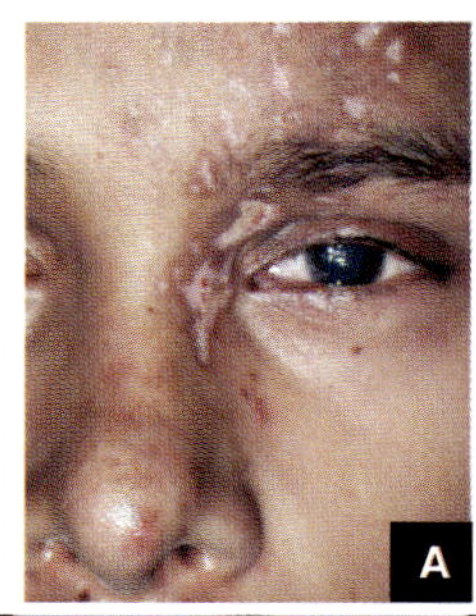 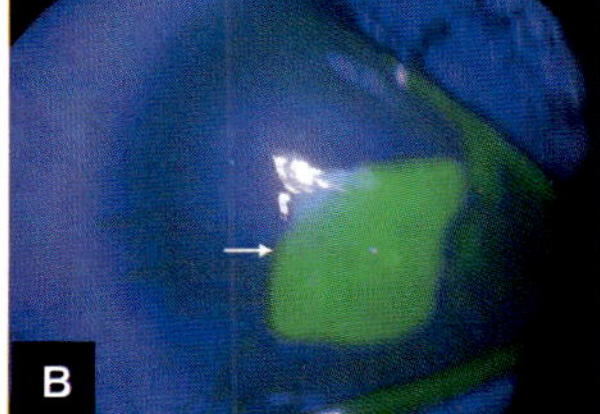 **Figures 8.4.4A and B:** (A) Herpes zoster ophthalmicus in a child with HIV infection; (B) Slit-lamp image shows active viral keratitis *Photo Courtesy*: Parul M Deshpande, Mumbai	Characterized by vesicular dermatitis along the fifth cranial nerve dermatome followed by scarring and postherpetic neuralgia (Figs 8.4.4A and B). Conjunctivitis, episcleritis, scleritis and iridocyclitis are more frequently seen eye manifestations than keratitis.	Systemic acyclovir, valacyclovir or famciclovir. Local lubricant therapy is given. Local and systemic steroids required in uveitis.

Picture	Note	Management

8.5 RETINAL AND POSTERIOR SEGMENT INFECTIONS

Toxoplasma Retinitis

Picture	Note	Management
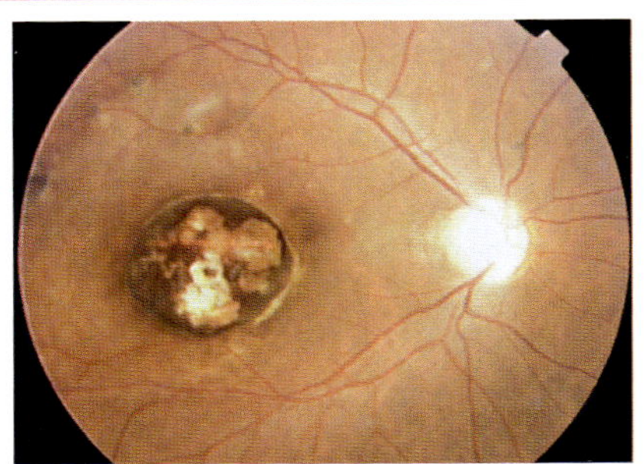 **Figure 8.5.1:** Fundus photograph of toxoplasma retinochoroiditis in a 5-year-old child *Photo Courtesy*: Mihir Kothari, Thane	Note punched out old retinal toxoplasmosis scar at the macula (Fig. 8.5.1). Child had squint and poor vision since childhood. Reactivation may sometimes occur next to an old congenital toxoplasmosis scar.	Systemic antitoxoplasma treatment with systemic steroids given only in cases of active disease or reactivation.

Cytomegalovirus Retinitis

Picture	Note	Management
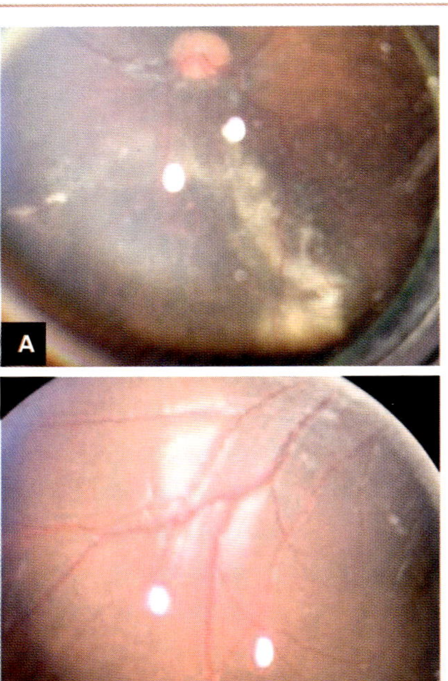 **Figures 8.5.2A and B:** (A) Fundus image of CMV retinitis in a 9-month-old HIV infected child pretreatment; (B) Resolution following treatment *Photo Courtesy*: Mamta V Manglani, Mumbai	Note the classical patchy hemorrhagic retinal necrosis along retinal vessels. Cytomegalovirus (CMV) retinitis is associated with low CD4 counts [< 50 cells/mm^3 (Figs 8.5.2A and B)]. Scarred CMV retinitis may develop a retinal detachment.	Intravenous ganciclovir and/or foscarnet therapy.

Section 9

Ear, Nose and Throat Infections

Section Editor

Pradip Uppal

Contributors

Pradip Uppal, Amol S Khale, Kamal Ghanshamnani

Section Outline

9.1 Ear

- Early Acute Otitis Media
- Acute Otitis Media
- Resolving Acute Otitis Media
- Acute Otitis Media with Perforation (Acute Suppurative Otitis Media)
- Acute Bullous Myringitis
- Otitis Media with Effusion
- Atelectasis
- Myringotomy Tube (Grommet and Ventilating Tube)
- Perforation
- Subtotal Perforation
- Primary Acquired Cholesteatoma
- Cholesteatoma
- Facial Palsy
- Aural Polyp
- Otitis Externa
- Infected Wax Granuloma
- Otomycosis
- Impetigo
- Mastoid Abscess
- Preaurical Sinus
- Preauricular Abscess

9.2 Nose

- Epistaxis from Little's Area
- Granuloma in Little's Area
- Nasal Vestibulitis
- Early Vestibulitis
- Vestibular Abscess
- Allergic Rhinosinusitis
- Septal Hematoma/Septal Abscess
- Orbital Abscess
- Rhinosporidiosis
- Lacrimal Fistula

9.3 Throat

- Tonsils
- Follicular Tonsillitis
- Membranous Tonsillitis
- Quinsy (Peritonsillar Abscess)
- Granular Pharyngitis
- Diphtheria
- Adenoids
- Radiology Adenoid Hypertrophy
- Preauricular Abscess
- Cold Abscess Neck
- Laryngeal Papillomatosis
- Erythema Multiforme
- Palatal Perforation

9.1 EAR

Early Acute Otitis Media

Picture	Note	Management
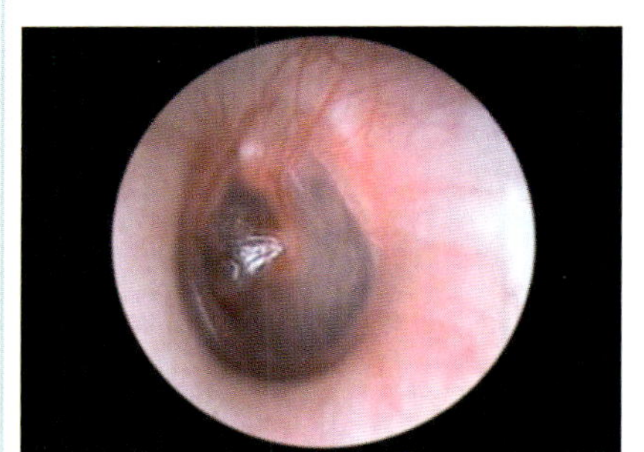 **Figure 9.1.1:** Early acute otitis media *Photo Courtesy:* Pradip Uppal, Thane	In this case, otoscopy reveals congestion of the eardrum with blood vessels seen, usually preceded by upper respiratory tract infection (URTI) (Fig. 9.1.1).	*Treatment* is systemic and local decongestants, analgesics steam inhalation.

Acute Otitis Media

Picture	Note	Management
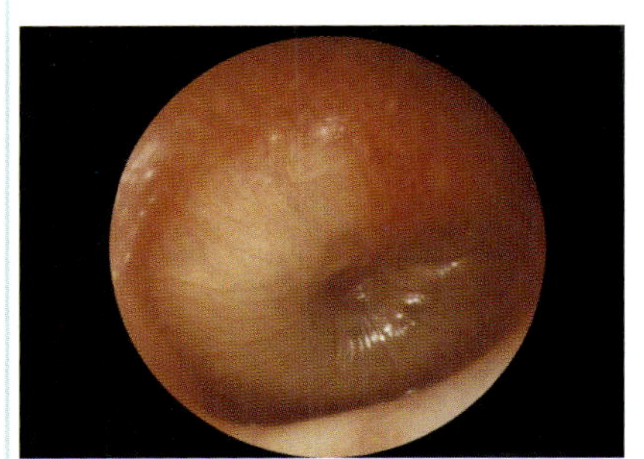 **Figure 9.1.2:** Acute otitis media *Photo Courtesy:* Pradip Uppal, Thane	In this case of acute otitis media, patient complaints of severe pain with URTI, otoscopy reveals bulging ear drum due to purulent middle ear effusion, prominent blood vessels are seen (Fig. 9.1.2).	*Treatment* is antibiotics, decongestants and analgesics.

Resolving Acute Otitis Media

Picture	Note	Management
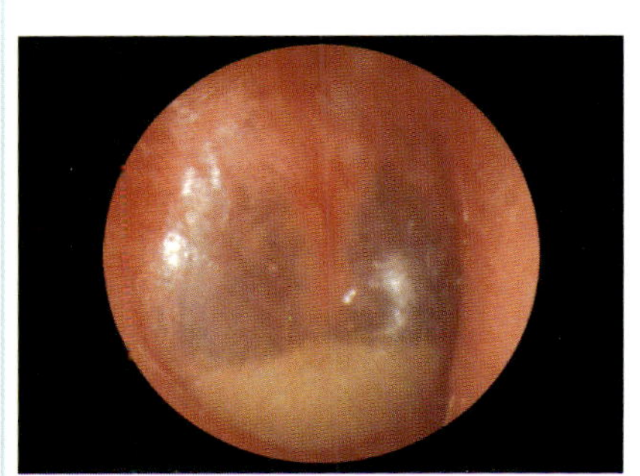 **Figure 9.1.3:** Resolving acute otitis media *Photo Courtesy:* Pradip Uppal, Thane	Resolving acute otitis media pus can be seen in hypotympanum (Fig. 9.1.3).	*Treatment* is antibiotics, decongestants and analgesics.

Picture	Note	Management

Acute Otitis Media with Perforation (Acute Suppurative Otitis Media)

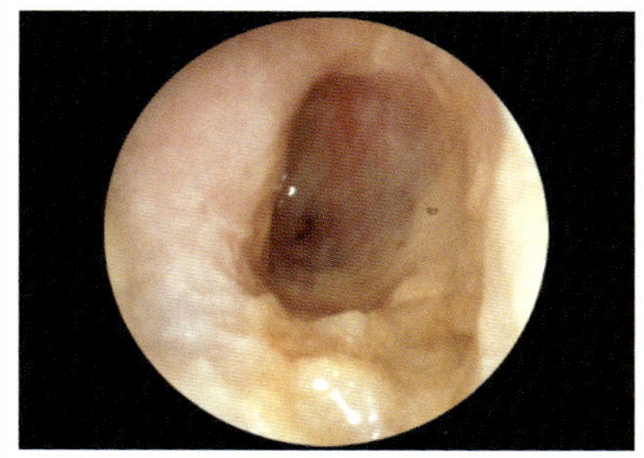 **Figure 9.1.4:** Acute otitis media with perforation acute suppurative otitis media (ASOM) *Photo Courtesy:* Pradip Uppal, Thane	In this stage, pain and discomfort disappear as pressure is released after tympanic membrane ruptures with ear discharge (Fig. 9.1.4).	*Treatment* is antibiotics, decongestants and analgesics. Antibiotic eardrops can be added.

Acute Bullous Myringitis

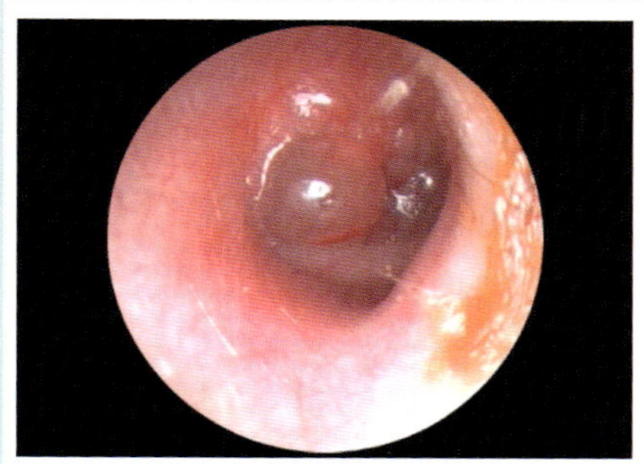 **Figure 9.1.5:** Acute bullous myringitis *Photo Courtesy:* Pradip Uppal, Thane	Patient complaints of acute onset of severe pain, usually self-limiting disorder, is due to viral infection (Fig. 9.1.5).	*Treatment*: Symptomatic treatment, analgesic and antipyretic SOS decongestant.

Otitis Media with Effusion

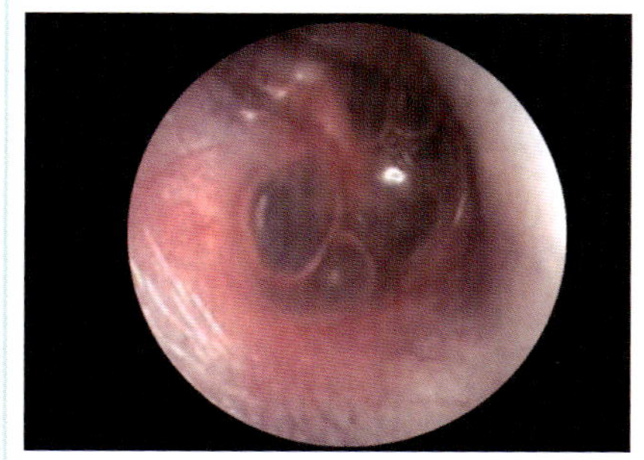 **Figure 9.1.6:** Otitis media with effusion *Photo Courtesy:* Pradip Uppal, Thane	Otitis media with effusion (OME) (serous otitis media) is often seen as a sequela of acute otitis media. Multiple bubbles of sterile fluid are seen. Mechanical obstruction of the Eustachian tube (e.g. adenoids, cleft palate) can lead to a middle-ear effusion (Fig. 9.1.6).	*Treatment*: Steroids with decongestants. If not responding grommet can be considered.

Picture	Note	Management

Atelectasis

Picture	Note	Management
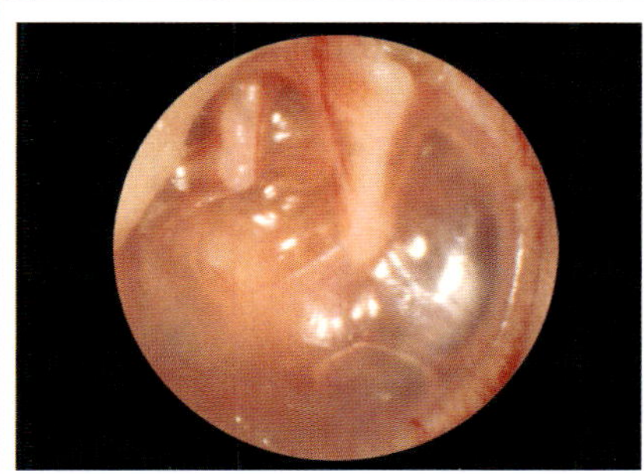 Figure 9.1.7: Atelectasis *Photo Courtesy:* Pradip Uppal, Thane	This is a sequeale of recurrent otitis media. This tympanic membrane is severely retracted to the extent that there is very little middle-ear space present. As the eardrum becomes adherent to the structures of the medial wall of the tympanic cavity, the condition is termed "atelectasis" (Fig. 9.1.7).	*Treatment*: Valsalva maneuver and steroids can be tried. Results are not good.

Myringotomy Tube (Grommet and Ventilating Tube)

Picture	Note	Management
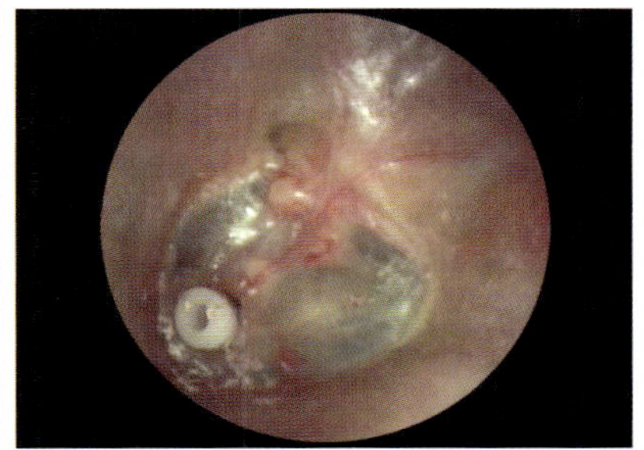 **Figure 9.1.8:** Myringotomy tube (Grommet and ventilating tube) *Photo Courtesy:* Pradip Uppal, Thane	Myringotomy tube is seen in antero-inferior compartment. This 4-year-old boy had history of persistent otitis media with effusion. Indications include persistent otitis media with effusion, recurrent otitis media and tympanic membrane retraction (Fig. 9.1.8).	Myringotomy with grommet (Ventilation tube) insertion is the treatment for persistent otitis media with effusion, recurrent otitis media and tympanic membrane retraction. In small children, even adenoidectomy with the said surgery will increase the efficacy of treatment.

Perforation

Picture	Note	Management
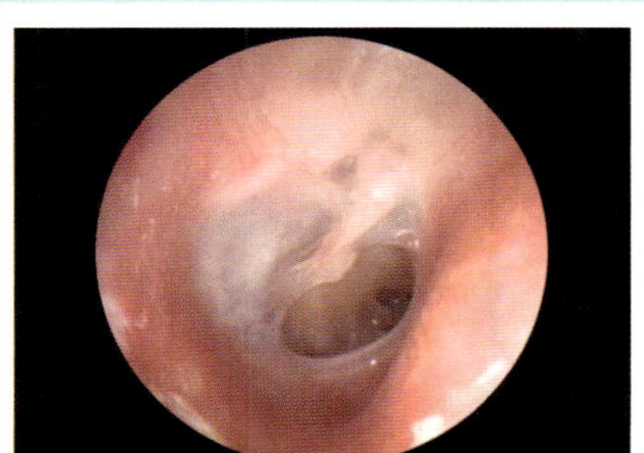 **Figure 9.1.9:** Perforation *Photo Courtesy:* Pradip Uppal, Thane	Perforation is seen in anterior half of drum, commonest cause is repeated otitis media or trauma. Audiogram will show conductive hearing loss (Fig. 9.1.9).	*Treatment*: Tympanoplasty procedure for closure of the perforation.

Picture	Note	Management

Subtotal Perforation

Picture	Note	Management
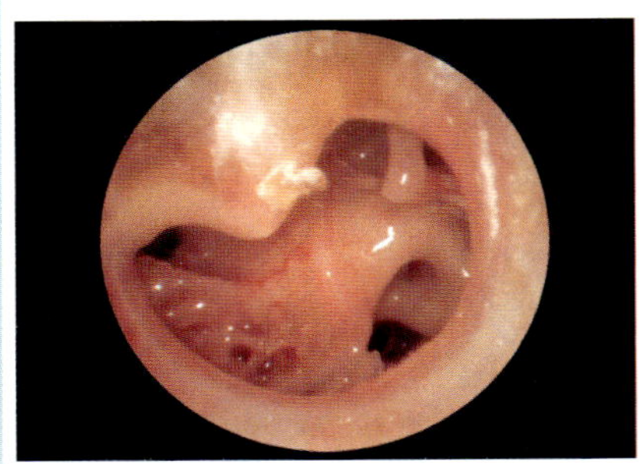 **Figure 9.1.10:** Subtotal perforation *Photo Courtesy:* Pradip Uppal, Thane	Through the perforation incus, hypotympanic air cell and round window is seen (Fig. 9.1.10).	*Treatment*: Tympanoplasty procedure for closure of the perforation.

Primary Acquired Cholesteatoma

Picture	Note	Management
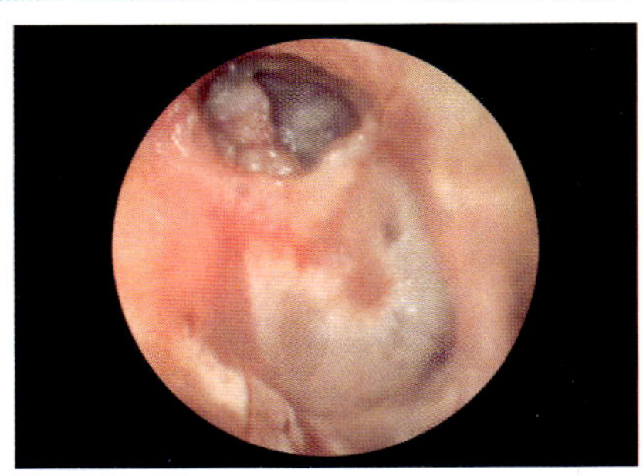 **Figure 9.1.11:** Primary acquired cholesteatoma *Photo Courtesy:* Pradip Uppal, Thane	A large cholesteatoma is seen arising from the pars flaccida of this tympanic membrane. The cholesteatoma has extensively eroded the superior canal wall and is filled with typical keratin debris (Fig. 9.1.11).	*Treatment*: Mastoidectomy with tympanoplasty

Cholesteatoma

Picture	Note	Management
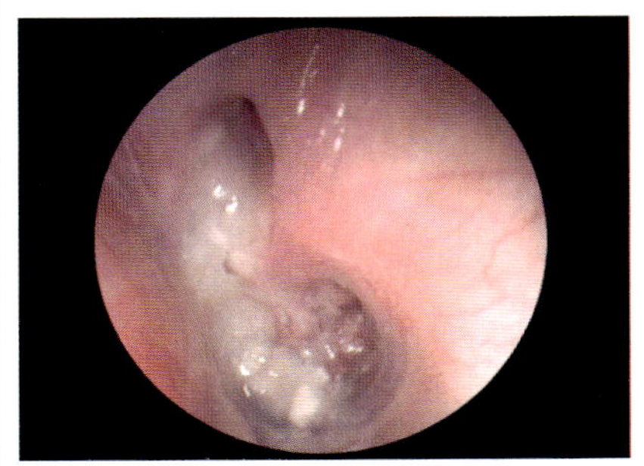 **Figure 9.1.12:** Cholesteatoma *Photo Courtesy:* Pradip Uppal, Thane	Unsafe chronic otitis media with cholesteatoma with superadded infection. If not treated, it can lead to intracranial complications (Fig. 9.1.12).	*Treatment*: Antibiotics followed by mastoidectomy

Picture	Note	Management

Facial Palsy

Picture	Note	Management
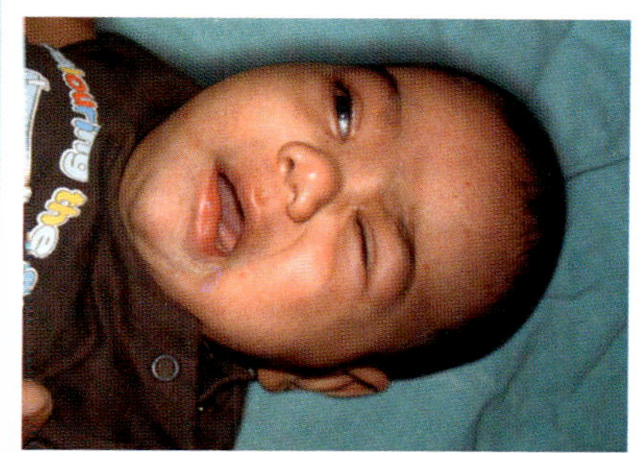 **Figure 9.1.13:** Facial palsy *Photo Courtesy:* Pradip Uppal, Thane	It is one of the complications of cholesteatoma. The disease process may involve facial nerve directly (Fig. 9.1.13).	*Treatment*: Urgent mastoidectomy with decompression of facial nerve.

Aural Polyp

Picture	Note	Management
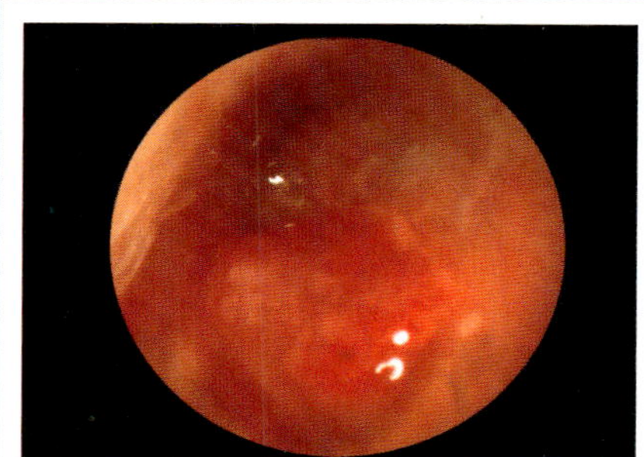 **Figure 9.1.14:** Aural polyp *Photo Courtesy:* Pradip Uppal, Thane	Sequale to injury with buds or pins, c/o of pain and ear discharge (Fig. 9.1.14).	*Treatment*: Antibiotics and eardrops. Surgical excision if medical treatment fails.

Otitis Externa

Picture	Note	Management
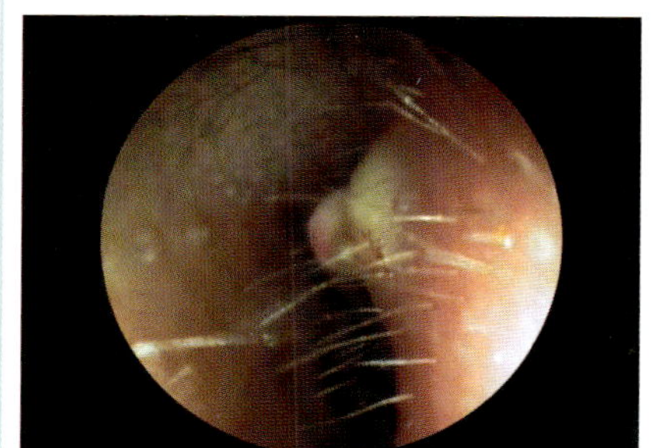 **Figure 9.1.15:** Otitis externa *Photo Courtesy:* Pradip Uppal, Thane	This picture reveals a boil in the external auditory canal, the condition is usually painful and the ear is very tender to touch (Fig. 9.1.15).	*Treatment*: Antibiotics with analgesics.

Picture	Note	Management

Infected Wax Granuloma

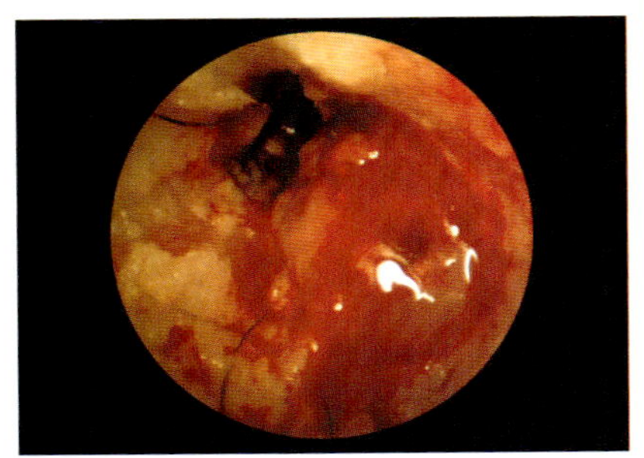 **Figure 9.1.16:** Infected wax granuloma *Photo Courtesy:* Pradip Uppal, Thane	Patient presents with severe pain, a long-standing wax leads to pressure necrosis with secondary infection and granuloma formation (Fig. 9.1.16).	*Treatment*: Antibiotics and analgesics. If pain is unbearable, the wax granuloma is removed under GA.

Otomycosis

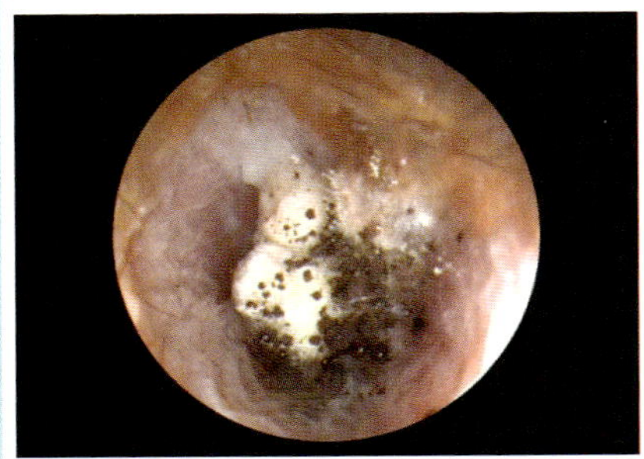 **Figure 9.1.17:** Otomycosis *Photo Courtesy:* Pradip Uppal, Thane	This picture represents the typical fungal infection of *A. niger*. The patient usually complains of otorrhea with severe itching (Fig. 9.1.17).	*Treatment*: Besides antibiotics would be local antifungal drops. Steroid eardrops should be avoided.

Impetigo

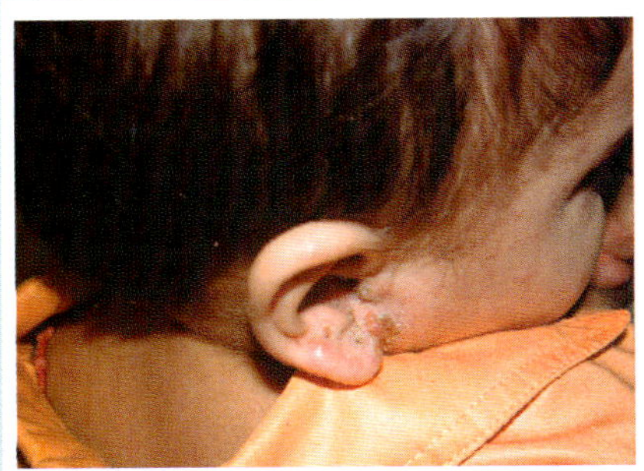 **Figure 9.1.18:** Impetigo *Photo Courtesy:* Pradip Uppal, Thane	Patient presents with pruritus and variable degree of pain characterized by pustule and crusts. It is caused by group A Streptococci or *Staphylococcus aureus* (Fig. 9.1.18).	*Treatment* consists of local and systemic antibiotics and anti-inflammatory drugs.

Picture	Note	Management

Mastoid Abscess

Picture	Note	Management
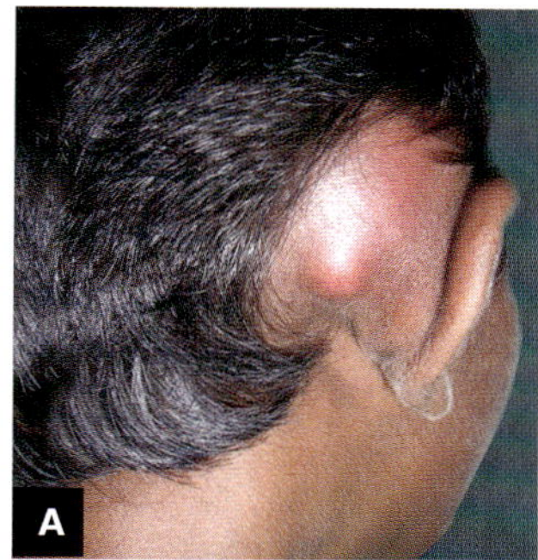 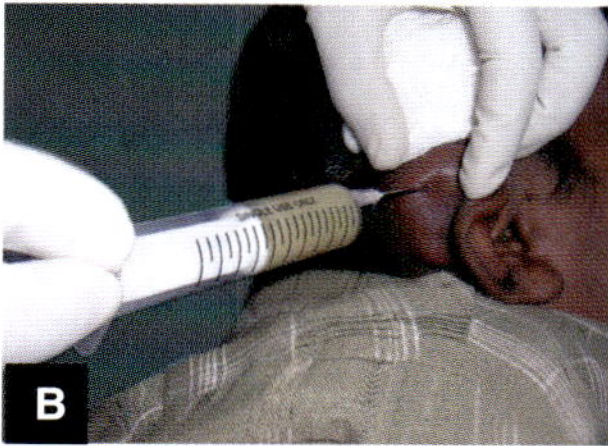 **Figures 9.1.19A and B:** (A) Mastoid abscess (B) Mastoid abscess aspiration *Photo Courtesy:* Pradip Uppal, Thane	Mastoid abscess is a common extra-cranial complication of unsafe otitis media. It manifests by earache, profuse foul-smelling discharge from the ear, postaural swelling and constitutional symptoms (Fig. 9.1.19A).	Treatment is incision and drainage. Aspiration (with a wide-bore) needle is done only to have a sample for culture and sensitivity (Fig. 9.1.19B). Definitive treatment in the form of mastoidectomy may be performed simultaneously or at a later date.

Preaurical Sinus

Picture	Note	Management
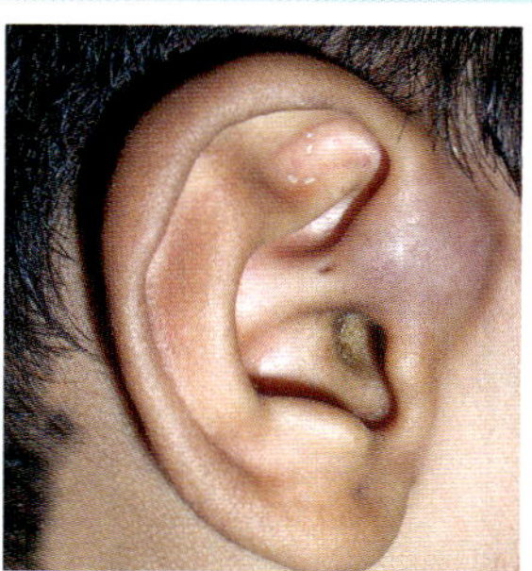 **Figure 9.1.20:** Preaurical sinus *Photo Courtesy:* Pradip Uppal, Thane	It is a congenital anomaly which may be either unilateral or bilateral. Sometimes, it is asymptomatic and is best left alone. But the one which gets repeatedly infected needs a complete excision at the earliest (Fig. 9.1.20).	Control of infection followed by surgical excision is required. Sometimes, a small amount of diluted methylene blue may be injected into the tract to identify it completely and ensure a complete excision.

Preauricular Abscess

Picture	Note	Management
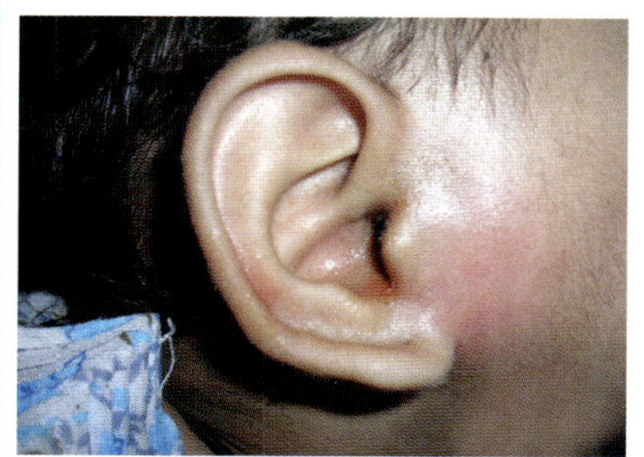 **Figure 9.1.21:** Preauricular abscess *Photo Courtesy:* Pradip Uppal, Thane	Infection of preauricular lymph nodes followed by suppuration may occur due to infections arising in the external auditory canal or facial skin (Fig. 9.1.21). It may be confused with a parotid abscess. parotid abscess will cause raised lobule of pinna.	Treatment is incision and drainage along with treatment of the primary cause.

Picture	Note	Management

9.2 NOSE

Epistaxis from Little's Area

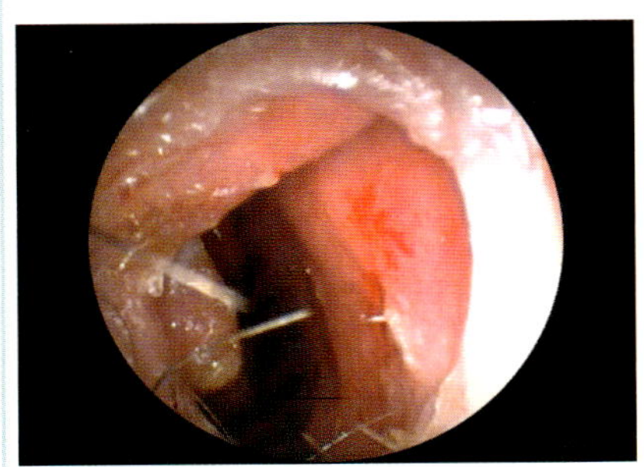 **Figure 9.2.1:** Epistaxis from Little's area *Photo Courtesy:* Amol S Khale, Thane	The commonest cause is nose picking due to dryness and scab formation. It is the area of nasal arterial anastomosis and hence trivial trauma causes profuse bleeding (Fig. 9.2.1).	Treatment includes local ointment application, external ice application and if required chemical cautery and nasal packing.

Granuloma in Little's Area

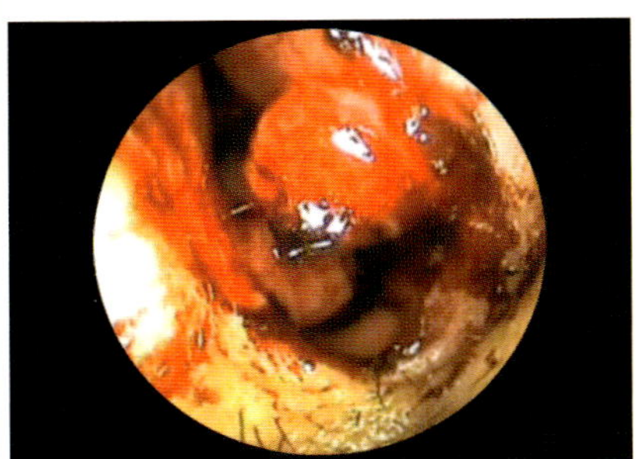 **Figure 9.2.2:** Granuloma in Little's area *Photo Courtesy:* Amol S Khale, Thane	When crusts and scabs in Little's area are not cleaned, it forms vicious cycle of crusts-dryness-itching-bleeding-crusts and ultimately it leads to infection and granuloma formation (Fig. 9.2.2).	Excision and bipolar cauterization.

Nasal Vestibulitis

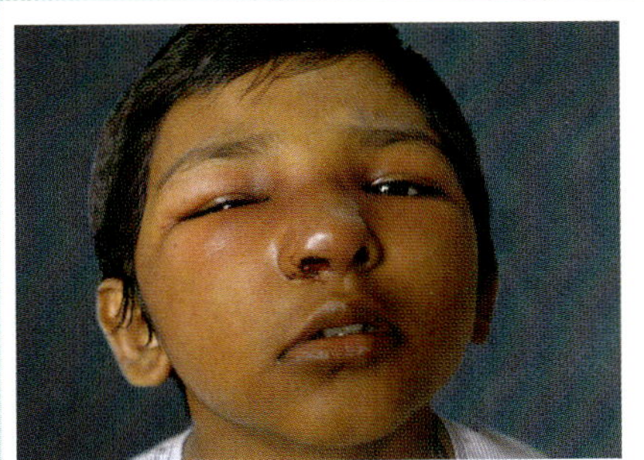 **Figure 9.2.3:** Nasal vestibulitis *Photo Courtesy:* Amol S Khale, Thane	This occurs due to infection of hair follicles of nasal vestibular skin leading to furuncles. Infection spreads to surrounding areas (as seen above) giving rise to pain, swelling and redness (Fig. 9.2.3).	*Management* includes antibiotics, analgesics and anti-inflammatory drugs and avoidance of nose picking.

Picture	Note	Management

Early Vestibulitis

Picture	Note	Management
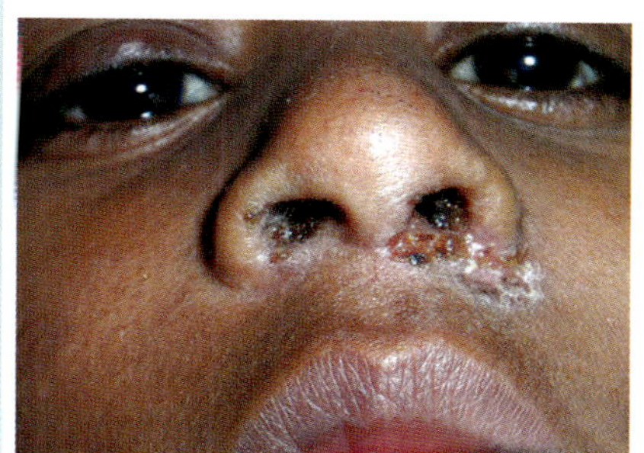 **Figure 9.2.4:** Early vestibulitis *Photo Courtesy:* Amol S Khale, Thane	Nasal crusts in early vestibulitis are usually caused by *Staphylococcus aureus* and may result from excessive nose picking or excessive nose blowing. The crusts may bleed on sloughing off.	This can be treated with local ointment like mupirocin (Fig. 9.2.4). Maintaining personal hygiene (like cutting nails) and a good immunity will go a long way in preventing recurrences. Small children, elderly people (who may be immunocompromised) and health care professionals need special attention in this apparently innocuous condition.

Vestibular Abscess

Picture	Note	Management
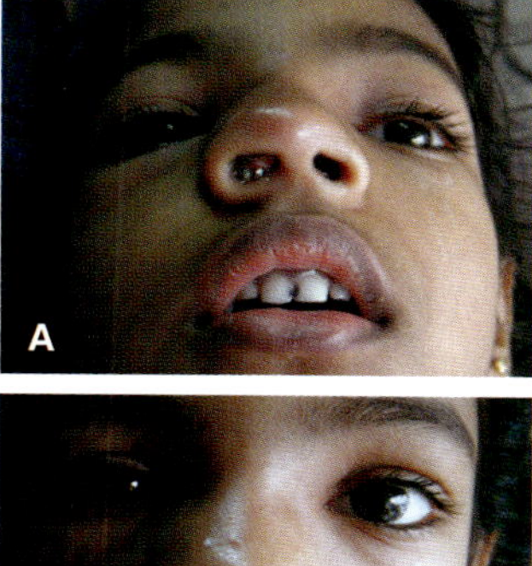 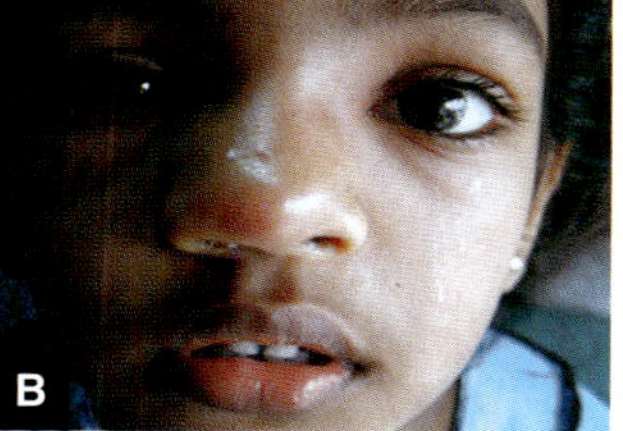 **Figures 9.2.5A and B:** Vestibular abscess *Photo Courtesy:* Amol S Khale, Thane	If left untreated, vestibulitis can lead to abscess formation. Since this is the "danger area" of face, abscess may spread retrograde into cavernous sinus leading to its thrombosis. Patients present with frontal headache, fever with chills and diplopia (Figs 9.2.5A and B) (Danger area of face-veins here is valveless and communicates freely with cavernous sinus).	Drainage of vestibular abscess is deferred till at least 24 hours of antimicrobial therapy to prevent any further spread of infection to cavernous sinus. Combination therapy of penicillins and clindamycin is recommended. Even during incision and drainage, undue pressure to express out pus should be avoided to prevent the (theoretical) possibility of retrograde spread of infection.

Allergic Rhinosinusitis

Picture	Note	Management
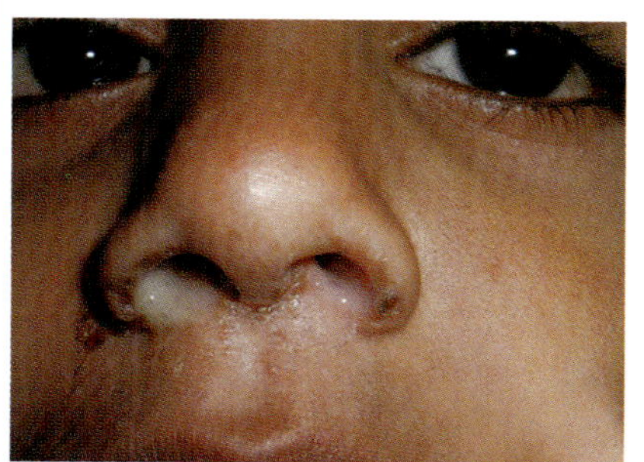 **Figure 9.2.6:** Allergic rhinosinusitis *Photo Courtesy:* Amol S Khale, Thane	Child suffers from recurrent attacks of allergic rhinitis. Discharge is watery to begin with then becomes mucoid and eventually turns purulent (Fig. 9.2.6).	Symptomatic treatment is in the form of antihistamines and decongestant. Between the attacks, nasal steroid sprays can be tried.

Picture	Note	Management

Septal Hematoma/Septal Abscess

Picture	Note	Management
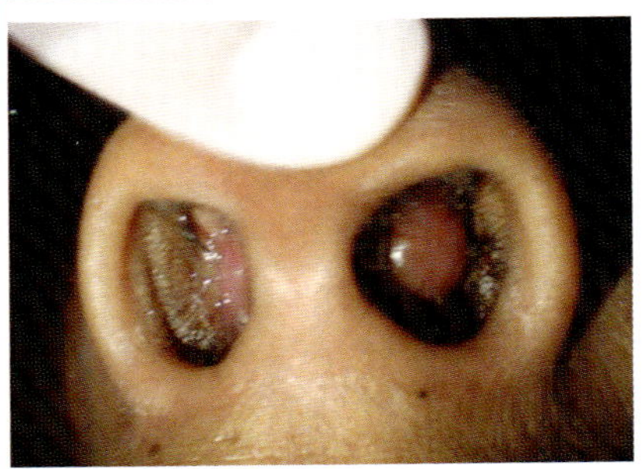 **Figure 9.2.7:** Septal hematoma/septal abscess *Photo Courtesy:* Amol S Khale, Thane	It is the collection of blood between two layers of perichondrium. If left untreated can get infected and form septal abscess (Fig. 9.2.7). This occurs due to nasal trauma.	*Management* is done by incision and drainage followed by nasal packing and also antibiotics, analgesics and anti-inflammatory drugs. When abscess is formed patients present with fever with chills, and frontal headache.

Orbital Abscess

Picture	Note	Management
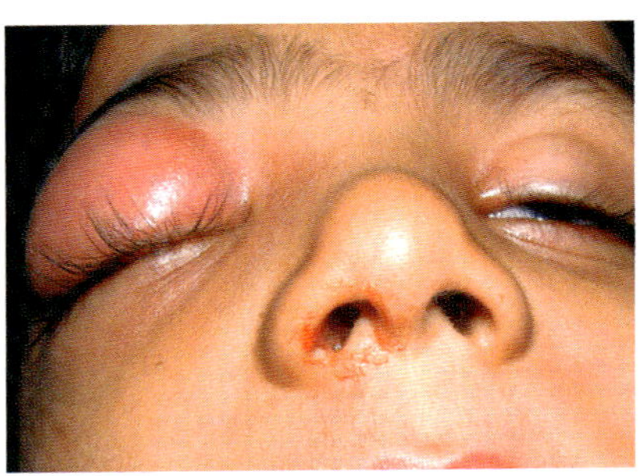 **Figure 9.2.8A:** Orbital abscess *Photo Courtesy:* Amol S Khale, Thane	This condition is due to ethmoidal sinusitis where lamina papyracea is breached. It can cause orbital cellulitis and if not treated in time, leads to orbital abscess (Fig. 9.2.8A) and sometimes blindness.	*Management* includes antibiotics, analgesics and anti-inflammatory drugs. If not responding to it, then endonasal endoscopic drainage and decompression of orbit is required.
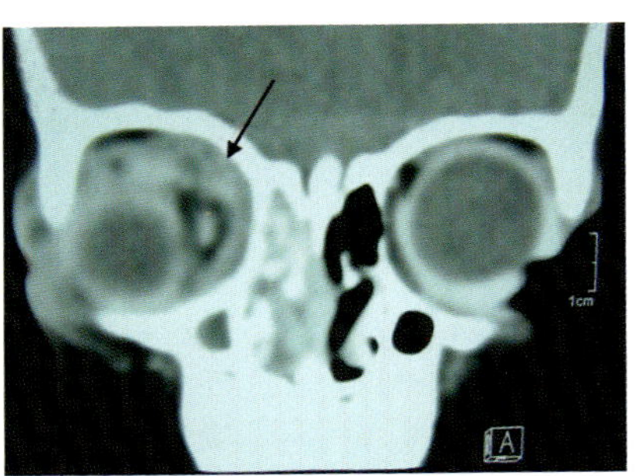 **Figure 9.2.8B:** CT scan *Photo Courtesy:* Amol S Khale, Thane	It shows wall of the orbit is breached. Periorbital abscess is pushing the eyeball (Fig. 9.2.8B).	The CT scan being of the same patient as above, treatment is the same as above.

Picture	Note	Management

Rhinosporidiosis

Picture	Note	Management
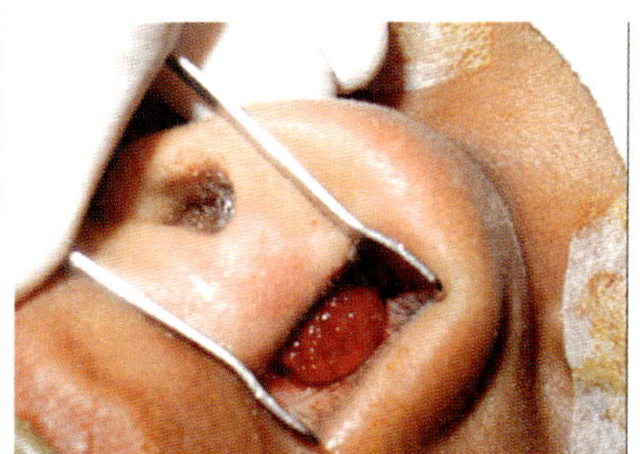 **Figure 9.2.9:** Rhinosporidiosis *Photo Courtesy:* Amol S Khale, Thane	It is a chronic infection caused by fungus rhinosporidium seeberi that mainly affects the nasal mucosa. It is clinically presented as friable polyp; common symptoms are nasal blockage and epistaxis (Fig. 9.2.9).	Its treatment is eminently surgical with resection and electrocoagulation of its base.

Lacrimal Fistula

Picture	Note	Management
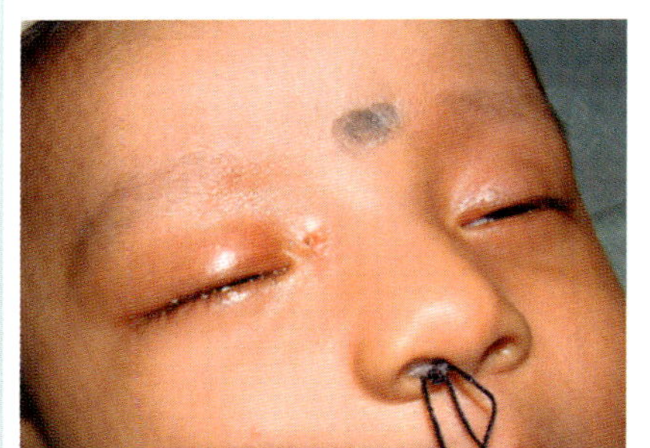 **Figure 9.2.10:** Lacrimal fistula *Photo Courtesy:* Amol S Khale, Thane	It occurs when there is congenital (as above) or inflammatory narrowing of lacrimal duct, which causes obstruction to flow of tears. Left untreated it causes infection and when pus develops inside sac, it finds its way on to the skin surface, leaving behind a fistula (as seen above) (Fig. 9.2.10).	Unilateral affection should remind the attending physician of probably an old and forgotten foreign body.

9.3 THROAT

Tonsils

Picture	Note	Management
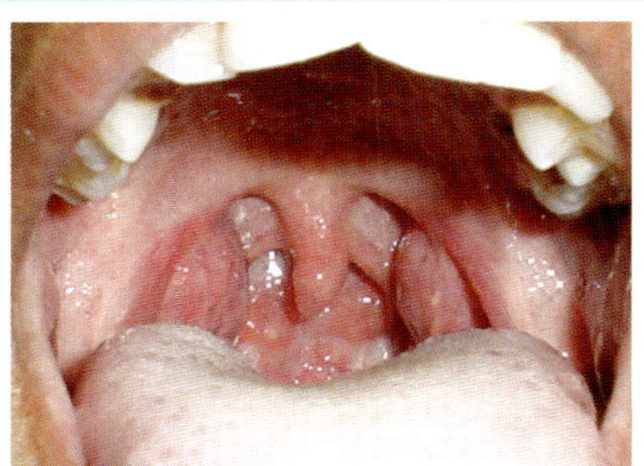 **Figure 9.3.1:** Tonsils *Photo Courtesy:* Kamal Ghanshamnani, Thane	They are part of Waldeyer's ring—an aggregate of lymphoid tissue. Recurrent infection causes tonsillar enlargement (Fig. 9.3.1).	Tonsillitis needs to be treated with appropriate antibiotics like beta lactams, macrolides. In case of repeated tonsillitis (> 7/year), tonsils may be removed by dissection method, cryosurgery or radiofrequency ablation.

Picture	Note	Management

Follicular Tonsillitis

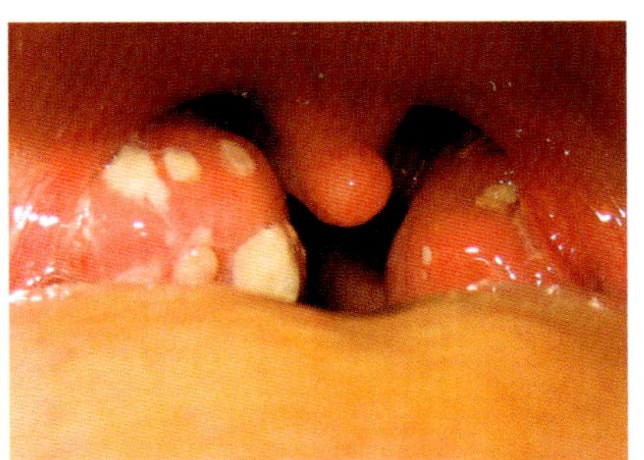 **Figure 9.3.2:** Follicular tonsillitis *Photo Courtesy:* Kamal Ghanshamnani, Thane	Tonsillar crypts get infected in this condition. Most common organism responsible is beta hemolytic streptococci. Others are staphylococci, pneumococci, and *H. influenzae* (Fig. 9.3.2).	*Treatment*: Antibiotics, analgesics and anti-inflammatory drugs.

Membranous Tonsillitis

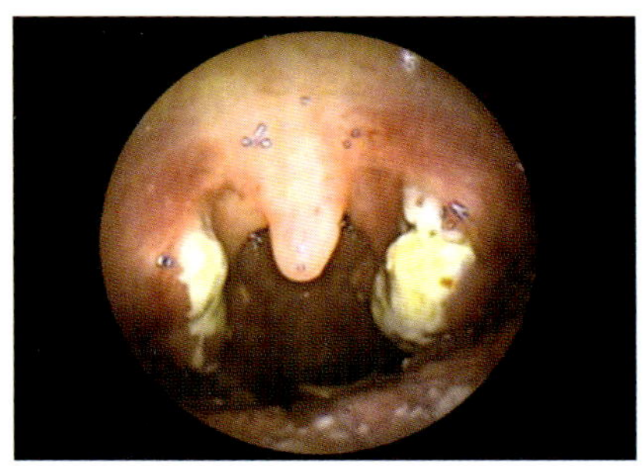 **Figure 9.3.3:** Membranous tonsillitis *Photo Courtesy:* Kamal Ghanshamnani, Thane	Organisms are responsible—same as follicular tonsillitis. If white patches is seen (as above), then send swab for smear and culture for removal of diphtheria (Fig. 9.3.3).	*Treatment*: Antibiotics, analgesics and anti-inflammatory drugs.

Quinsy (Peritonsillar Abscess)

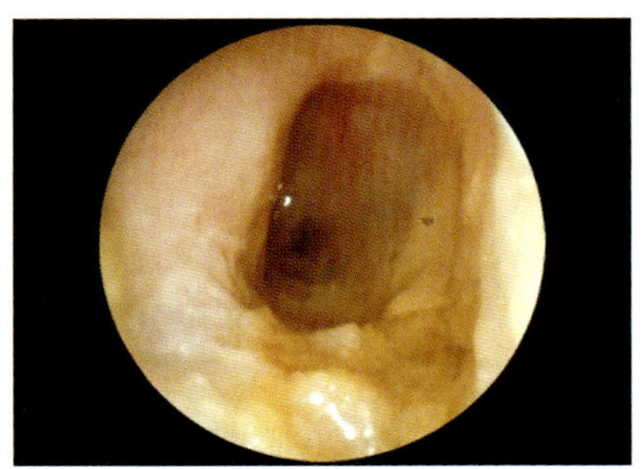 **Figure 9.3.4:** Quinsy (peritonsillar abscess) *Photo Courtesy:* Kamal Ghanshamnani, Thane	It is the collection of pus in peritonsillar space. Results from untreated tonsillitis, uvula gets pushed to opposite side (Fig.. 9.3.4).	*Treatment*: Intraoral incision and drainage and antibiotics, analgesics and anti-inflammatory drugs.

Picture	Note	Management

Granular Pharyngitis

Picture	Note	Management
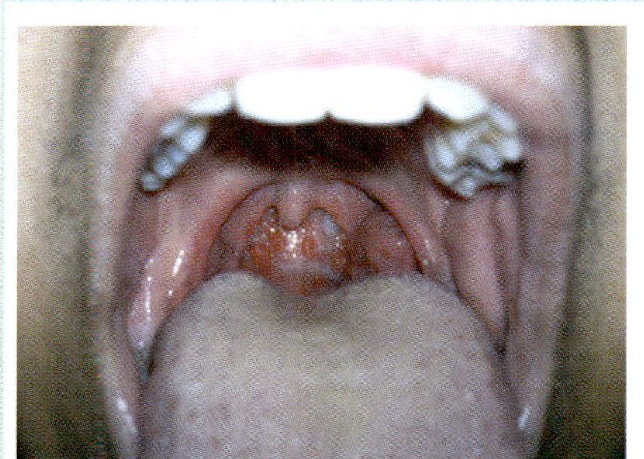 **Figure 9.3.5:** Granular pharyngitis *Photo Courtesy:* Kamal Ghanshamnani, Thane	It is characterized by hypertrophy of mucosa, seromucinous glands and subepithelial lymphoid follicles. Causative factors include persistant rhinosinusitis, allergy and gastro-esophageal reflux disease (GERD) (Fig. 9.3.5).	*Treatment*: Anti-allergic and antacids, SOS steroids and removal of etiological factors.

Diphtheria

Picture	Note	Management
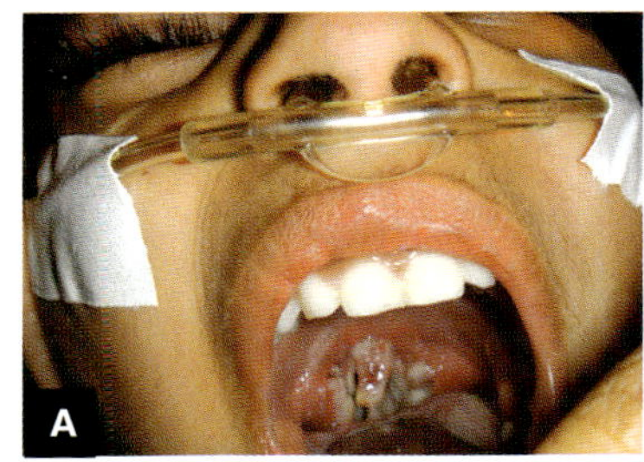 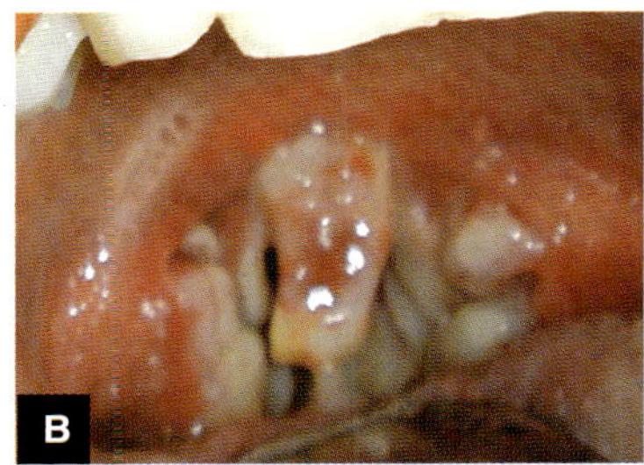 **Figures 9.3.6A and B:** Diphtheria *Photo Courtesy:* Kamal Ghanshamnani, Thane	The exudates in crypts form tough membrane over tonsils (as above). It is adherent and its removal leaves a bleeding surface. The membrane tends to extend beyond tonsils, on to the soft palate and its dirty gray in color (Figs 9.3.6A and B).	*Treatment*: Antibiotics, analgesics and anti-inflammatory drugs as well as antidiphtheric serum.

Adenoids

Picture	Note	Management
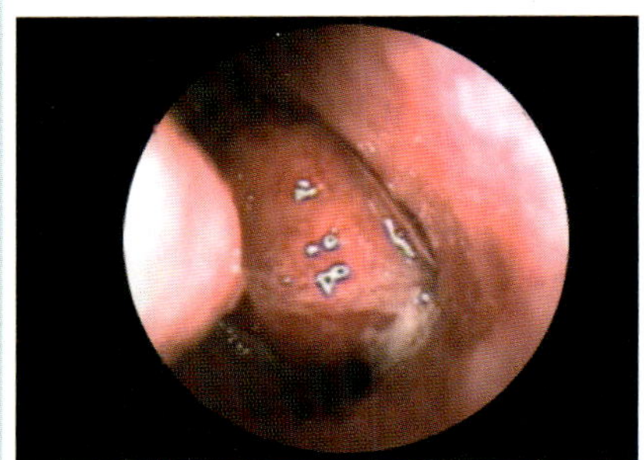 **Figure 9.3.7:** Adenoids *Photo Courtesy:* Kamal Ghanshamnani, Thane	They are part of Waldeyer's ring—an aggregate of lymphoid tissue. It is present at birth, shows physiological enlargement up to age of 6 years and tends to atrophy at puberty and almost completely disappears by age of 20 years (Fig. 9.3.7). Chief complaint is snoring and mouth breathing. It can lead to recurrent ear affections. And in extreme cases, it presents with adenoid facies.	*Treatment*: Removal by curettage, microdebrider, if compromising airway.

Picture	Note	Management

Radiology Adenoid Hypertrophy

Picture	Note	Management
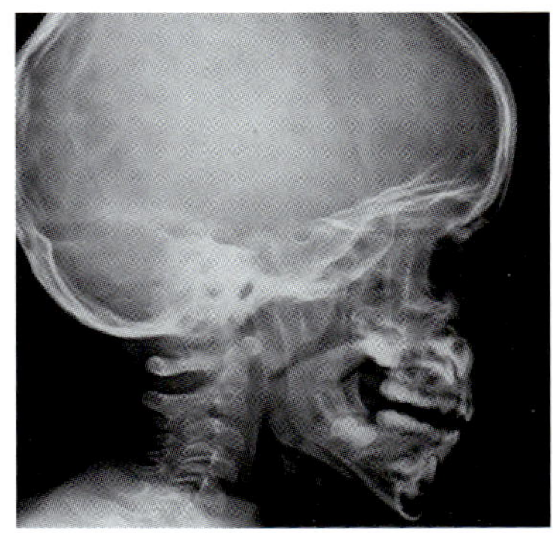 **Figure 9.3.8:** Radiology adenoid hypertrophy *Photo Courtesy:* Kamal Ghanshamnani, Thane	Soft tissue lateral radiograph of nasopharynx reveals the size of adenoids and also the extent to which nasopharyngeal air space has been compromised. Preferably the X-ray should be taken with mouth open (Fig. 9.3.8).	*Treatment:* Removal by curettage, microdebrider, if compromising airway.

Preauricular Abscess

Picture	Note	Management
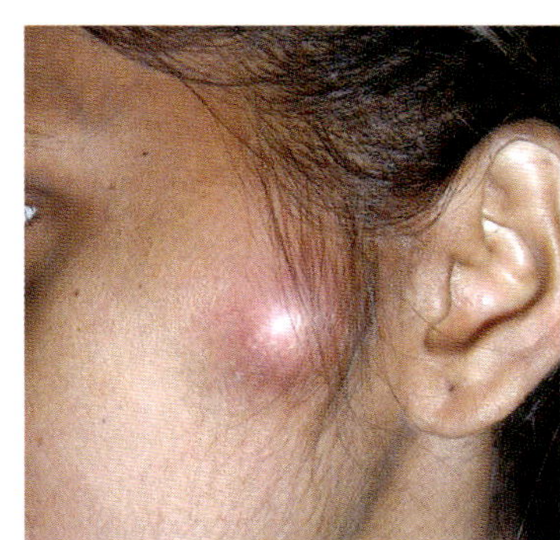 **Figure 9.3.9:** Preauricular abscess *Photo Courtesy:* Kamal Ghanshamnani, Thane	Lymphadenitis or suppuration of preauricular lymph nodes can be secondary to infection of the facial skin, sinus infection or otitis externa. It can be confused with parotid abscess which is more painful and can cause severe trismus (Fig. 9.3.9).	*Treatment*: Mainly involves addressing the cause as well as incision and drainage.

Cold Abscess Neck

Picture	Note	Management
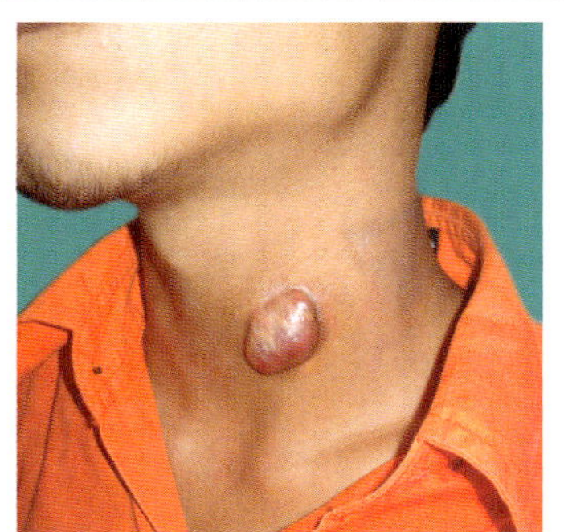 **Figure 9.3.10:** Cold abscess neck *Photo Courtesy:* Kamal Ghanshamnani, Thane	Tuberculous affection of the lymph nodes in the neck is a common manifestation of extrapulmonary form of tuberculosis (Fig. 9.3.10). It is called "cold" because it is usually devoid of acute signs of inflammation pain, local rise of temperature.	*Treatment*: Aspiration of the abscess and/or incision and drainage has to be done with caution and in a "nondependent" position to prevent fistula formation. Anti-TB treatment.

Picture	Note	Management

Laryngeal Papillomatosis

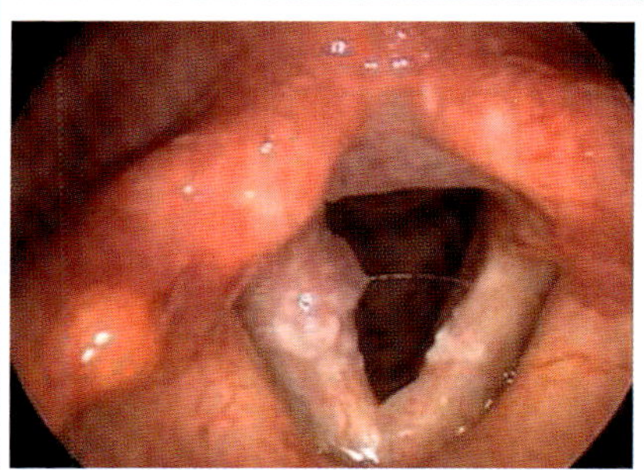 **Figure 9.3.11:** Laryngeal papillomatosis *Photo Courtesy:* Kamal Ghanshamnani, Thane	Juvenile onset laryngeal papillomas are caused by human papilloma virus. They are multiple and often involving infants and young children who present with hoarseness and stridor. Mostly they are seen on true and false cords and epiglottis. They tend to disappear spontaneously after puberty (Fig. 9.3.11).	*Treatment*: Endoscopic removal with cup forceps, cryotherapy, microelectrocautery, CO_2 laser and interferon therapy.

Erythema Multiforme

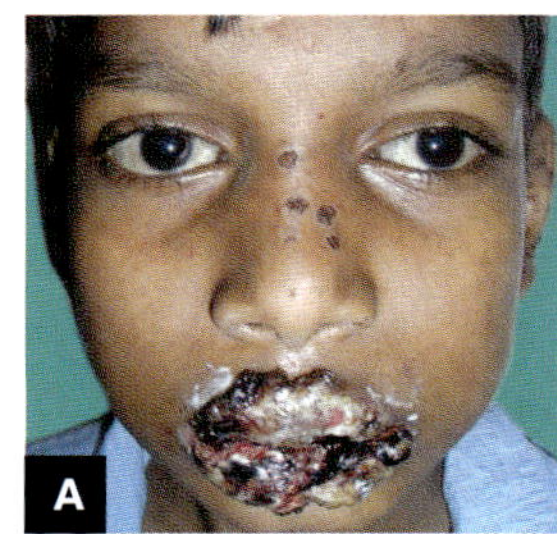 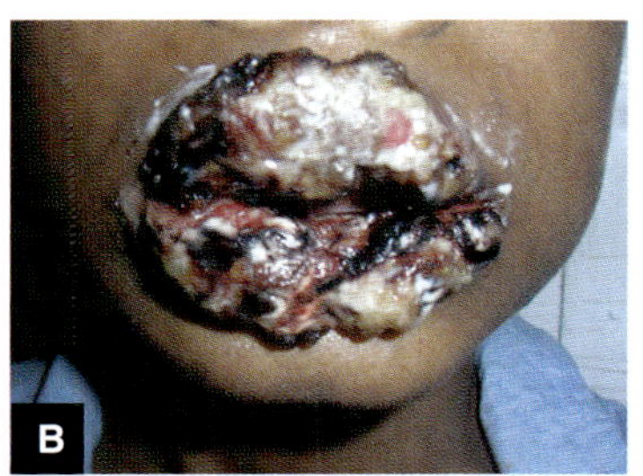 **Figures 9.3.12A and B:** Erythema multiforme *Photo Courtesy:* Kamal Ghanshamnani, Thane	Secondary to human immunodeficiency virus (HIV) otolaryngological symptoms occur in more than 40% of patients with acquired immunodeficiency syndrome (AIDS). Herpes simplex of the lips, mouth and pharynx (Figs 9.3.12A and B).	*Treatment*: Symptomatic and antiretroviral treatment.

Picture	Note	Management

Palatal Perforation

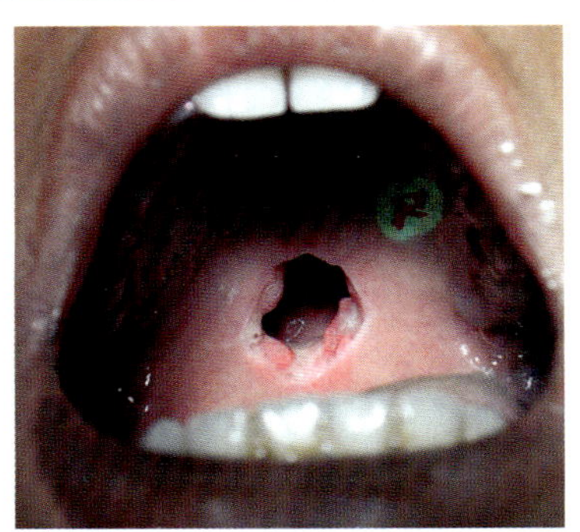 **Figure 9.3.13:** Palatal perforation *Photo Courtesy:* Kamal Ghanshamnani, Thane	This photograph shows perforation in palate. Patient presents with excessive nasal twang, nasal regurgitation of eaten food, excessive nasal crusting and sometimes bloody nasal discharge (Fig. 9.3.13). Differential diagnosis includes: • Secondary to cleft palate repair • Wegener's granulomatosis • Tuberculosis • Post-HIV palatal ulceration. This was the case of tuberculosis.	*Treatment*: Transoral repair of fistula with or without prosthesis.

Section 10

Infections in Musculoskeletal System

Section Editor
Alaric Aroojis

Contributors
Alaric Aroojis, Rujuta Mehta, John Mukhopadhaya

Section Outline

10.1 Acute Septic Arthritis

- Acute Septic Arthritis of Right Hip Joint
- Neonatal Hip Joint Infection
- Treatment of Hip Joint Septic Arthritis
- Late Presentation of Hip Septic Arthritis
- Shoulder Joint Septic Arthritis

10.2 Acute Hematogenous Osteomyelitis

- Acute Osteomyelitis Left Proximal Femur
- Acute Osteomyelitis Left Distal Femur

10.3 Sequelae of Acute Osteomyelitis

- Chronic Osteomyelitis with Sequestration and Gap Nonunion of Femur
- Chronic Osteomyelitis with Sequestrum
- Bone Loss of the Tibia following Osteomyelitis
- Bone Loss and Gap Nonunion of Humerus following Osteomyelitis

10.4 Sequelae of Septic Arthritis

- Complete Destruction of Proximal Femoral Epiphysis following Osteomyelitis and Septic Arthritis
- Dislocation of the Hip Joint following Septic Arthritis
- Tom Smith's Arthritis causing Bilateral Loss of Capital Femoral Epiphysis
- Reconstructive Options for Tom Smith's Arthritis of Right Hip
- Sequel of Septic Arthritis of Knee

Picture	Note	Management

10.1 ACUTE SEPTIC ARTHRITIS

Acute Septic Arthritis of Right Hip Joint

Picture	Note	Management
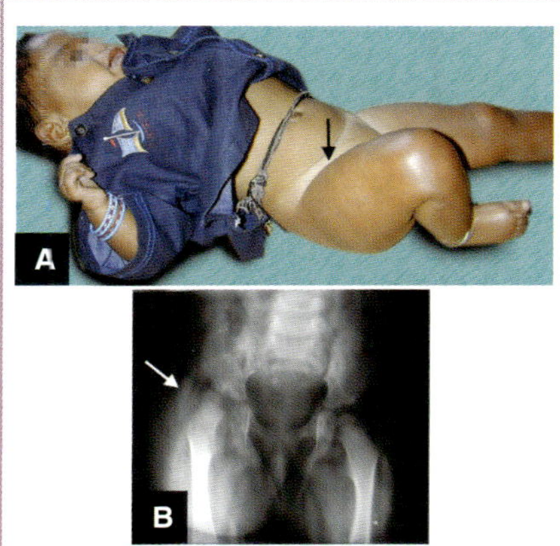 **Figures 10.1.1A and B:** Acute septic arthritis of right hip joint *Photo Courtesy:* Alaric Aroojis, Mumbai	A 6-month-old child with painful movements of the right hip associated with high-grade fever and irritability since 3 days. Note the flexion deformity of the right hip joint and associated swelling in the buttock and groin which is usually diagnostic of joint infection. Passive movements of the affected joint are painful and severely restricted (Fig. 10.1.1A). X-ray of both hips shows a marked capsular distension and subluxation of the right hip joint (Fig. 10.1.1B).	Early diagnosis and emergent treatment is the key to ensure a good outcome. High-grade fever, irritability and refusal to move the affected limb are the earliest signs of joint infection. *Staphylococcus aureus* is the commonest community—acquired infection, though Group A Streptococci, methicillin resistant *Staphylococcus aureus* (MRSA) and gram-negative infections can also occur. Hematological work-up must include complete blood count, C-reactive protein (CRP), erythrocyte sedimentation rate (ESR) and blood culture.

Neonatal Hip Joint Infection

Picture	Note	Management
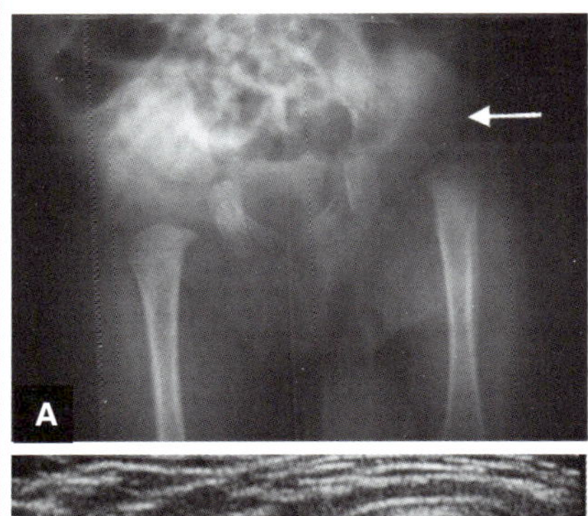 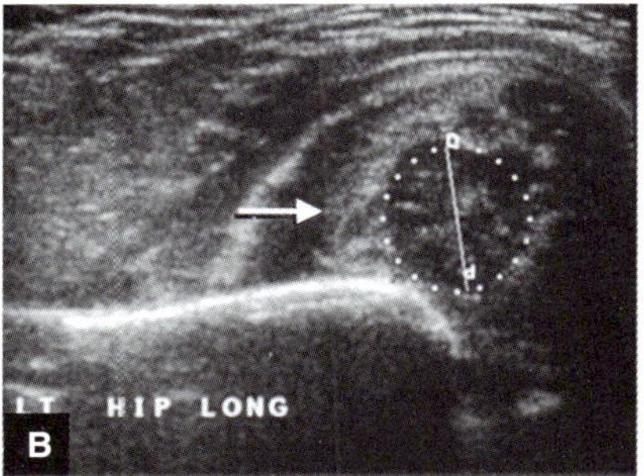 **Figures 10.1.2A and B:** Neonatal hip joint infection *Photo Courtesy:* Alaric Aroojis, Mumbai	X-ray of a 10-day-old neonate in the ICU showing capsular distension and septic subluxation of left hip joint. X-rays are often difficult to interpret due to nonossification of capital femoral epiphysis, and the diagnosis is often missed or delayed (Fig. 10.1.2A). Hip ultrasound is usually diagnostic and shows evidence of joint effusion, dislocation and cartilage destruction within first 48 hours (Fig. 10.1.2B).	High-risk neonates in the ICU are especially prone to silent joint sepsis and a high index of suspicion must be maintained in any neonate with irritability, refusal to feed and decreased joint movements. Fever and overt signs of infection are frequently absent in this age group. X-rays are misleading and usually not very helpful in coming to a diagnosis. Ultrasound is a cheap and readily available imaging modality in diagnosing joint effusion, but must be interpreted with caution.

Picture	Note	Management

Treatment of Hip Joint Septic Arthritis

Picture	Note	Management
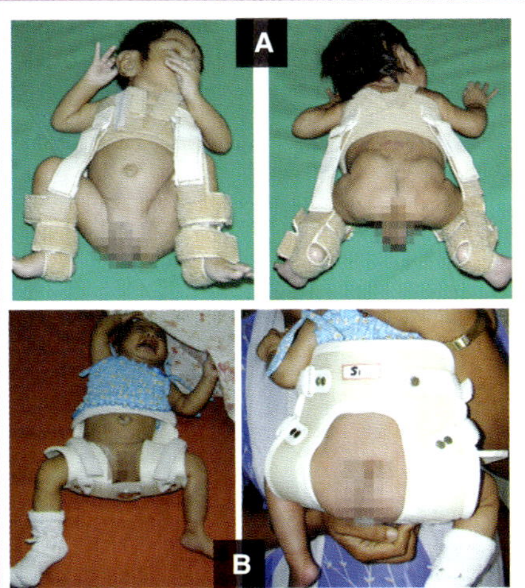 **Figures 10.1.3A and B:** Treatment of hip joint septic arthritis *Photo Courtesy:* Alaric Aroojis, Mumbai	Aspiration of hip joint followed by immobilization in Pavlik harness (Fig. 10.1.3A). Arthrotomy of hip joint and immobilization in a hip spica brace (Fig. 10.1.3B).	When in doubt—aspirate. Aspiration should be performed in a sterile environment and the aspirate is sent for urgent smear and culture. Aspiration and lavage may be adequate for superficial joints like the shoulder, but deep joints such as the hip should always undergo urgent arthrotomy and joint decompression once the diagnosis is confirmed on clinical, laboratory and imaging modalities. Following arthrotomy, the hip must be immobilized in a harness, brace or plaster spica for 4–6 weeks. Broad spectrum antibiotics must be administered intravenously for 7–10 days awaiting the culture report, followed by oral antibiotics for 3–4 weeks.

Late Presentation of Hip Septic Arthritis

Picture	Note	Management
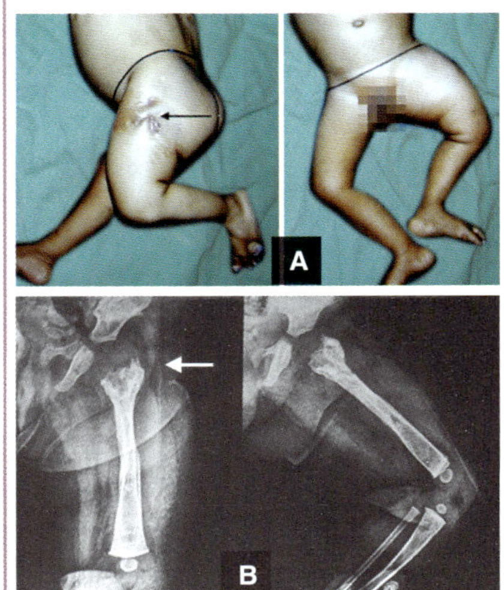 **Figures 10.1.4A and B:** Late presentation of hip septic arthritis *Photo Courtesy:* Alaric Aroojis, Mumbai	Left hip-joint swelling and discharging sinus (Fig. 10.1.4A). X-ray showing destruction of the capital femoral epiphysis and extensive osteomyelitis of the proximal femur (Fig. 10.1.4B).	Hip-joint infection is commonly missed in the sick neonate, with disastrous consequences. Delayed diagnosis is frequent in our country and can result in destruction of the capital femoral epiphysis, avascular necrosis, growth disturbances, hip instability and limb shortening (Tom Smith's arthritis).

Picture	Note	Management

Shoulder Joint Septic Arthritis

Picture	Note	Management
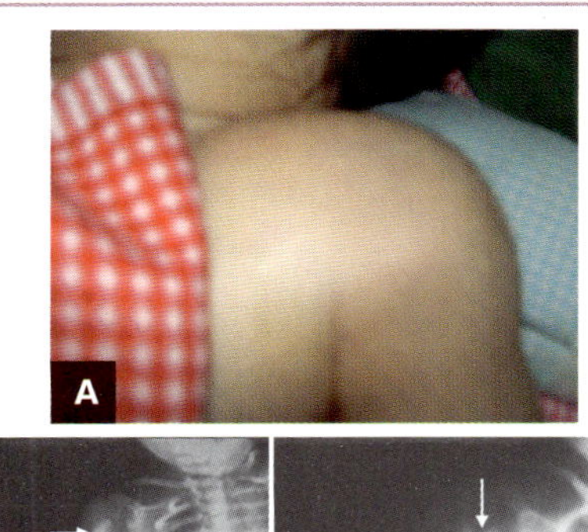 Figures 10.1.5A and B: Shoulder joint septic arthritis *Photo Courtesy:* Rujuta Mehta, Mumbai	Neonate in ICU with multifocal joint swelling involving left shoulder and both knee joints. Note the swelling and redness over left shoulder joint (Fig. 10.1.5A). X-ray showing osteomyelitis of proximal humerus and accompanying septic arthritis of the shoulder (Fig. 10.1.5B).	Acute hematogenous osteomyelitis often occurs concurrently with adjacent joint sepsis. Multifocal osteomyelitis and septic arthritis are occasionally seen in the immunocompromised septicemic neonate in the ICU and multiple joints involvement must be looked for in sick neonates. *Candida albicans* and other fungi are frequent pathogens especially in the ICU setting due to long-term hyperalimentation, prolonged intravenous access, use of potent broad spectrum antibiotics and ventilatory support for critically ill neonates.

10.2 ACUTE HEMATOGENOUS OSTEOMYELITIS

Acute Osteomyelitis Left Proximal Femur

Picture	Note	Management
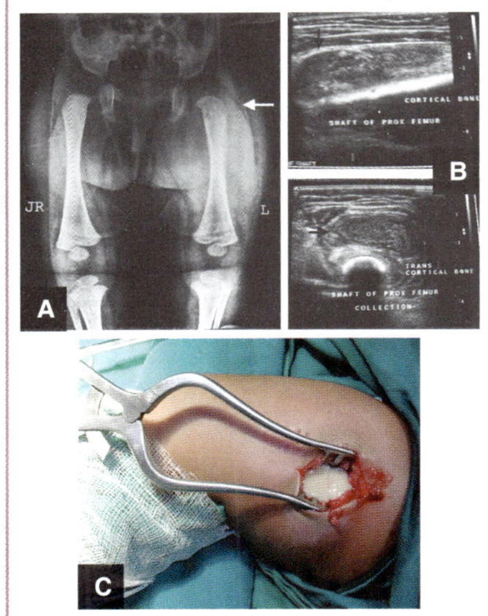 Figures 10.2.1A to C: Acute osteomyelitis left proximal femur *Photo Courtesy:* Rujuta Mehta, Mumbai	An 8-month-old child with high-grade fever, irritability and refusal to move left lower limb since 2 days. X-rays of both lower limbs shows a suspicious lytic area in the left proximal femoral metaphysis and soft tissue swelling of the left thigh, but are otherwise unremarkable (Fig. 10.2.1A). Ultrasound of the left thigh shows a large soft-tissue collection adjacent to the bone which has elevated the periosteum and escaped into the intramuscular compartment (Fig. 10.2.1B). Urgent incision and drainage revealed a large pus collection in the proximal thigh, which was drained (Fig. 10.2.1C).	• Acute hematogenous osteomyelitis is an orthopedic emergency and prompt diagnosis and management is essential to prevent long-term sequelae. • Basic investigations required to confirm the diagnosis are WBC count, ESR, CRP and blood cultures. Imaging modalities are bone scan, ultrasound or MRI. Ultrasound is an excellent imaging modality to confirm periosteal elevation and soft-tissue pus collection. • Urgent treatment must be initiated in the form of broad-spectrum parenteral antibiotics and urgent decompression of subperiosteal and soft-tissue abscess.

Picture	Note	Management

Acute Osteomyelitis Left Distal Femur

Picture	Note	Management
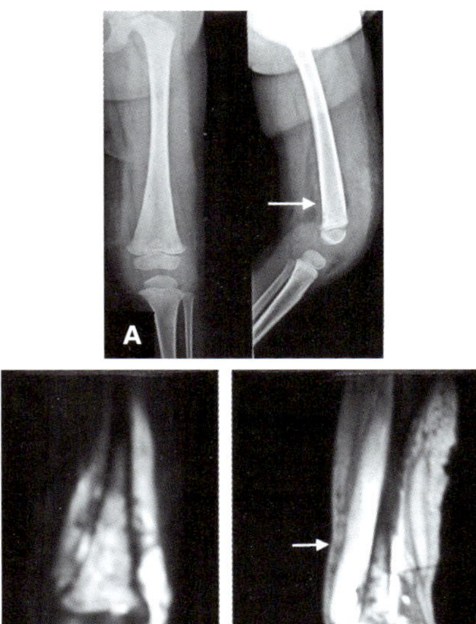 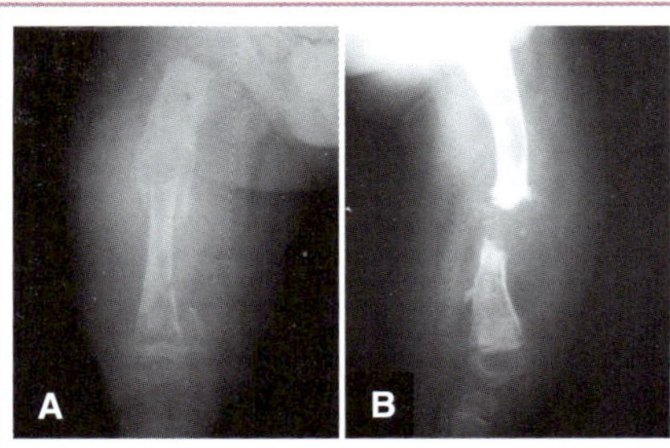 **Figures 10.2.2A and B:** Acute osteomyelitis left distal femur *Photo Courtesy:* Alaric Aroojis, Mumbai	A 5-year-old child presented with fever and refusal to bear weight on the left lower limb. X-rays are unremarkable except for a mild soft-tissue swelling posteriorly (Fig. 10.2.2A). MRI of the left knee shows marrow edema of the distal femur and an extensive subperiosteal pus collection suggestive of acute hematogenous osteomyelitis (Fig. 10.2.2B).	• X-ray changes are not seen till 7–10 days and are thus not useful in confirming the diagnosis of osteomyelitis. • MRI is the most sensitive and specific (> 90%) imaging modality to diagnose acute osteomyelitis but its usefulness for routine use is offset by its high-cost and the need for GA in the young child.

10.3 SEQUELAE OF ACUTE OSTEOMYELITIS

Chronic Osteomyelitis with Sequestration and Gap Nonunion of Femur

Picture	Note	Management
Figures 10.3.1A and B: Chronic osteomyelitis with sequestration and gap nonunion of femur *Photo Courtesy:* Rujuta Mehta, Mumbai	X-ray of the right femur of a 3-year-old child showing extensive diaphyseal osteomyelitis with sequestration of the entire lower half of the femur (Fig. 10.3.1A). X-ray showing a gap nonunion following removal of diaphyseal sequestrum (Fig. 10.3.1B).	Failure to diagnose and treat acute osteomyelitis emergently can lead to disastrous consequences such as sequestration, pathological fracture, bone loss with gap nonunion, growth arrest with residual deformities or limb shortening.

Picture	Note	Management

Chronic Osteomyelitis with Sequestrum

Picture	Note	Management
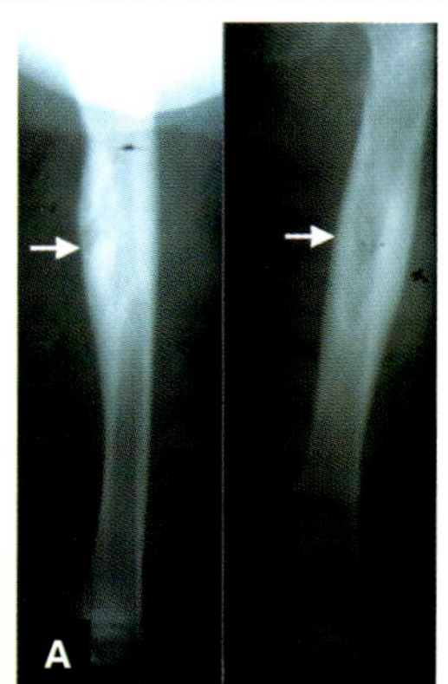 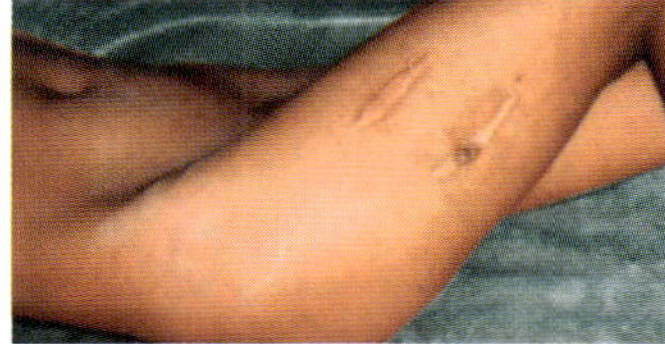 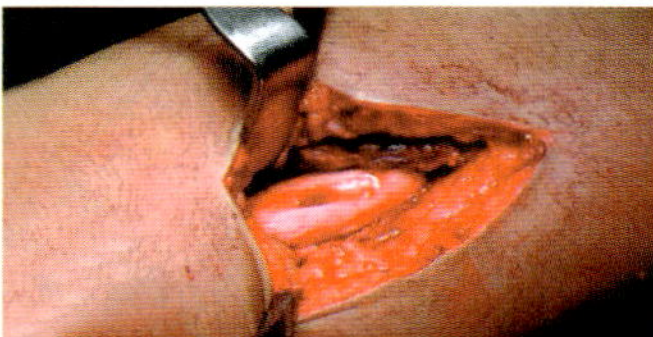 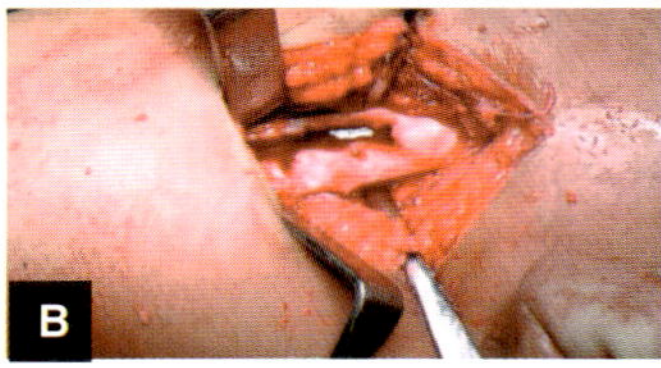 **Figures 10.3.2A and B:** Chronic osteomyelitis with sequestrum *Photo Courtesy:* Alaric Aroojis, Mumbai	X-rays of the right femur with sequestrum contained within a good involucrum (Fig. 10.3.2A) Clinical picture showing a discharging sinus in the middle third of the thigh. Scar of prior debridement is also seen. Sequestrectomy was performed after saucerization of the osteomyelitic cavity (Fig. 10.3.2B).	Late diagnosis or inadequate treatment of acute osteomyelitis can lead to formation of sequestrae (nonviable bone) and chronic osteomyelitis, with recurrent episodes of pain, swelling and seropurulent discharge. Treatment involves surgical debridement and saucerization of the osteomyelitic cavity with removal of nonviable bone and debris (sequestrectomy). Prolonged oral antibiotic cover is required for 6–8 weeks to sterilize the bone and prevent relapses.

Bone Loss of the Tibia following Osteomyelitis

Picture	Note	Management
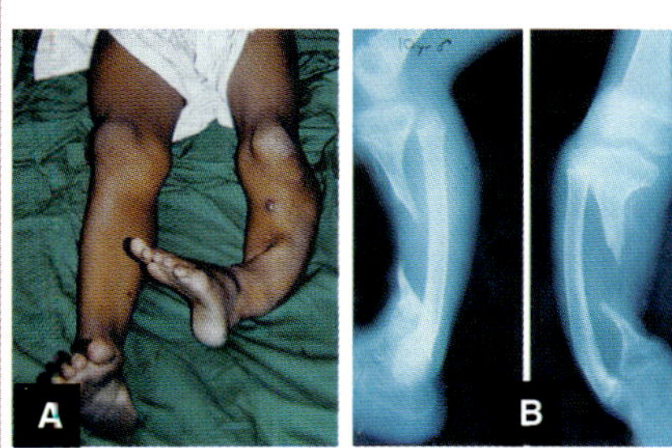 **Figures 10.3.3A and B:** Bone loss of the tibia following osteomyelitis *Photo Courtesy:* Alaric Aroojis, Mumbai	Clinical photo showing shortening and varus deformity of the left leg (Fig. 10.3.3A). X-ray of left leg showing bone loss and varus deformity following osteomyelitis of the tibia (Fig. 10.3.3B).	One of the disastrous consequences of osteomyelitis is sequestration of the entire long-bone diaphysis resulting in bone loss, gap nonunion, growth disturbances and severe limb deformity with shortening. Treatment involves fixator-assisted deformity correction and restoration of bone defect with nonvascularized or free fibular bone graft.

Picture	Note	Management

Bone Loss and Gap Nonunion of Humerus following Osteomyelitis

Picture	Note	Management
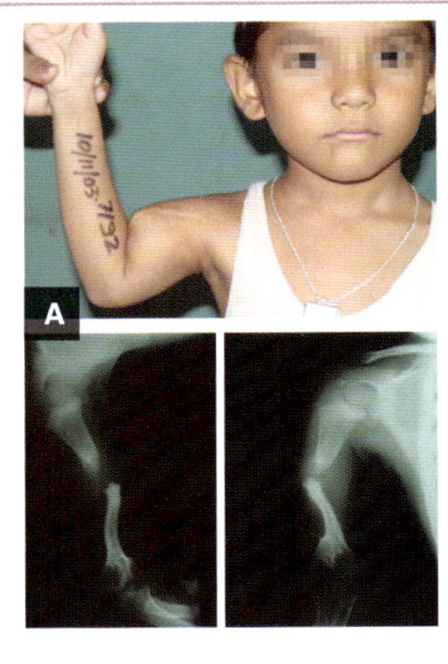 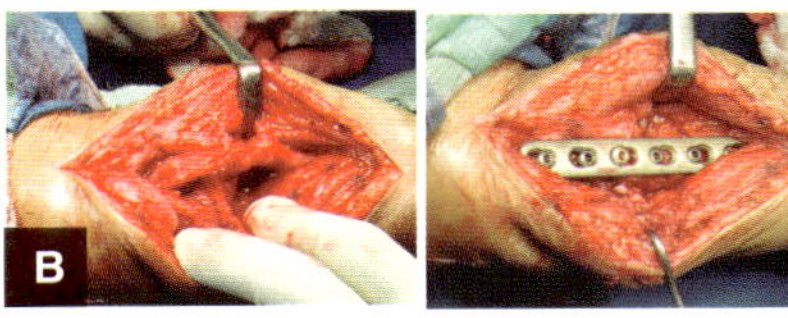 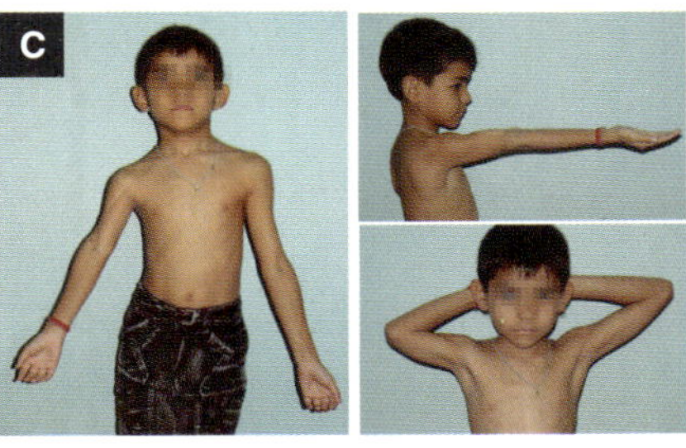 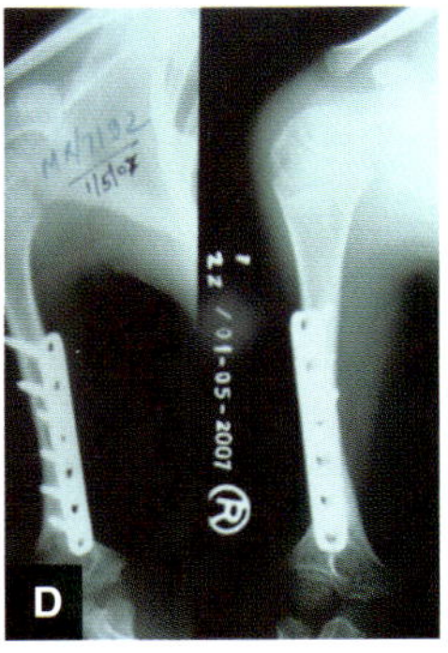 **Figures 10.3.4A to D:** Bone loss and gap nonunion of humerus following osteomyelitis *Photo Courtesy:* John Mukhopadhaya, Patna	Clinical photo and X-rays showing gap nonunion of right humerus following childhood osteomyelitis (Fig. 10.3.4A). Intraoperative photo showing resection of bone edges, bone grafting and stabilization with a locking plate and screws (Fig. 10.3.4B). Postoperative clinical photo showing correction of deformity and full range of shoulder and elbow movements (Fig. 10.3.4C). Postoperative X-ray showing successful healing and a successful outcome (Fig. 10.3.4D).	Management of sequelae of osteomyelitis requires a high degree of expertise using various reconstructive options. Various procedures such as freshening of sclerotic bone edges, deformity correction, bone grafting and stabilization with external or internal fixation need to be combined to ensure a successful outcome.

10.4 SEQUELAE OF SEPTIC ARTHRITIS

Complete Destruction of Proximal Femoral Epiphysis following Osteomyelitis and Septic Arthritis

<table>
<tr>
<td>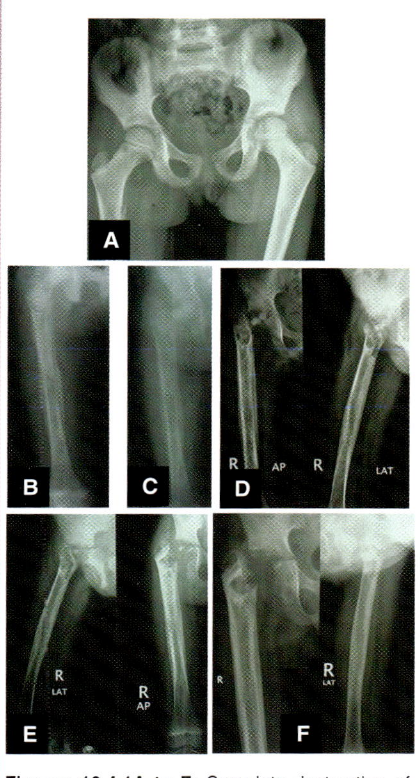

Figures 10.4.1A to F: Complete destruction of proximal femoral epiphysis following osteomyelitis and septic arthritis
Photo Courtesy: John Mukhopadhaya, Patna</td>
<td>Serial X-rays showing untreated osteomyelitis of the femur resulting in destruction and complete disappearance of the proximal femoral epiphysis over a period of 2 months (Figs 10.4.1A to F).</td>
<td>Osteomyelitis of the femur can spread to the hip joint due to the intracapsular nature of the proximal femoral metaphysis. Infection can also spread to the hip joint due to presence of transphyseal blood vessels in children which carry the infection from the metaphysis to the epiphysis. Tamponade on the blood vessels due to intracapsular pus can cause avascular necrosis and destruction of the entire capital femoral epiphysis.</td>
</tr>
</table>

Dislocation of the Hip Joint following Septic Arthritis

<table>
<tr>
<td>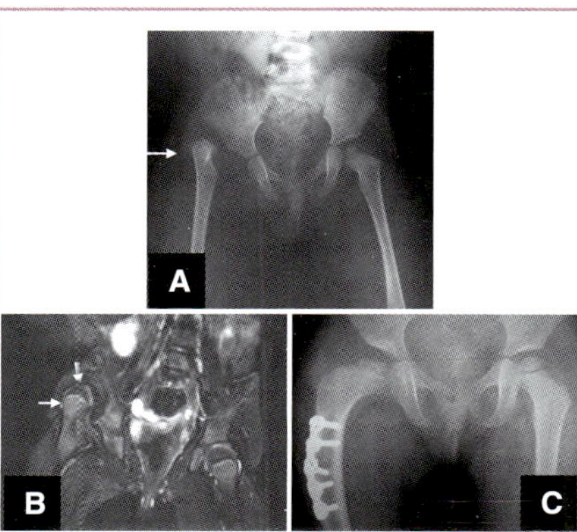

Figures 10.4.2A to C: Dislocation of the hip joint following septic arthritis
Photo Courtesy: Alaric Aroojis, Mumbai</td>
<td>A 3-year-old child presenting with dislocation of the right hip joint following neonatal hip joint sepsis (Fig. 10.4.2A).
MRI showing the dislocation and presence of fibrous tissue and debris within the acetabulum (Fig. 10.4.2B).
Postoperative X-ray showing a good outcome following open reduction, acetabular clearance and femoral osteotomy (Fig. 10.4.2C).</td>
<td>Late hip dislocation can occur as a consequence of neonatal hip joint septic arthritis. It is essential to immobilize the hip in a hip spica cast or brace following arthrotomy for septic hip drainage, to avoid this complication.</td>
</tr>
</table>

Picture	Note	Management

Tom Smith's Arthritis causing Bilateral Loss of Capital Femoral Epiphysis

Picture	Note	Management
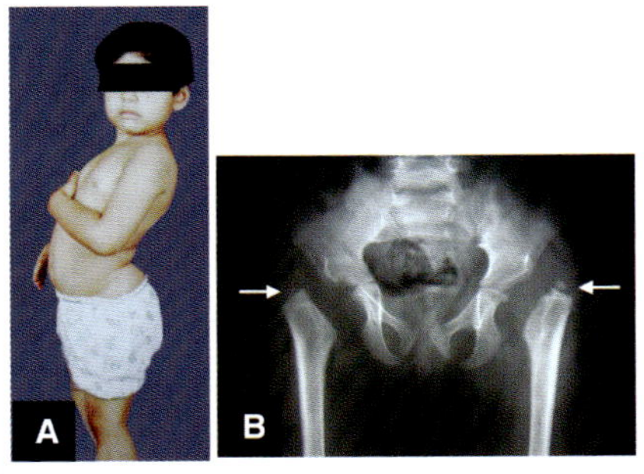 **Figures 10.4.3A and B:** Tom Smith's arthritis causing bilateral loss of capital femoral epiphysis *Photo Courtesy:* Alaric Aroojis, Mumbai	Clinical photo showing typical hyperlordotic gait due to bilateral hip instability (Fig. 10.4.3A). X-rays show bilateral disappearance of capital femoral epiphysis. Arrows point to the trochanteric apophysis which should not be confused with the femoral epiphysis (Fig. 10.4.3B).	Tom Smith's arthritis is an eponymous name given to silent septic arthritis of the hip joint usually occurring in the very sick septicemic neonate in the NICU. Hip joint infection is commonly missed due to other morbid medical conditions in this vulnerable population. Late diagnosis results in destruction and gradual resorption of the entire cartilaginous capital femoral epiphysis causing limp, deformity and instability at an older age. Neonates in the NICU should be carefully monitored for swelling or inability to move a limb and orthopedic advice should be sought urgently in order to avoid this disastrous complication.

Reconstructive Options for Tom Smith's Arthritis of Right Hip

Picture	Note	Management
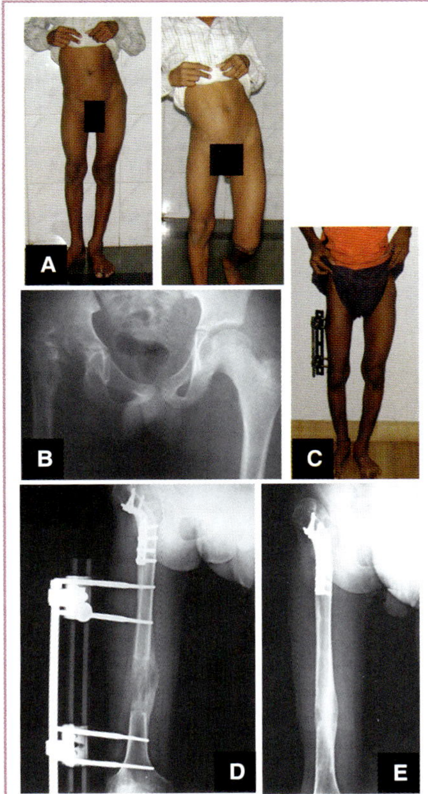 **Figures 10.4.4A to E:** Reconstructive options for Tom Smith's arthritis of right hip *Photo Courtesy:* Alaric Aroojis, Mumbai	Clinical photos of a 12-year-old boy with sequel of neonatal septic arthritis of right hip joint. Note the deformity, shortening and instability on weight-bearing (Fig. 10.4.4A). X-ray showing destruction of right hip capital epiphysis as a sequel of neonatal sepsis (Fig. 10.4.4B). Clinical photo showing limb lengthening being achieved by use of an external fixator (Fig. 10.4.4C). X-ray showing femoral valgus osteotomy to provide pelvic support and lengthening being achieved by an external fixator (Fig. 10.4.4D). Final postoperative X-ray showing good pelvic support and lengthened bone (Fig. 10.4.4E).	Consequences of Tom Smith's arthritis include deformity, limb length discrepancy, hip instability, vertical telescopy, Trendelenburg lurch and occasional pain. Reconstructive options should provide for hip stability by pelvic support and limb lengthening by distraction osteogenesis to overcome limb length discrepancy.

Picture	Note	Management

Sequel of Septic Arthritis of Knee

Picture	Note	Management
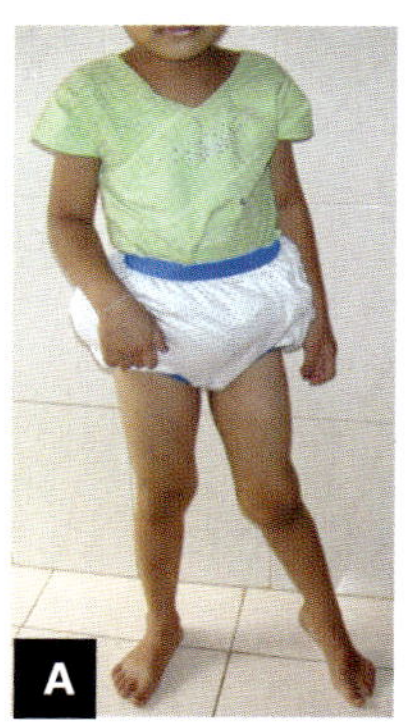 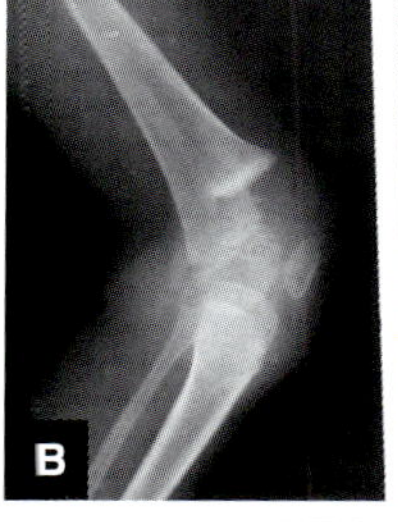 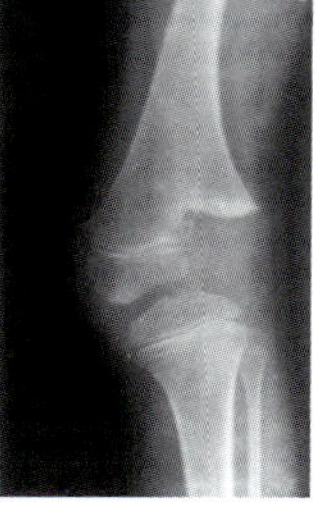 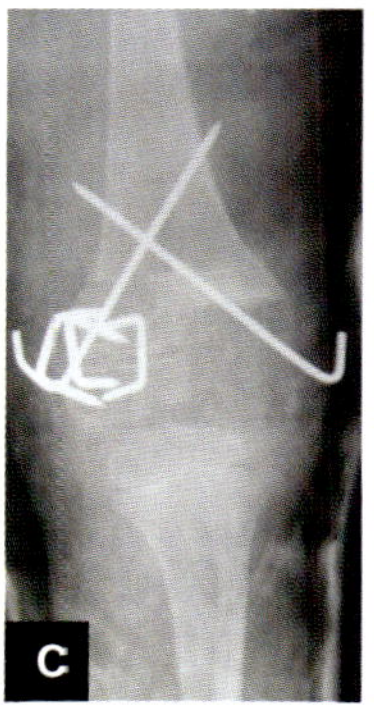 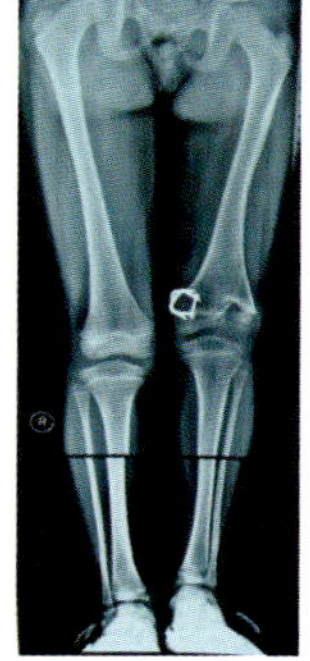 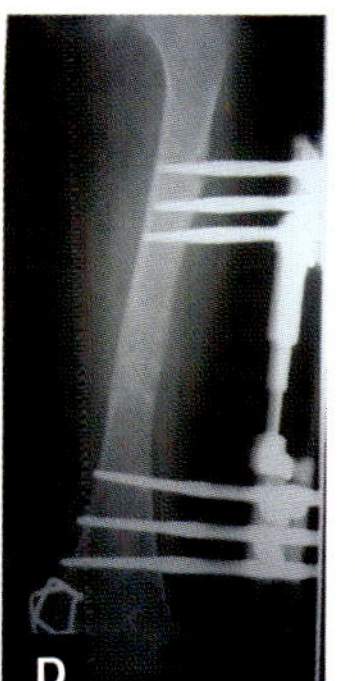 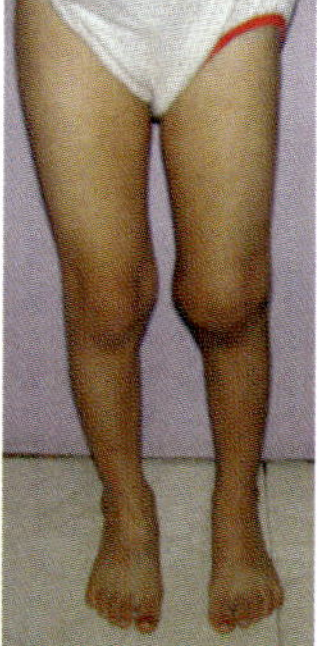 **Figures 10.4.5A to D:** Sequel of septic arthritis of knee *Photo Courtesy:* Alaric Aroojis, Mumbai	A 6-year-old girl with valgus deformity of left knee and shortening following neonatal knee joint septic arthritis (Fig. 10.4.5A). X-rays showing destruction and disappearance of lateral condyle of femur due to neonatal infection (Fig. 10.4.5B). In the first stage, supracondylar femoral corrective osteotomy with staple epiphysiodesis of medial femoral growth plate was performed to correct the valgus deformity (Fig. 10.4.5C). X-ray and clinical picture after second stage surgery to restore limb length (Fig. 10.4.5D).	Untreated or late-diagnosed neonatal knee sepsis can result in enzymatic destruction of cartilage by pus, causing damage to the femoral condyle and articular cartilage. This can result in intra-articular adhesions causing knee stiffness or growth disturbances causing severe deformities and limb shortening. The distal femoral physis contributes significantly to growth, so damage to this physis can result in severe deformities and limb length discrepancy.

Section 11

Infections Requiring Surgical Care

Section Editor
Arbinder Kumar Singal

Contributor
Arbinder Kumar Singal

Section Outline

11.1 General Infections

- Scalp Abscess
- Breast Abscess
- Axillary Abscess
- Infected Branchial Cyst
- Infected Thyroglossal Cyst
- Umbilical Sepsis (Omphalitis)
- Necrotizing Fasciitis

11.2 Chest and Thorax

- Chest Wall Abscess
- Pneumatocele
- Empyema
- Lung Abscess
- Hydatid Cyst
- Bronchiectasis

11.3 Gastrointestinal Infections

- Necrotizing Enterocolitis
- Appendicitis
- Peritonitis
- Ascariasis
- Amebic Liver Abscess

11.4 Urological Conditions causing Urinary Infections

- Antenatally Diagnosed Hydronephrosis
- Pelvi-ureteric Junction Obstruction
- Duplex System
- Ureterocele
- Vesico-ureteric Reflux
- Posterior Urethral Valves
- Bladder Diverticulum
- Neuropathic Bladder
- Dysfunctional Voiding
- Epididymo-orchitis
- Phimosis
- Labial Adhesions
- Urolithiasis

Picture	Note	Management

11.1 GENERAL INFECTIONS

Scalp Abscess

Picture	Note	Management
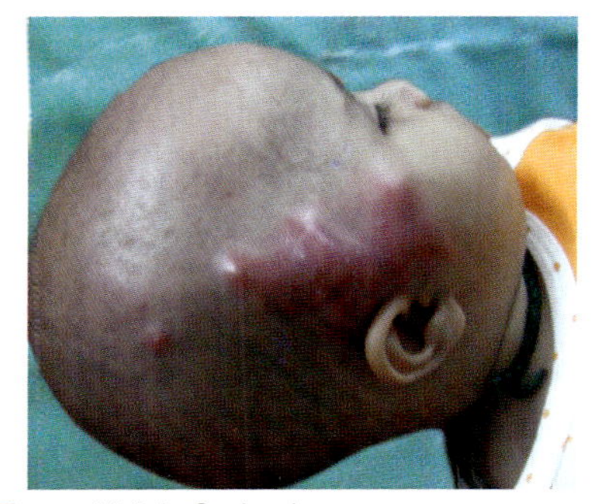 **Figure 11.1.1:** Scalp abscess *Photo Courtesy*: Arbinder Kumar Singal, Navi Mumbai	*Causes:* • Extension of furuncle, or skin injury or abrasion or idiopathic • Organism: *Streptococcus* or *Staphylococcus* *Symptoms and Signs:* • Painful, red swelling generally with fever (Fig. 11.1.1) • Initial stages fluctuation may be absent.	• Large abscesses, associated cellulitis or newborn babies—may need admission and intravenous antibiotics else oral antibiotics, warm fomentation, analgesics and antipyretics. • Drainage under sedation or anesthesia followed by daily dressings.

Breast Abscess

Picture	Note	Management
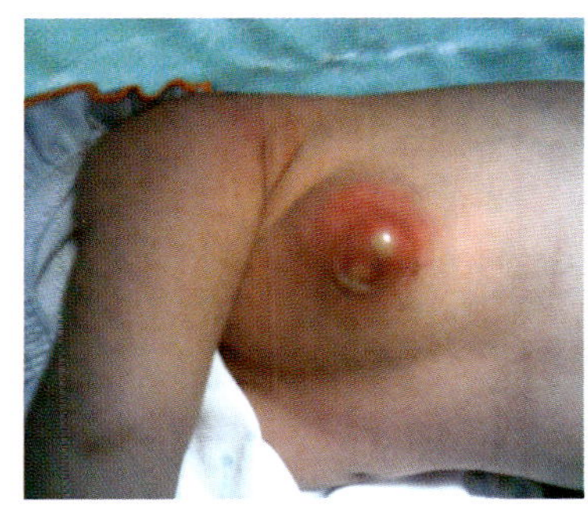 **Figure 11.1.2:** Breast abscess *Photo Courtesy*: Arbinder Kumar Singal, Navi Mumbai	*Causes:* • Mostly occur in newborn babies and infants • Breast massage may predispose to abscess *Symptoms:* • Tender, red breast swelling (Fig. 11.1.2) • Fluctuation heralds pus formation.	• Large abscesses, associated cellulitis or newborn babies—may need admission and intravenous antibiotics else oral antibiotics, warm fomentation, analgesics and antipyretics. • Drainage using a radial incision at margin of nipple mostly under anesthesia.

Axillary Abscess

Picture	Note	Management
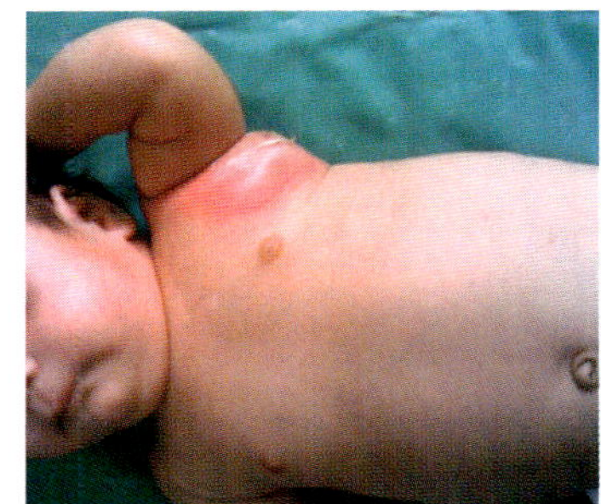 **Figure 11.1.3:** Axillary abscess *Photo Courtesy*: Arbinder Kumar Singal, Navi Mumbai	*Causes:* Suppuration of axillary nodes due to extension of infection from upper limb or sometimes primary origin in axillary area *Symptoms and Signs:* • Tender, red axillary swelling limiting movements of upper limb (Fig. 11.1.3) • Fluctuation develops once abscess liquefies.	• Large abscesses, associated cellulitis or newborn babies—may need admission and intravenous antibiotics else oral antibiotics, warm fomentation, analgesics and antipyretics • Drainage under sedation/anesthesia and then dressings.

Picture	Note	Management

Infected Branchial Cyst

Picture	Note	Management
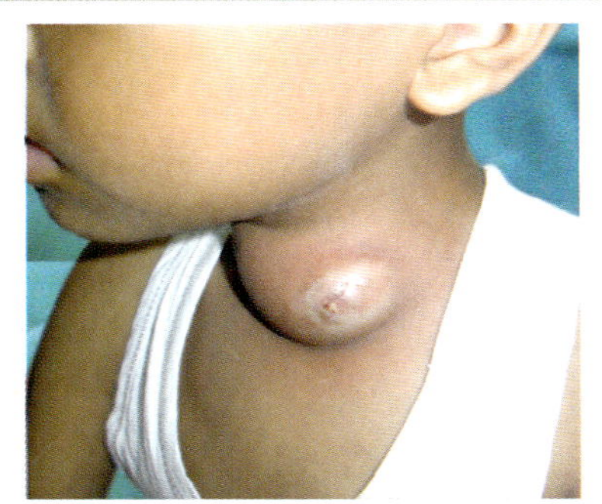 **Figure 11.1.4:** Infected branchial cyst *Photo Courtesy*: Arbinder Kumar Singal, Navi Mumbai	*Causes:* Underlying branchial cyst noted in early childhood. *Symptoms and Signs:* • Characteristic location in neck along anterior border of sternomastoid muscle either in middle or upper one third (Fig. 11.1.4). • Tender/red swelling with fluctuation.	• Antibiotics, warm fomentation, analgesics and antipyretics • Excision of cyst after inflammation subsides, generally after 6–8 weeks.

Infected Thyroglossal Cyst

Picture	Note	Management
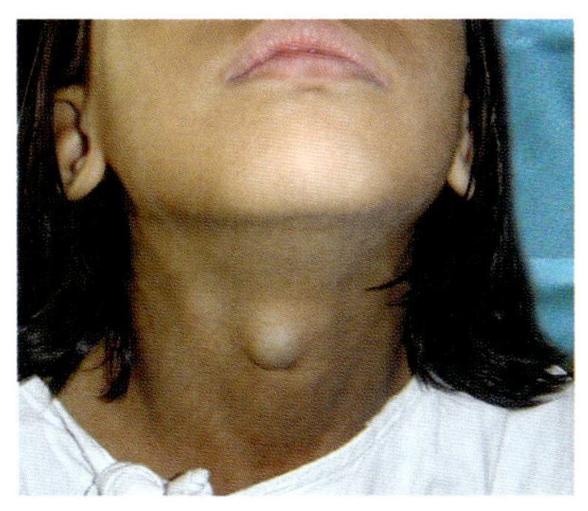 **Figure 11.1.5:** Infected thyroglossal cyst *Photo Courtesy*: Arbinder Kumar Singal, Navi Mumbai	*Causes:* Thyroglossal cyst develops from a remnant of the thyroglossal tract. *Symptoms and Signs* • Mostly asymptomatic swelling in the midline or slightly off midline of neck (Fig. 11.1.5) which moves with deglutition and protrusion of tongue • If infected, there is redness, tenderness and fever. Rarely it may burst and discharge pus and heal as a thyroglossal fistula.	• Infected cysts should undergo a needle aspiration and antibiotics, analgesics should be prescribed. • Once infection is fully clear, elective surgery—Sistrunk's procedure should be planned.

Umbilical Sepsis (Omphalitis)

Picture	Note	Management
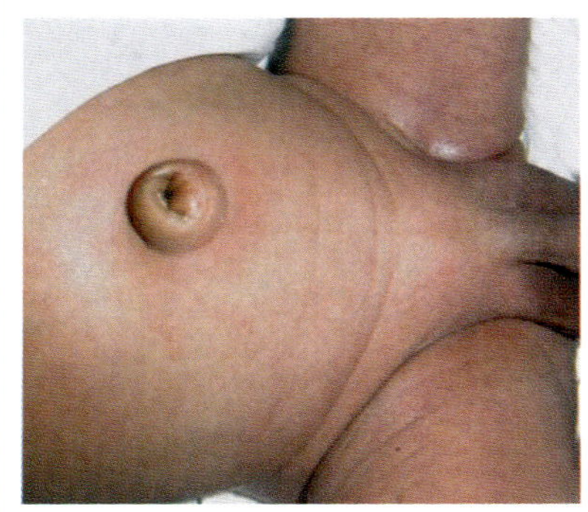 **Figure 11.1.6:** Umbilical sepsis (Omphalitis) *Photo Courtesy*: Arbinder Kumar Singal, Navi Mumbai	*Causes:* • Cellulitis and subcutaneous infection of the umbilical skin and periumbilical area. • Occurs in newborns and infants especially in premature babies, having sepsis or weakened immune system • Organisms include *Staphylococcus*, *Streptococcus*, *E. coli* in order of prevalence. *Symptoms:* • Redness and cellulitis around umbilicus (Fig. 11.1.6) • Severe cases may have tachycardia, hypotension and generalized sepsis.	• Newborn babies need intravenous antibiotics directed towards both gram-positive and gram-negative organisms and general measures for sepsis • Local application of muciprocin and warm fomentation may help • Drainage is rarely needed.

Picture	Note	Management

Necrotizing Fasciitis

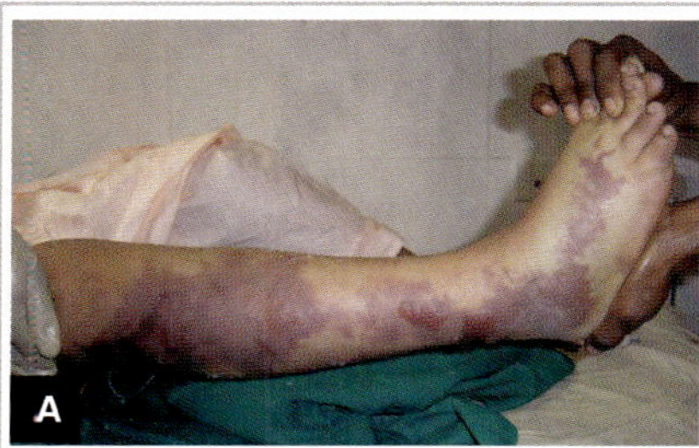 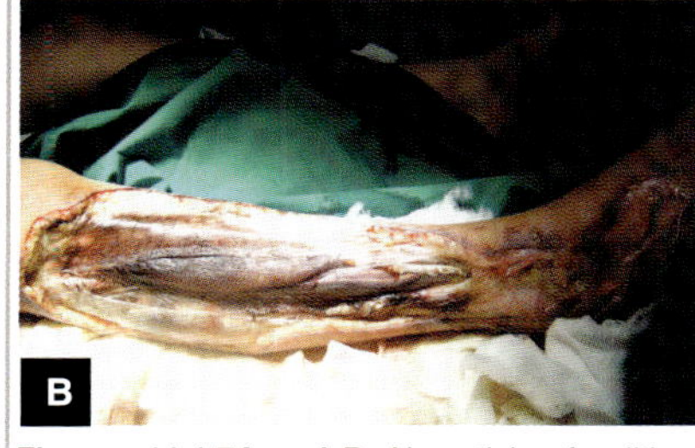 **Figures 11.1.7A and B:** Necrotizing fasciitis *Photo Courtesy*: Arbinder Kumar Singal, Navi Mumbai	*Causes:* • Necrotizing fasciitis is a fast spreading, polymicrobial, life-threatening infection of the deeper layers of skin and subcutaneous tissues. Bacteria include Group A *Streptococcus*, *Staphylococcus aureus*, *Clostridium perfringens*, *Bacteroides fragilis*. • Predisposing factors—cuts, puncture wounds, surgical incisions, or insect bites *Signs and Symptoms:* • Erythema, swelling, pain, fever and chills, early skin changes may resemble those of cellulitis, but later skin ulceration, bullae, necrotic scars (black scabs), gas formation and fluid drainage from the site can occur (Fig. 11.1.7A) • Features of sepsis and shock.	• Urgent surgical exploration and aggressive surgical debridement is the only treatment available. Diagnosis is confirmed by visual examination of the tissues (Fig. 11.1.7B—note gangrenous muscles) and by tissue samples sent for microscopic evaluation. • Intravenous antibiotics including penicillin, vancomycin and clindamycin should be instituted. • Hyperbaric oxygen treatment can be a valuable adjunctive therapy. • Amputations, repeat exploration and skin grafting may be often required.

11.2 CHEST AND THORAX

Chest Wall Abscess

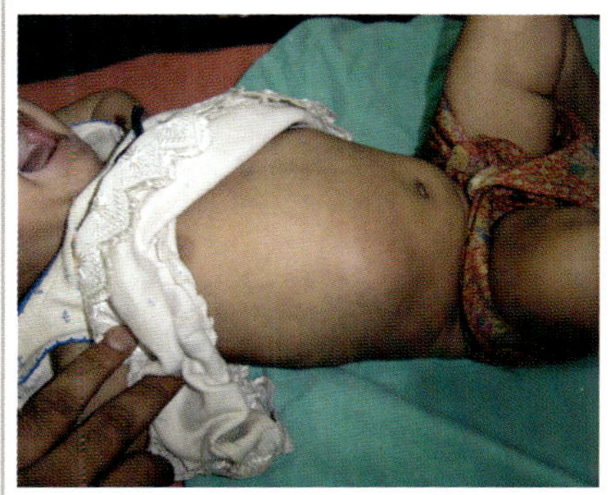 **Figure 11.2.1:** Chest wall abscess *Photo Courtesy*: Arbinder Kumar Singal, Navi Mumbai	*Causes:* • Mostly occur in infants • Local injury, cuts, puncture wounds, etc. may predispose to abscess formation. *Symptoms:* • Tender, red swelling (Fig. 11.2.1) • Fluctuation heralds pus formation • Chest X-ray and a clinical examination is a must to rule out intrathoracic extension.	• Drainage under sedation or anesthesia followed by daily dressings • Large abscesses, associated cellulitis or newborn babies—may need admission and intravenous antibiotics else oral antibiotics, warm fomentation, analgesics and antipyretics.

Picture	Note	Management

Pneumatocele

Picture	Note	Management
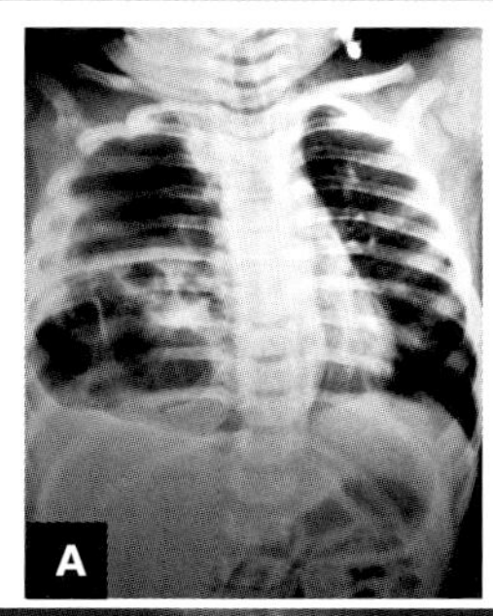 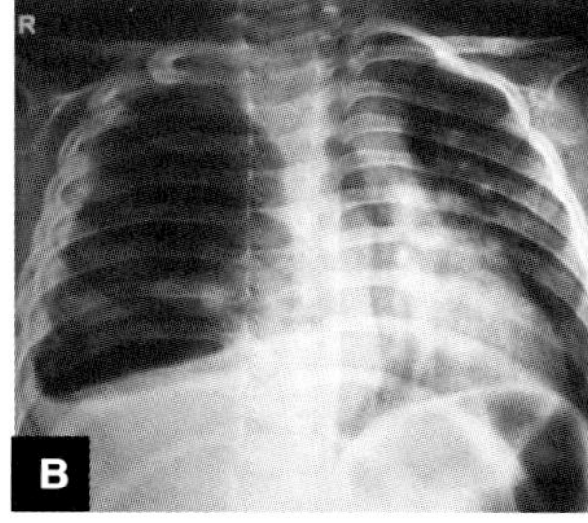 **Figures 11.2.2A and B:** (A) Pneumatocele in right lower lobe; (B) Tension pneumothorax *Photo Courtesy*: Arbinder Kumar Singal, Navi Mumbai	*Causes:* Severe necrotizing pneumonias as caused by *Staphylococcus* and *Klebsiella*. *Symptoms and Signs:* • Features of pneumonitis such as respiratory distress, fever, conducted sounds etc. • Chest X-ray shows typical bullous translucencies (Fig. 11.2.2A—note pneumatoceles in right-lower zone) • High chances of bullae rupturing to form tension pneumothorax (Fig. 11.2.2B).	• Intravenous antibiotics, oxygen and supportive treatment. • Daily X-ray to monitor progress and urgently if pneumothorax is suspected due to sudden deterioration. • ICU care, intercostal drainage set and tube should be kept ready for chest tube insertion whenever needed.

Empyema

Picture	Note	Management
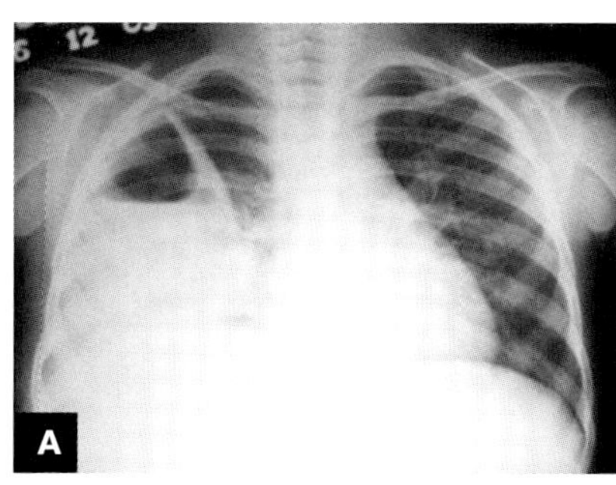 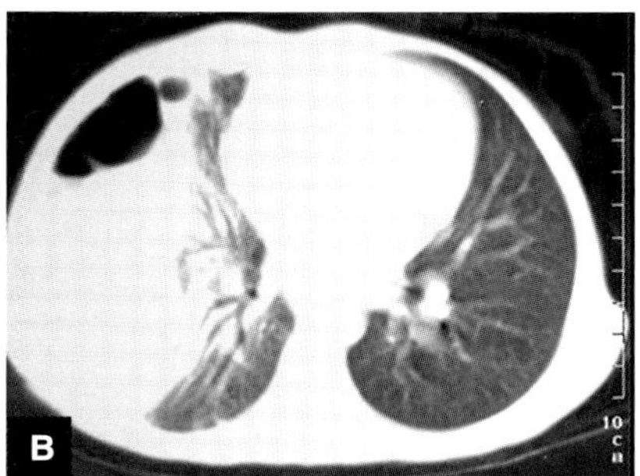 **Figures 11.2.3A and B:** (A) Chest X-ray showing hydropneumothorax; (B) CT chest showing collapsed lung with empyema *Photo Courtesy*: Arbinder Kumar Singal, Navi Mumbai	*Causes:* • Mostly pneumonic–extension of bacteria beyond lung tissue into pleural space. • Common organisms: *Staphylococcus, Pneumococcus, Streptococcus* and *Hemophilus*. *Symptoms and Signs:* • Nonresponsive fever and worsening distress, dullness to percussion and decreased air entry on affected side. • Chest X-ray—blunted costophrenic angle initially which progresses to evident fluid collection and then sometimes complete whiteout (Fig. 11.2.3A—shows right-sided empyema with a fluid level) • Diagnosis confirmed by contrast enhanced computed tomography (CECT) which shows fluid collection, compression of lung and thick enhancing walls (Fig. 11.2.3B).	• Needle aspiration of pus (thoracocentesis) to establish empyema. • Antibiotics and chest physiotherapy. • Stage 1: Exudative phase (5–7 days)—Antibiotics plus intercostal tube. • Stage 2: Fibrino-purulent stage (5–10 days)—Antibiotics plus thoracoscopic debridement. • Stage 3: Organizing stage—Thoracoscopy may be difficult—thoractomy and decortication may be needed.

Lung Abscess

Picture	Note	Management
Figure 11.2.4: CT scan showing lung abscess in the right lower lobe *Photo Courtesy*: Arbinder Kumar Singal, Navi Mumbai	*Causes:* Primary lung abscesses result from severe pneumonias while secondary results from underlying diseases such as tuberculosis, congenital heart disease and hematologic disorders. Symptoms: • Fever, distress and chest pain • Sometimes, the abscess may rupture and cause massive expectoration or hemoptysis.	• Chest X-ray shows rounded lesion and after a cavity is formed these may show an air-fluid level (Fig. 11.2.4). • CECT shows a thick-walled cavity • Ultrasonography or CT guided aspiration, pig tail catheter drainage and antibiotics is the first-line of treatment. • Rarely lobectomy may be needed.

Hydatid Cyst

Picture	Note	Management
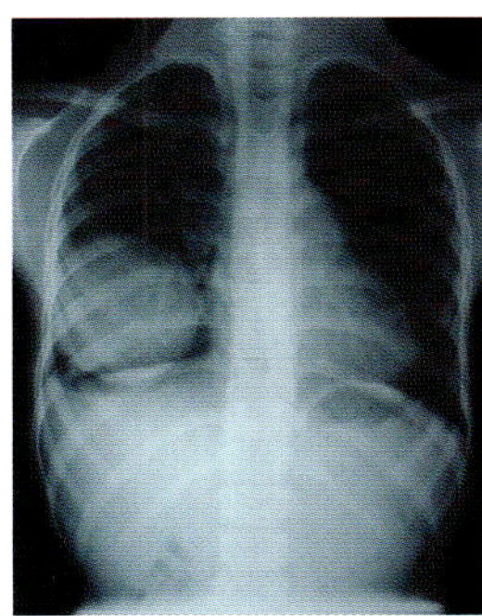 **Figure 11.2.5:** Hydatid cyst in the right lower lobe *Photo Courtesy*: Arbinder Kumar Singal, Navi Mumbai	*Causes:* Infestation with larval form of Echinococcus which travels through blood and lodges in various organs. Lungs are a common location in children. *Symptoms and Signs:* • Initially asymptomatic but symptoms may be chest pain, cough and expectoration due to bronchial fistulization. • Dullness percussion and decreased air entry on the affected side.	• Ultrasonography, computed tomography, and magnetic resonance imaging can lead to diagnosis (Fig. 11.2.5) • Serologic diagnosis is done with immunoglobulin G enzyme-linked immunosorbent assay and immunoelectrophoresis. • Treatment is essentially surgical. In general, chemotherapy is used as a complement to operative treatment to avoid recurrence.

Bronchiectasis

Picture	Note	Management
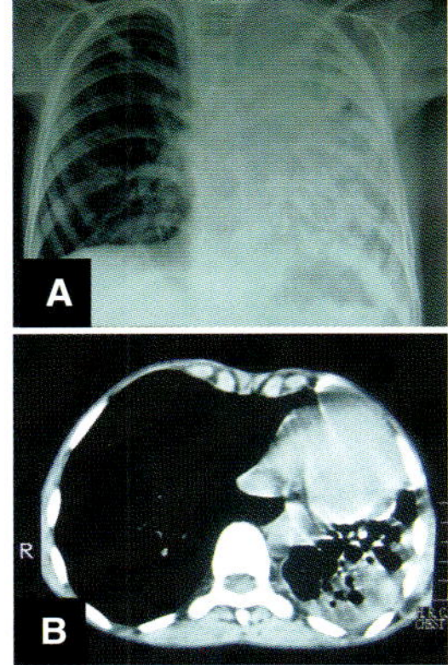 **Figures 11.2.6A and B:** (A) Chest X-ray showing left destroyed lung secondary to bronchiectasis; (B) CT scan showing left bronchiectasis *Photo Courtesy*: Arbinder Kumar Singal, Navi Mumbai	*Causes:* • Congenital airway abnormalities, foreign body • Mostly segmental, affects lower lobes of lung most commonly, especially right side. *Symptoms and Signs:* • Malaise, failure to thrive, repeated LRTI and productive cough • Chest X-ray (Fig. 11.2.6A) shows volume loss, crowding of ribs and shifting of mediastinum • CECT chest (Fig. 11.2.6B) shows honey combed kind of destroyed lung parenchyma.	• Chest physiotherapy and antibiotics • Most of the cases require resection of the affected lobe (lobectomy). • If the whole lung is affected, pneumonectomy may be needed.

Picture	Note	Management

11.3 GASTROINTESTINAL INFECTIONS

Necrotizing Enterocolitis

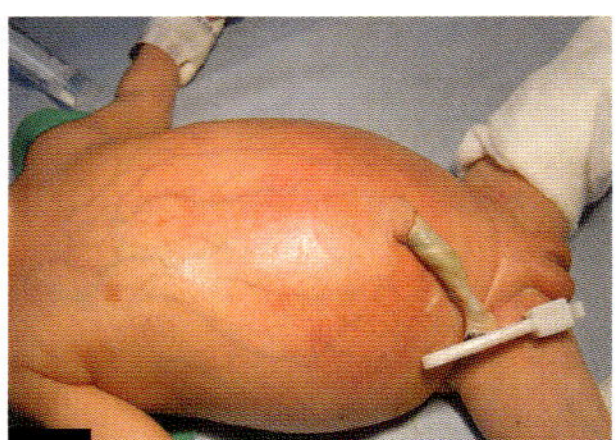

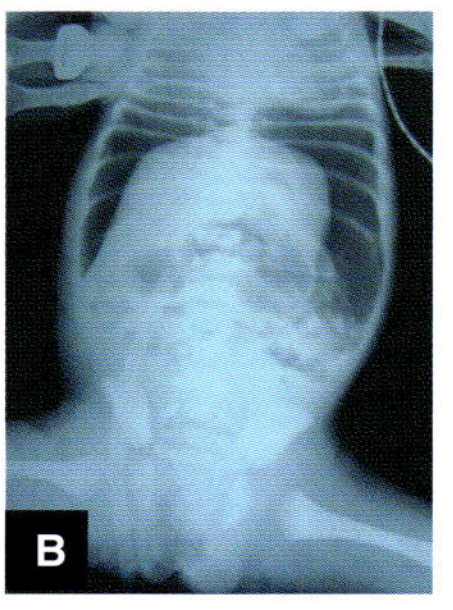

Figures 11.3.1A and B: (A) Tense, erythematous and shiny abdomen of a newborn with NEC; (B) Erect X-ray of the abdomen showing free air
Photo Courtesy: Arbinder Kumar Singal, Navi Mumbai

Causes:

Prematurity, rapid increase of feeds, perinatal stress conditions and sepsis.

Symptoms and Signs:

- Begins with abdominal distension, vomiting and later redness of abdominal wall (Fig. 11.3.1A), tenderness, edema, distress, features of generalized sepsis and bleeding per rectum.
- Abdominal X-rays may show pneumatosis intestinalis, fixed loop or free air (Fig. 11.3.1B).

- Early stages—conservative measures such as antibiotics, bowel rest, etc.
- If there is perforation, massive GI bleed or fixed loop sign—surgical exploration may be needed.

Appendicitis

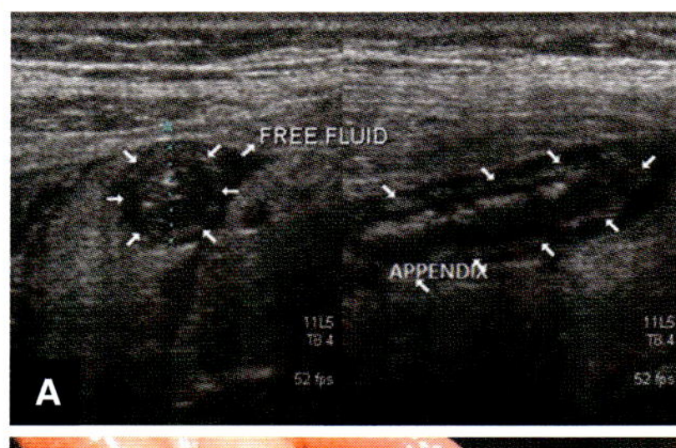

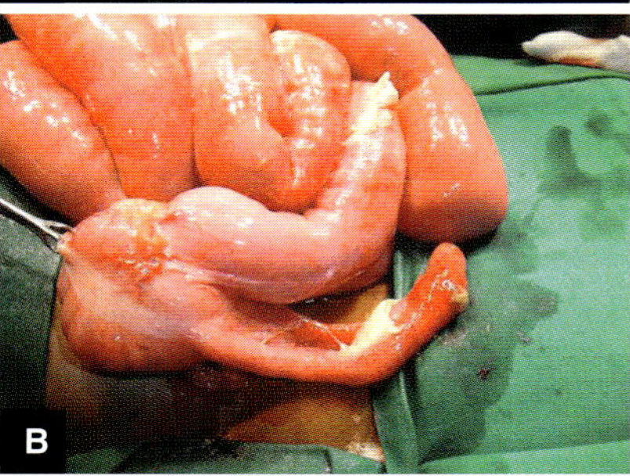

Figures 11.3.2A and B: (A) USG showing distended appendix with free fluid in right iliac fossa; (B) Inflamed turgid appendix as seen at surgery
Photo Courtesy: Arbinder Kumar Singal, Navi Mumbai

Causes:

Inflammation of appendix mostly due to impaction of fecolith.

Symptoms and Signs:

- Fever, abdominal pain and vomiting in early stages.
- Appendicular perforation can lead to distension, rigidity and guarding.

- Diagnosis is based on clinical findings, blood counts, USG (Fig. 11.3.2A—note distended appendix) and sometimes CECT abdomen may be needed.
- Appendicectomy (done via conventional open or laparoscopic technique)—(Fig. 11.3.2B shows inflamed appendix with perforation).

Picture	Note	Management

Peritonitis

Picture	Note	Management
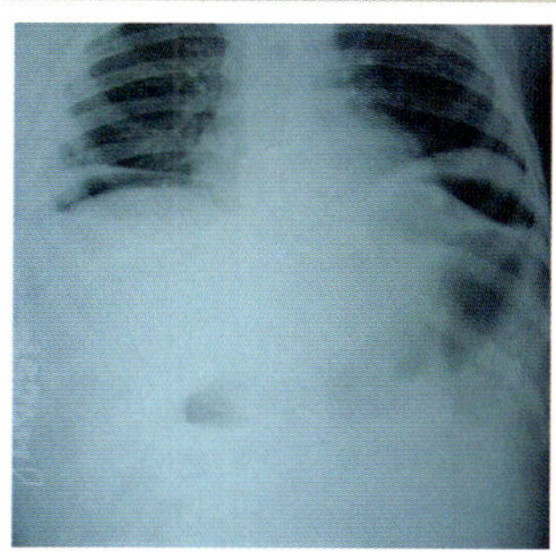 **Figure 11.3.3:** Note free air under both domes of diaphragm *Photo Courtesy*: Arbinder Kumar Singal, Navi Mumbai	*Causes:* • Perforation due to enteric fever, volvulus, appendicular perforation (most common) • Rarely primary peritonitis *(Pneumococcus)* may occur in children. *Symptoms and Signs:* • Abdominal pain, fever, distension, bilious vomiting and constipation. • Tenderness, redness, guarding, rigidity rebound tenderness, absent or diminished tinkling bowel sounds.	• X-ray: Fluid levels, ground glass appearance with fluid between bowel loops and free air under diaphragm (Fig. 11.3.3) • Hydration, IV antibiotics, supportive measures • Exploration either by laparoscopy or by laparotomy.

Ascariasis

Picture	Note	Management
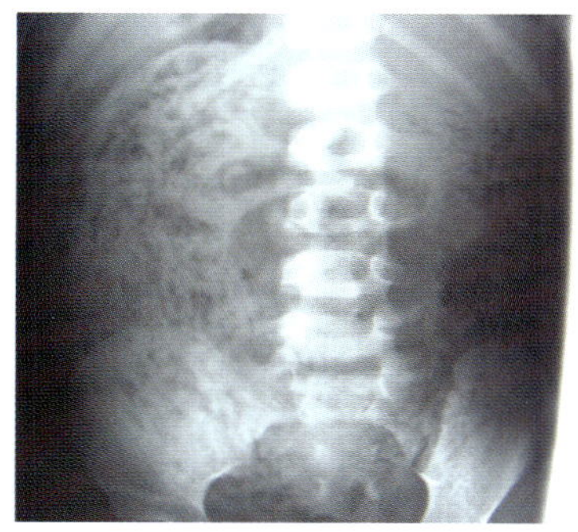 **Figure 11.3.4:** Ascariasis: Abdomen X-ray showing cigar bundle appearance *Photo Courtesy*: Arbinder Kumar Singal, Navi Mumbai	*Causes:* Infestation by roundworms (ascariasis) in small intestine. *Symptoms and Signs:* • Mostly asymptomatic but sometimes massive load may produce an obstructing ball of worms • Distension, vomiting and palpable lump.	• Abdominal X-ray and USG are diagnostic (Fig. 11.3.4). • Conservative treatment with bowel rest, piperazine, saline enemas and then deworming once obstruction is relieved. • Rarely, if there is perforation surgery may be needed.

Amebic Liver Abscess

Picture	Note	Management
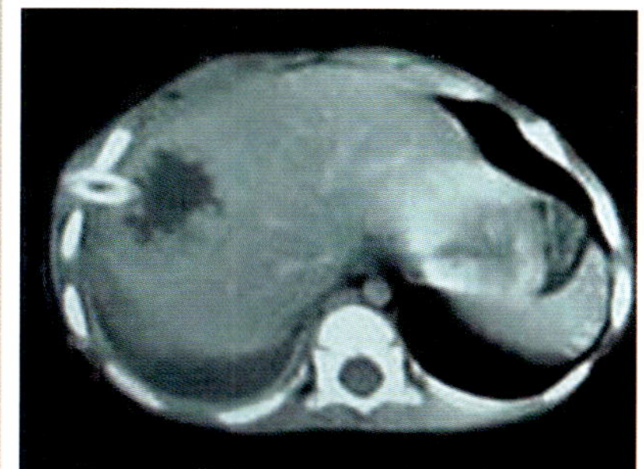 **Figure 11.3.5:** CT scan showing liver abscess in right lobe of liver *Photo Courtesy*: Arbinder Kumar Singal, Navi Mumbai	*Causes:* Localization of *Entamoeba histolytica* into abscess in liver. Right lobe is more common than left (Fig. 11.3.5). *Symptoms:* • Fever, abdominal pain, distension, vomiting and hepatomegaly. • Rarely, a superficial abscess may rupture and lead to signs of peritonitis • Ultrasonography and CECT are diagnostic	• Intravenous metronidazole, antibiotics, analgesics and antipyretics • Ultrasonography guided wide bore needle aspiration is the first-line of treatment and can be repeated if collects again • Rarely, a superficial abscess may rupture and require laparotomy.

11.4 UROLOGICAL CONDITIONS CAUSING URINARY INFECTIONS

Antenatally Diagnosed Hydronephrosis

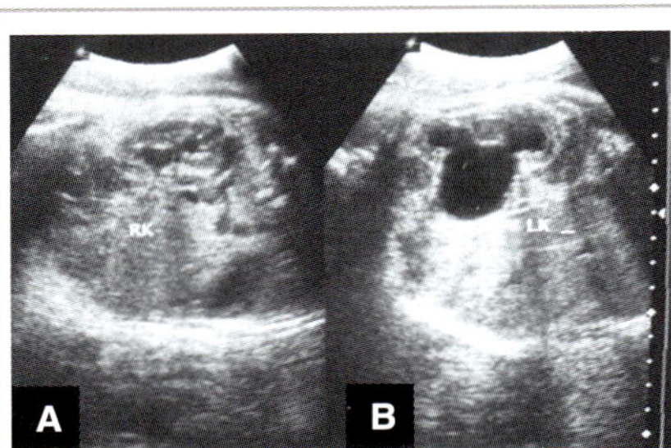

Figures 11.4.1A and B: (A) Normal antenatal appearance of kidney on USG; (B) Hydronephrotic left kidney with distended pelvis
Photo Courtesy: Arbinder Kumar Singal, Navi Mumbai

Causes:

- Occurs in 0.7–1% of all pregnancies
- Common causes are pelvi-ureteric junction obstruction (PUJO), vesico-ureteric reflux (VUR), posterior urethral valves (PUV), duplex system and ureterocele.

Symptoms and Signs:

- Antenatal hydronephrosis can be diagnosed on USG anytime after 16 weeks (Fig. 11.4.1A shows unilateral left hydronephrosis with pelvis and calyceal dilatation, right kidney is normal; Fig. 11.4.1B shows bilateral hydronephrosis in fetus, suspect posterior urethral valves)
- Children with antenatal hydronephrosis are prone to UTIs in infancy especially those with posterior urethral valves, ureterocele and reflux.

- Severity of hydronephrosis is assessed by measuring anteroposterior (AP) diameter of the pelvis and cortical thickness.
- Unilateral hydronephrosis is best dealt postnatally and does not require much antenatal follow-up
- Bilateral hydronephrosis (Fig. 11.4.1B) can lead to renal insufficiency and requires regular antenatal scans to check for impending renal insufficiency.
- Oligohydramnios is an ominous sign.
- Unilateral hydronephrosis—USG at 1 week postnatally and then decision.
- Bilateral hydronephrosis—immediate checkup and workup to rule out PUV.

Pelvi-ureteric Junction Obstruction

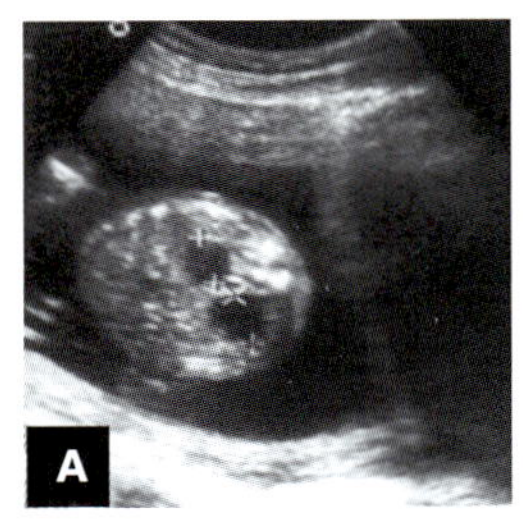

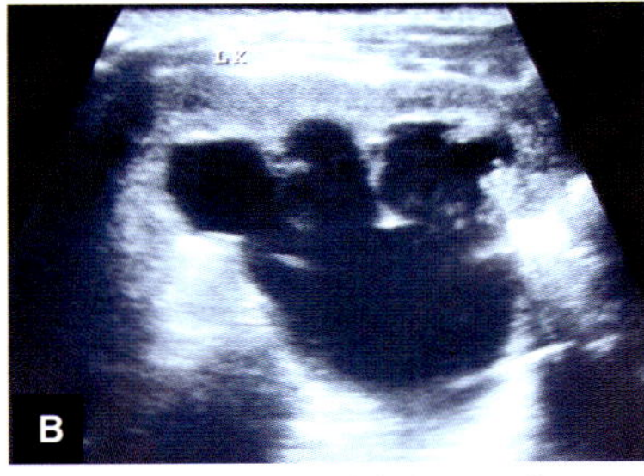

Figures 11.4.2A and B: (A) Antenatal scan showing bilateral hydronephrosis; (B) Gross hydronephrosis left kidney
Photo Courtesy: Arbinder Kumar Singal, Navi Mumbai

Causes:

Pelvi-ureteric junction obstruction (PUJO) is the most common cause of antenatal hydronephrosis

Symptoms and Signs:

- Lump (Fig. 11.4.2A), rarely UTI and pyonephrosis which is evidenced by high-grade fever, chills, flank tenderness and general features
- Ultrasonography shows pelvic and calyceal dilatation (Fig. 11.4.2B) while diuretic renal scan (EC or DTPA) is needed to determine differential renal function and decide for surgery.

- Children with PUJO need regular follow-up with USG every 3 months in first 2 years
- Around 60–70% do not need surgery as hydronephrosis gradually subsides, other pyeloplasty
- Pyonephrosis needs urgent management with IV antibiotics, drainage (DJ stenting or percutaneous nephrostomy) to save the kidney and later pyeloplasty is done.

Picture	Note	Management

Duplex System

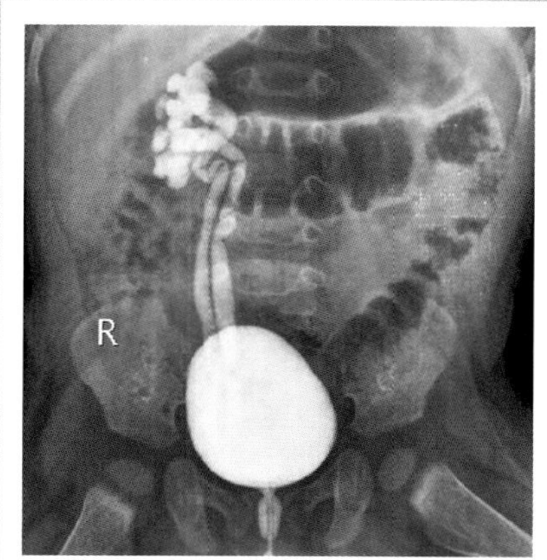 **Figure 11.4.3:** Duplex system as seen on MCU *Photo Courtesy*: Arbinder Kumar Singal, Navi Mumbai	*Cause:* Duplex system implies the presence of two draining systems and ureters instead of one ureter. *Symptoms and Signs:* • Duplex system is mostly asymptomatic except where one of the systems is associated with ureterocele, reflux (Fig. 11.4.3—Note right-sided double system with reflux), obstructive mega-ureter or pelvi-ureteric junction obstruction • Children with duplex system and associated reflux, obstruction or ureterocele are prone to UTIs.	• Diagnosis is based on USG, nuclear scan and micturating cystourethrogram (MCU). • Children with UTI and reflux who do not respond to conservative measures may require ureteric reimplantation or uretero-ureterostomy. • Children with PUJ or VUJ obstruction may need lower pole pyeloplasty or ureteric reimplantation.

Ureterocele

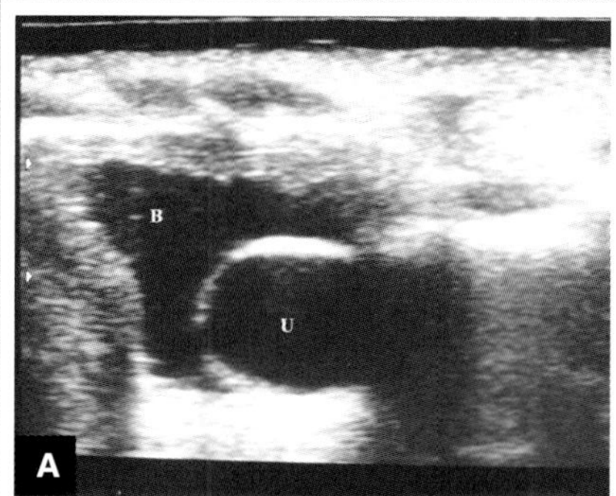 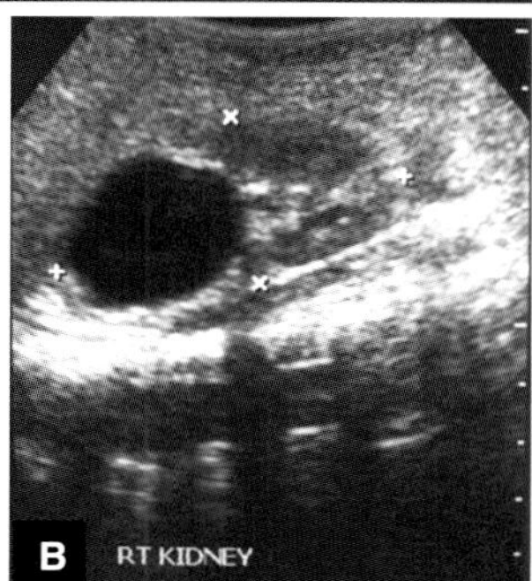 **Figures 11.4.4A and B:** (A) USG of bladder showing large ureterocele; (B) USG showing hydronephrosis of upper pole in a duplex system *Photo Courtesy*: Arbinder Kumar Singal, Navi Mumbai	*Causes:* • Dilatation of the terminal intramural segment of ureter which projects into the bladder lumen (Fig. 11.4.4A) • Mostly associated with upper ureter of a duplex system (Fig. 11.4.4B) but may occur in a single system as well. *Symptoms and Signs:* Children with ureterocele mostly present with repeated UTIs or rarely obstructive symptoms if the ureterocele is big and blocks the bladder outlet.	• Diagnosis is based on USG (Figs 11.4.4A and B) and MCU. A diuretic renal scan is done to see the function of the affected kidney/moiety. • Cystoscopy and deroofing of the ureterocele is the first-line of therapy • Some children may require a formal ureteric reimplantation if the symptoms continue even after cystoscopy.

Picture	Note	Management

Vesico-ureteric Reflux

Picture	Note	Management
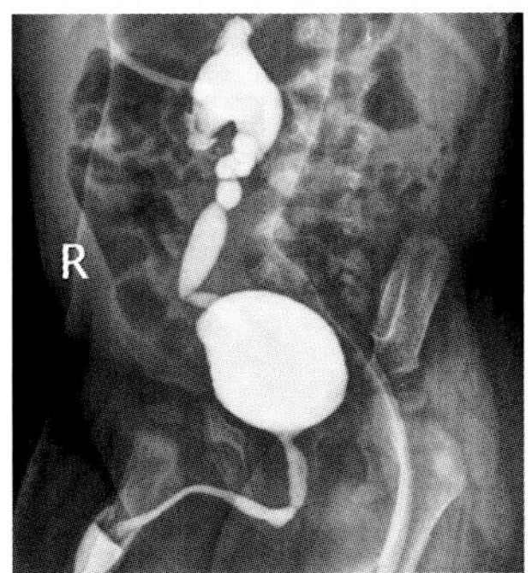 **Figure 11.4.5:** MCU showing Grade 5 right-sided VUR *Photo Courtesy*: Arbinder Kumar Singal, Navi Mumbai	*Cause:* Congenital deficiency of submucosal tunnel at site of ureteric meatus in bladder leads to a refluxing system. *Symptoms and Signs* • Diagnosed antenatally as variable hydroureteronephrosis • May present with recurrent urinary infections and pyelonephritis in infancy.	• Reflux is diagnosed and graded on micturating cystourethrogram (Fig. 11.4.5 shows a Grade 5 VUR on right side) • Management consists of prevention of UTI by prophylactic antibiotics, double voiding and management of constipation. • Children with breakthrough UTI may require ureteric reimplantation surgery.

Posterior Urethral Valves

Picture	Note	Management
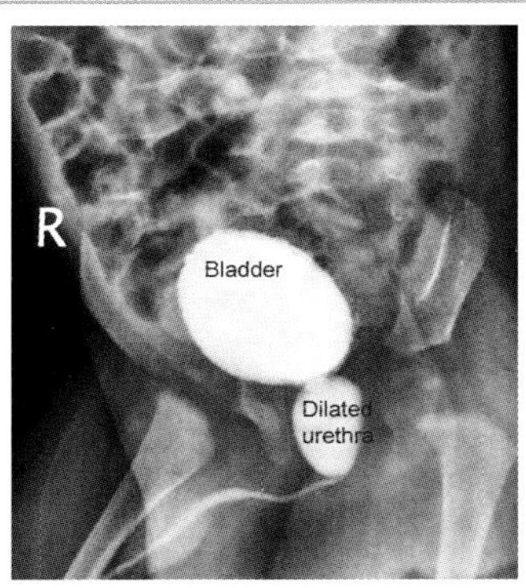 **Figure 11.4.6:** MCU showing classical features of posterior urethral valves *Photo Courtesy*: Arbinder Kumar Singal, Navi Mumbai	*Cause:* Congenital folds/membrane in posterior urethra causing lower urinary tract obstruction. *Symptoms and Signs:* • Most cases are diagnosed antenatally on USG. • Postnatal—urinary retention, poor stream, straining, urinary infections and renal failure.	• Features are bilateral hydroureteronephrosis, distended bladder, keyhole sign, severe cases may have oligohydramnios. • MCU is the diagnostic test (Fig. 11.4.6—note dilated posterior urethra with abrupt cutoff) • Cystoscopy and ablation of valves followed by pediatric nephrology annual checkups to watch for renal insufficiency.

Bladder Diverticulum

Picture	Note	Management
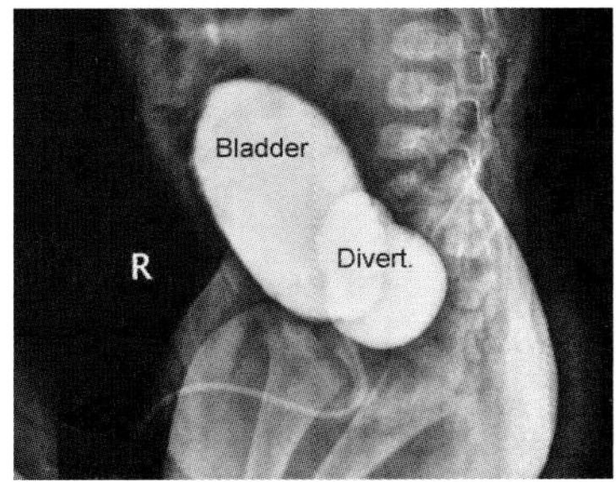 **Figure 11.4.7:** MCU showing large bladder diverticulum *Photo Courtesy*: Arbinder Kumar Singal, Navi Mumbai	*Cause:* Congenital defect in bladder muscle near ureteric hiatus. *Symptoms:* • Urinary infections, lower urinary obstructive symptoms such as urinary retention. • Detected on USG and MCU (Fig. 11.4.7).	• Smaller diverticuli can be managed conservatively with prophylactic antibiotics to prevent urinary infections • Larger or persistently symptomatic diverticuli require surgery in form of excision of diverticulum and reimplantation of ureter.

Picture	Note	Management

Neuropathic Bladder

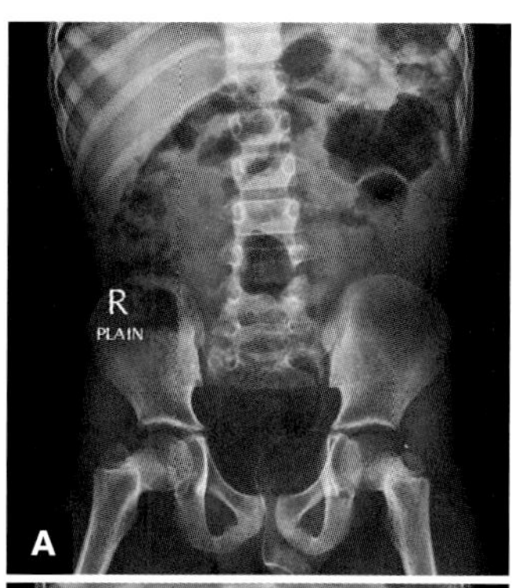 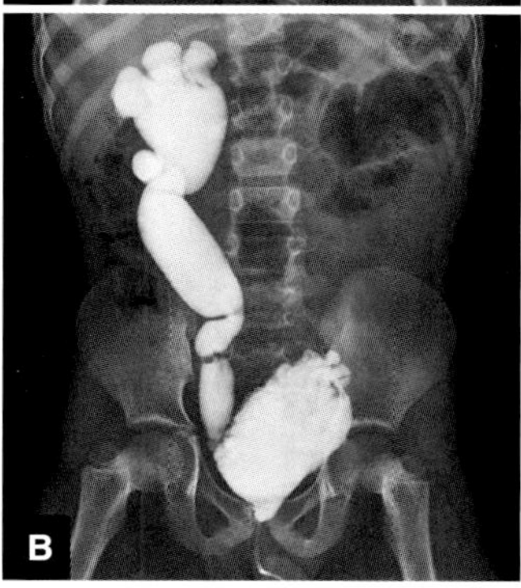 **Figures 11.4.8A and B:** (A) Plain X-ray spine of a child with partial sacral agenesis. Note only two pieces of sacrum are seen; (B) MCU showing small capacity trabeculated irregular bladder with gross right VUR *Photo Courtesy*: Arbinder Kumar Singal, Navi Mumbai	*Cause:* Spina bifida, postmeningitis, spinal injury, cerebral palsy and sacral agenesis (Fig. 11.4.8A—sacral agenesis—note only two pieces of sacrum) *Symptoms:* • Recurrent urinary infections, wetting, poor stream, partial retention episodes • Associated GI symptoms such as constipation, soiling, etc. • Associated lower limb deformities and gait abnormalities may be seen.	• USG, MCU (Fig. 11.4.8B—Note irregular bladder shape with high-grade VUR), urodynamic studies form the cornerstone of assessing bladder function • Combined methods such as clean intermittent catheterization, anticholinergics, prophylactic antibiotics • May need bladder augmentation and continence procedures.

Dysfunctional Voiding

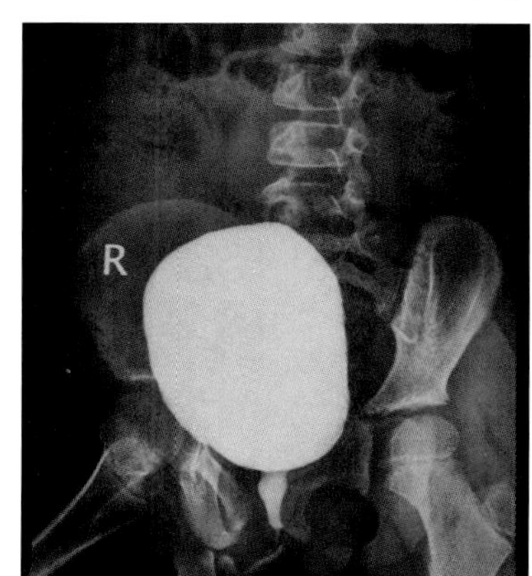 **Figure 11.4.9:** MCU showing funnel-shaped urethra in a girl with severe dysfunctional voiding *Photo Courtesy*: Arbinder Kumar Singal, Navi Mumbai	*Cause:* Constipation, urine retentive behavior and idiopathic *Symptom:* Urinary infections, wetting and incontinence.	• Diagnosis on clinical examination, USG and MCU (Fig. 11.4.9—Note spinning top urethra) • Regularizing bowel habits, regular voiding schedules, anticholinergics for overactive bladder and prophylactic antibiotics.

Picture	Note	Management

Epididymo-orchitis

Picture	Note	Management
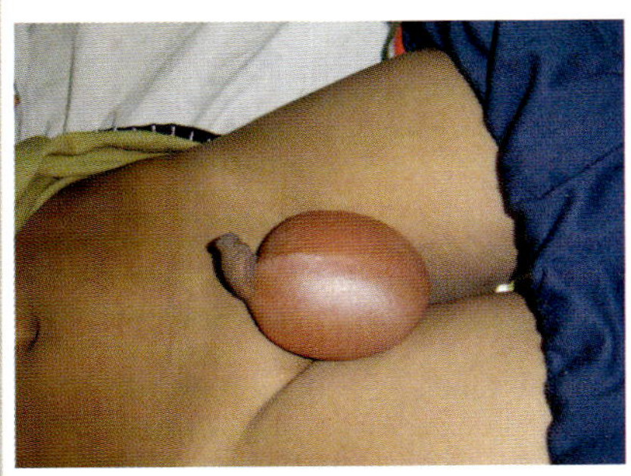 **Figure 11.4.10:** Gross scrotal edema in a child with epididymo-orchitis *Photo Courtesy*: Arbinder Kumar Singal, Navi Mumbai	*Cause:* Mumps (mostly postpubertal kids), urinary anomalies such as stricture, ectopic ureter, neuropathic bladder, urinary infections with *E. coli* and *Klebsiella*. *Symptoms:* • Red, tender swollen scrotum (Fig. 11.4.10) • Initially it is epididymis which is involved but in 50% testis also gets infected and inflamed. • Clinical distinction from testicular torsion is very important—cremasteric reflex is absent in torsion and Prehn's sign is positive (pain on lifting up the affected testis).	• Diagnosis is made on clinical examination and on USG Doppler which shows swollen tissues and increased blood supply. • Treatment is with oral antibiotics, analgesics, etc. • If in any doubt of torsion, urgent work up and exploration may be needed.

Phimosis

Picture	Note	Management
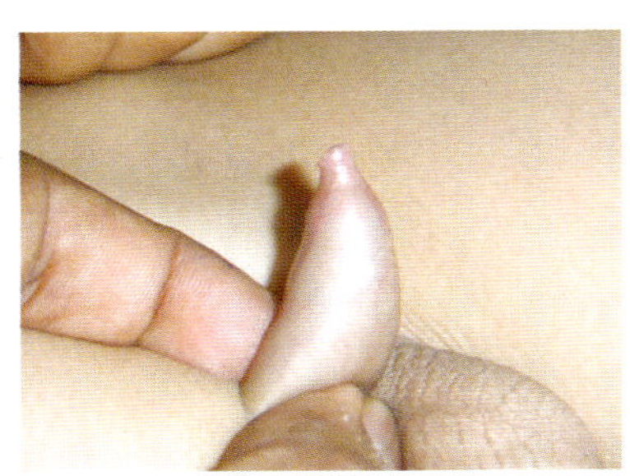 **Figure 11.4.11:** Phimosis *Photo Courtesy*: Arbinder Kumar Singal, Navi Mumbai	*Cause:* Common problem in prepubertal boys and physiological till 4–5 years of age (Fig. 11.4.11). *Symptoms:* • Ballooning, dysuria, local infections (balanoposthitis) or urinary infections • Whitish scarring of foreskin signifies balanitis xerotica obliterans (BXO).	• Asymptomatic children till 5 years do not need treatment. • Medical treatment with local betamethasone dipropionate • Nonresponders or children with BXO should be offered circumcision or preputioplasty (prepuce preserving surgery).

Labial Adhesions

Picture	Note	Management
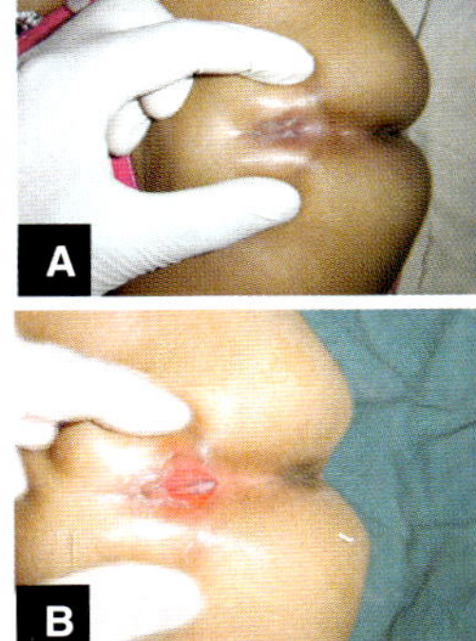 **Figures 11.4.12A and B:** (A) Labial adhesions; (B) After release in outpatient department *Photo Courtesy*: Arbinder Kumar Singal, Navi Mumbai	*Cause:* Superficial adhesions of labia minora seen in prepubertal girls; poor hygiene is one of the main reasons. *Symptoms and Signs:* • Mostly asymptomatic but can lead to vulvitis or dysuria. • Diagnosis is based on clinical examination alone (Fig. 11.4.12A) and no further tests are required.	• Home release can be taught to mother with earbud and vaseline jelly. • Separation in clinic under local anesthesia [Prilox/eutectic mixture of local anesthetics (EMLA)] and mild sedation (Fig. 11.4.12B) • Some cases may require general anesthesia if there is anxiety or recurrence. • Recurrence can be prevented by local estrogen ointment application post-release.

Urolithiasis

Picture	Note	Management
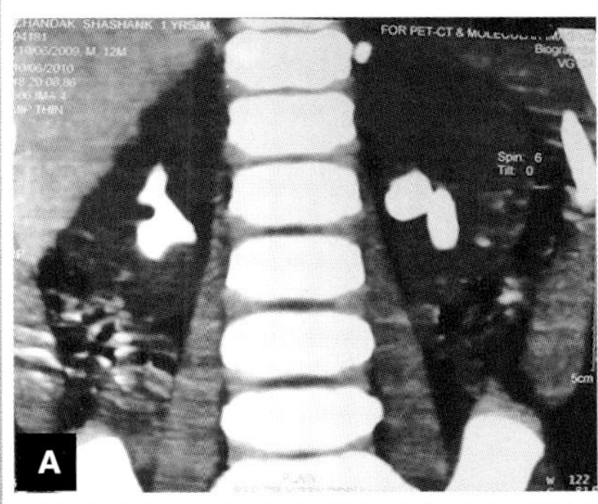 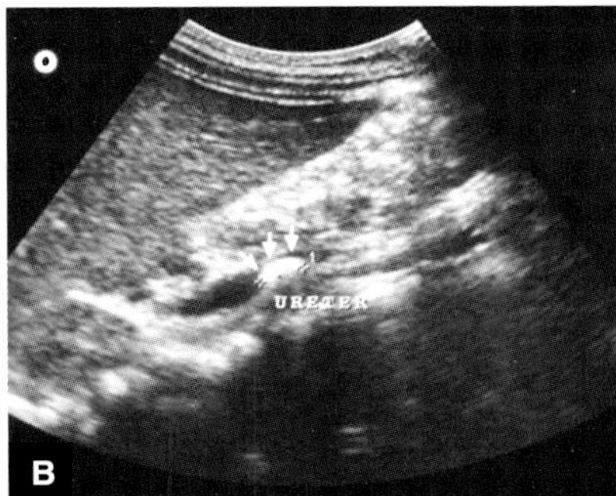 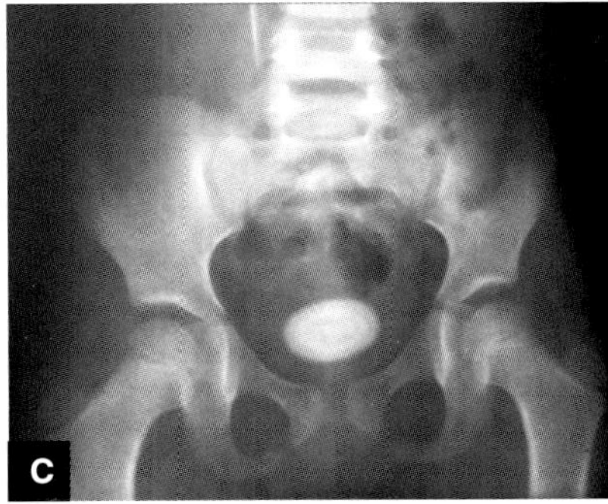 **Figures 11.4.13A to C:** (A) CT KUB showing bilateral staghorn renal calculi; (B) USG KUB showing a lower ureteric calculus; (C) Bladder calculus seen on plain X-ray of pelvis *Photo Courtesy*: Arbinder Kumar Singal, Navi Mumbai	*Cause:* Metabolic causes such as hypercalciuria, hypocitraturia and idiopathic. *Symptoms and Signs:* • Urinary infections, hematuria and pain • Pain—lumbar region due to renal or a pelvic calculus (Fig. 11.4.13A—Plain CT shows bilateral renal calculi) • Colicky pain with radiation from loin to groin—ureteric calculus (Fig. 11.4.13B—USG shows lower ureteric calculus) • Pain suprapubic with dysuria—bladder calculus (Fig. 11.4.13C—Plain X-ray pelvis shows bladder calculus).	*Diagnosis:* Plain X-ray KUB, noncontrast thin cut CT, USG KUB *Management:* • Renal calculi—lithotripsy (ESWL) or percutaneous nephrolithotomy • Ureteric calculi—less than 6 mm—wait and watch, alpha blockers; more than 6 mm—Ureterorenoscopy. • Bladder calculi: Percutaneous laser cystolithotripsy or open surgery. Metabolic workup is a must for all children.

Section 12

Infections in the Immunocompromised Child

Section Editor

Anita Shet

Contributors

Mukesh Desai, Anand Prakesh, Ira Shah, Preethy Harrison

Section Outline

- Bacille Calmette-Guérin Adenitis
- BCG Adenitis: Histopathology
- Disseminated BCGosis with Cutaneous Granulomatous Dermatitis
- Recurrent Pulmonary Infections
- Repeated Lower Respiratory Tract Infection and Absence of Thymic Shadow
- Hemorrhagic Varicella
- Liver and Skin Abscesses
- Griscelli Syndrome
- Severe Combined Immunodeficiency
- Large Skin Ulceration without Abscess Formation
- Recurrent Skin Abscesses
- Pneumatocele
- Persistent mucosal and Cutaneous Fungal Infections
- *Pneumocystis jiroveci* Pneumonia
- Scrofuloderma
- Herpes Zoster
- Axillary Lymphadenopathy
- Oral Candidiasis

Bacille Calmette-Guérin Adenitis

Picture	Note	Management
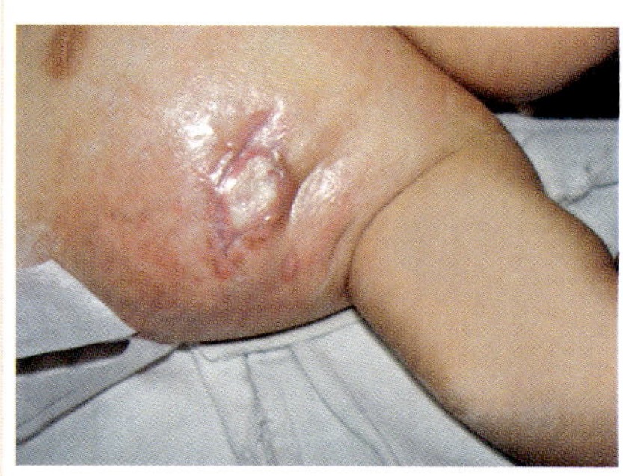 **Figure 12.1:** Bacille Calmette-Guérin adenitis *Photo Courtesy:* Mukesh Desai, Mumbai	Bacille Calmette-Guérin (BCG) adenitis (Fig. 12.1). • *Underlying immunodeficiency*: Mendelian susceptibility to mycobacterial diseases (MSMD). • Human immunodeficiency virus (HIV), chronic granulomatous disease.	Antimycobacterial therapy (INH + rifampicin − ethambutol + ethionamide or streptomycin) for 1 year.

BCG Adenitis: Histopathology

Picture	Note	Management
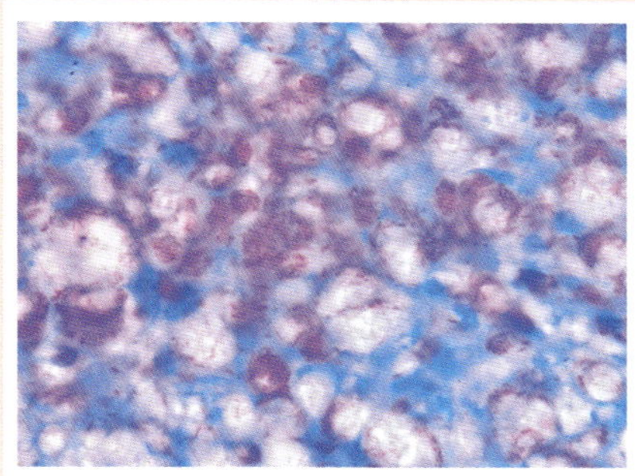 **Figure 12.2:** A diffuse histiocytic infiltrate with foci of necrosis *Photo Courtesy:* Mukesh Desai, Mumbai	BCG adenitis in a 2-month-old boy (Fig. 12.2). Histopathology shows a diffuse histiocytic infiltrate with foci of necrosis. The Ziehl-Neelsen stain was positive for numerous acid fast bacilli.	Conservative management if no underlying immunodeficiency.

Disseminated BCGosis with Cutaneous Granulomatous Dermatitis

Picture	Note	Management
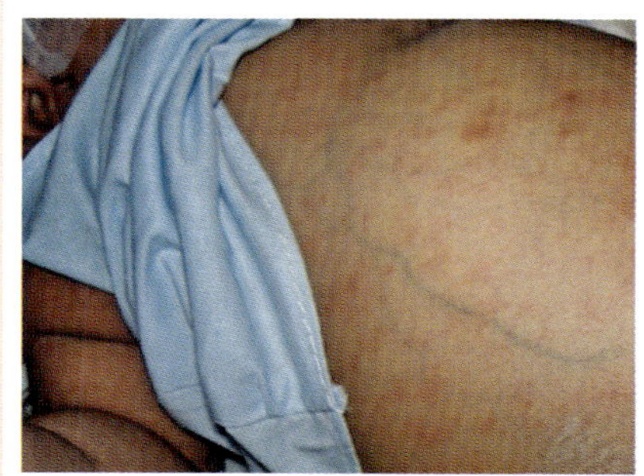 **Figure 12.3:** Disseminated BCGosis with cutaneous granulomatous dermatitis *Photo Courtesy:* Mukesh Desai, Mumbai	Disseminated BCGosis with cutaneous granulomatous dermatitis (Fig. 12.3). • *Underlying immunodeficiency*: Mendelian susceptibility to mycobacterial diseases (MSMD), e.g. IL2 receptor beta1 defect.	• Antimycobacterial therapy (HRE + ethionamide or streptomycin) for 1 year. • Additional gamma-interferon therapy. • Avoid BCG vaccine and other live vaccines.

Picture	Note	Management

Recurrent Pulmonary Infections

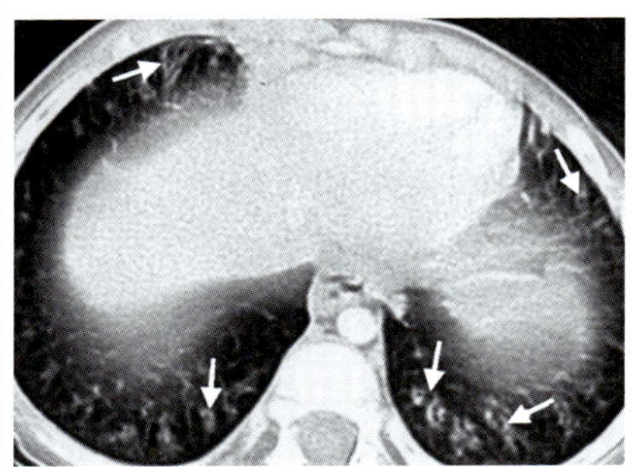 Figure 12.4: Recurrent pulmonary infections *Photo Courtesy:* Anand Prakash, Bengaluru	Recurrent pulmonary infections (Fig. 12.4) is described below. *Underlying immunodeficiency*: X-linked hypogammaglobulinemia. CT scan of lung shows bronchiectatic changes in the basilar regions of the lower lobe.	• Intravenous immunoglobulin (IVIG) every 3–4 weeks, given lifelong. • Supplementary antibiotics to treat underlying infection.

Repeated Lower Respiratory Tract Infection and Absence of Thymic Shadow

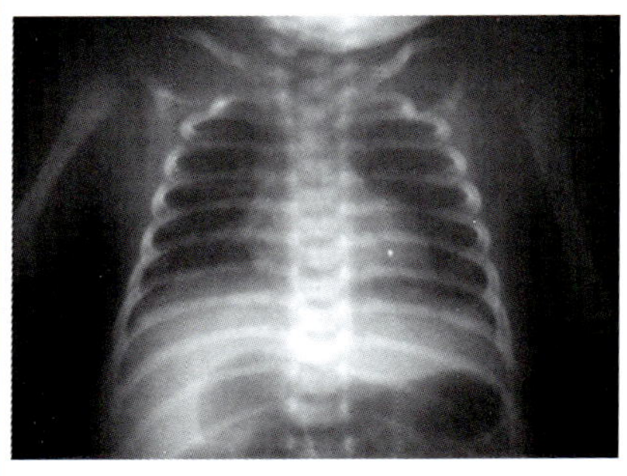 Figure 12.5: Repeated lower respiratory tract infection and absence of thymic shadow *Photo Courtesy:* Mukesh Desai, Mumbai	Repeated lower respiratory tract infection and absence of thymic shadow (Fig. 12.5). *Underlying immunodeficiency*: Di George syndrome. Also associated with hypoparathyroidism, congenital heart disease, low set notched ears and fish-shaped mouth.	Antibiotics and antifungal drugs for treatment of underlying infections.

Hemorrhagic Varicella

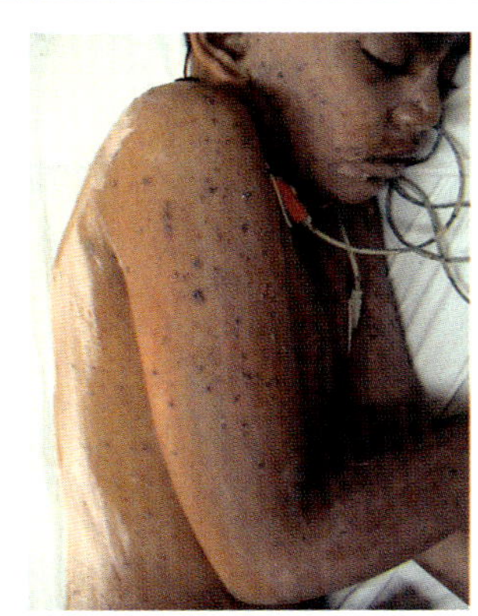 Figure 12.6: Hemorrhagic varicella *Photo Courtesy:* Mukesh Desai, Mumbai	Hemorrhagic varicella (Fig. 12.6) is described below. *Underlying immunodeficiency*: Natural killer (NK) cell disorders, characterized by susceptibility to severe and recurrent viral infections.	• Intravenous acyclovir in the case of varicella infection. • Treatment of underlying infection if NK cell deficiency is diagnosed.

Picture	Note	Management

Liver and Skin Abscesses

Picture	Note	Management
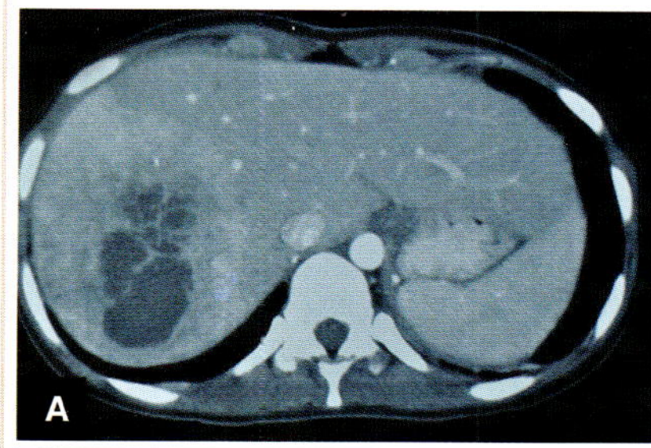 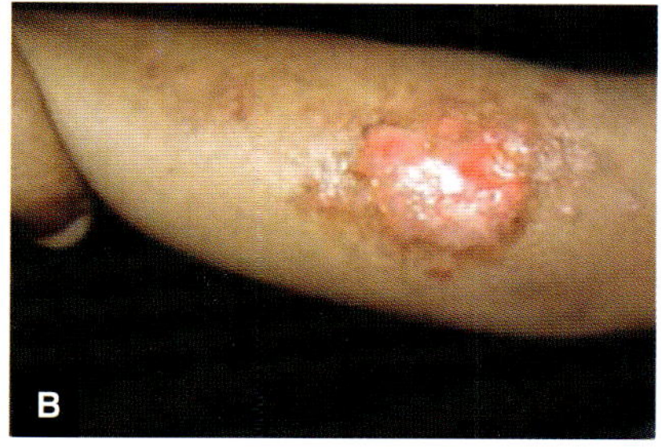 **Figures 12.7A and B:** Liver and skin abscesses *Photo Courtesy:* Mukesh Desai, Mumbai	Liver and skin abscesses (Figs 12.7A and B) is described below. • *Underlying immunodeficiency*: Chronic granulomatous disease (CGD). • CGD is also characterized by lymphadenopathy, hepatosplenomegaly and chronic draining lymph nodes. Leukocytes have poor intracellular killing due to deficiency of NADPH oxidase.	• These patients can be diagnosed by poor nitroblue tetrazolium (NBT) reduction which is a measure of respiratory burst. • Treatment consists of prophylactic antibiotics, therapy of specific infections, and interferon-gamma therapy. Cure can be achieved by a bone marrow transplant.

Griscelli Syndrome

Picture	Note	Management
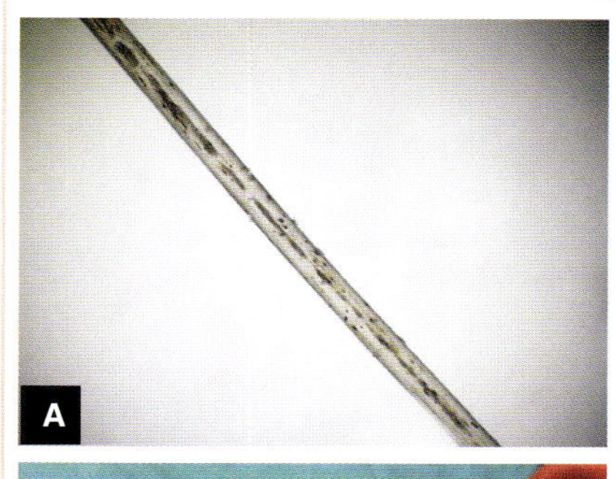 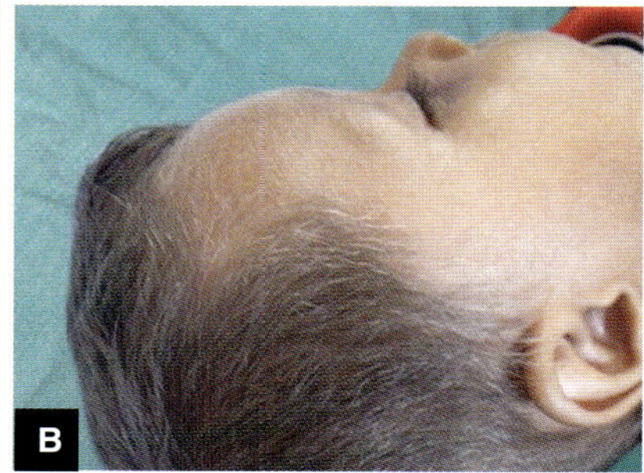 **Figures 12.8A and B:** Griscelli syndrome *Photo Courtesy:* Mukesh Desai, Mumbai	• Characterized by hypopigmentation (Fig. 12.8B) with frequent pyogenic infection, hepatosplenomegaly and pancytopenia. • Examination of the hair shaft under polarized light microscopy shows a monotonously white appearance (Fig. 12.8A).	• Treatment of associated infections. • Bone marrow transplant may be curative.

Picture	Note	Management

Severe Combined Immunodeficiency

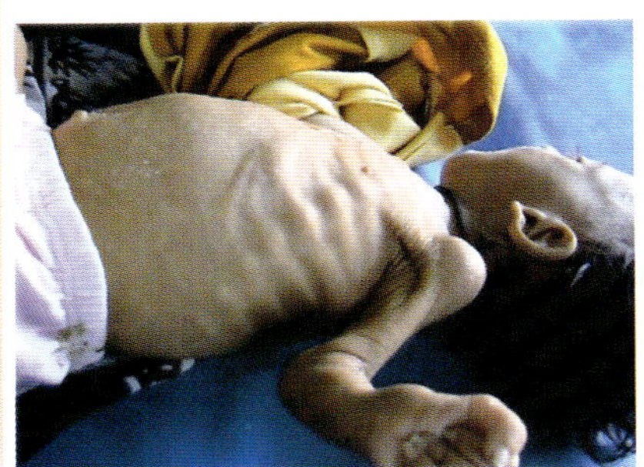 **Figure 12.9:** Severe combined immunodeficiency *Photo Courtesy:* Mukesh Desai, Mumbai	Combined B and T cell deficiency resulting in severe recurrent infections and marked failure to thrive (Fig. 12.9).	• Treatment of underlying infections. • Bone marrow transplantation.

Large Skin Ulceration without Abscess Formation

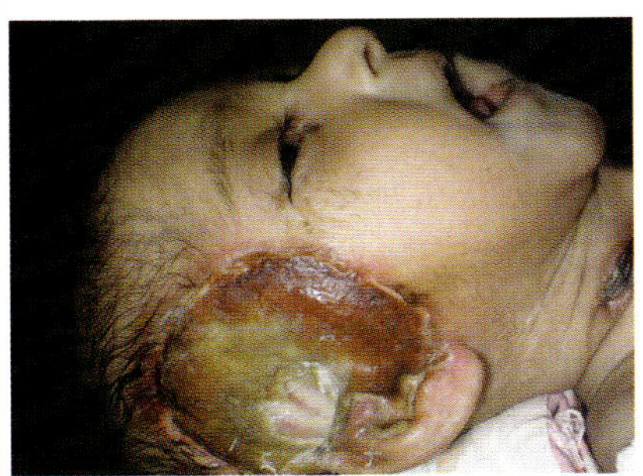 **Figure 12.10:** Large skin ulceration without abscess formation *Photo Courtesy:* Mukesh Desai, Mumbai	Large skin ulceration without abscess formation (Fig. 12.10) is described below. *Underlying immunodeficiency*: Leukocyte adhesion deficiency.	• *Specific diagnosis*: Flow cytometry for β_2 integrins. • Treatment of underlying infection. • Bone marrow transplantation.

Recurrent Skin Abscesses

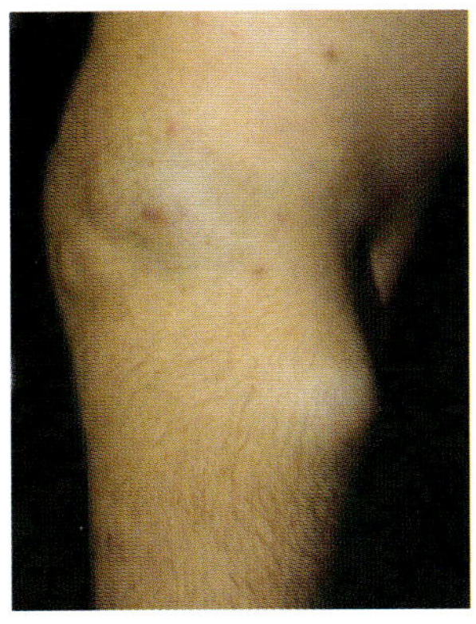 **Figure 12.11:** Recurrent skin abscesses *Photo Courtesy:* Mukesh Desai, Mumbai	Recurrent skin abscesses (Fig. 12.11) is described below. *Underlying immunodeficiency*: Hyper-immunoglobulin E (IgE) syndrome (Job syndrome)	• *Diagnosis*: Enumeration of immunoglobulins. • Antibiotics. • Surgery to drain abscesses.

Picture	Note	Management

Pneumatocele

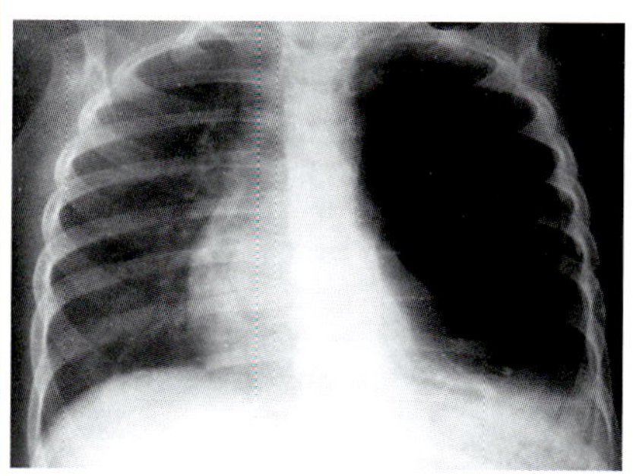 **Figure 12.12:** Pneumatocele *Photo Courtesy:* Mukesh Desai, Mumbai	Pneumatocele [usually caused by *Staphylococcus aureus* (Fig. 12.12)] is described below: • *Underlying immunodeficiency*: Hyper IgE syndrome (Job syndrome). • Other features include coarse facies, retained primary teeth and eczema.	• *Diagnosis*: Eosinophilia Elevated IgE (> 10 times normal levels). • *Treatment*: Antistaphylococcal antibiotics (cloxacillin, clindamycin, vancomycin) • Close respiratory monitoring.

Persistent Mucosal and Cutaneous Fungal Infections

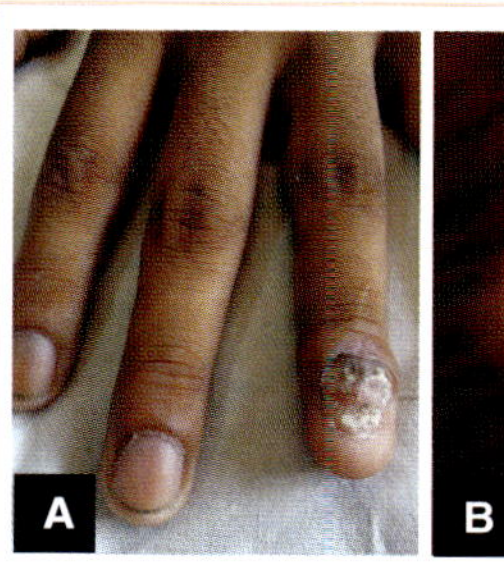 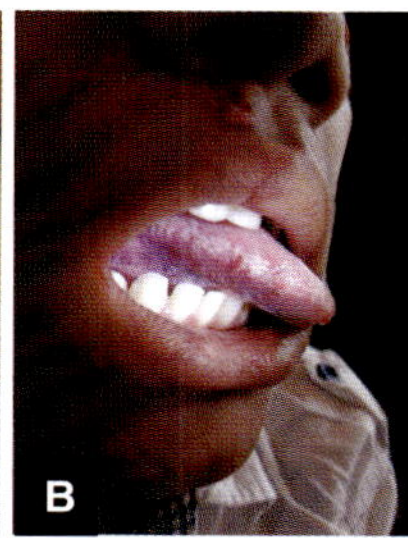 **Figures 12.13A and B:** Persistent mucosal and cutaneous fungal infections *Photo Courtesy:* Mukesh Desai, Mumbai	Persistent mucosal and cutaneous fungal infections (Figs 12.13A and B) is described below. *Underlying immunodeficiency*: Genetic disorder—Autoimmune polyendocrinopathy-candidiasis-ectodermal dystrophy (APECED).	*Onychomycosis (nail involvement)* *Oral terbinafine:* 6 weeks for fingernails; 12 weeks for toenails *Oral itraconazole:* 5 mg/kg daily, 2 months for fingernails; 3 months for toenails. *Adjunct therapy:* Topical treatment with antifungal nail lacquers incorporating ciclopirox and amorolfine.

Pneumocystis jiroveci Pneumonia

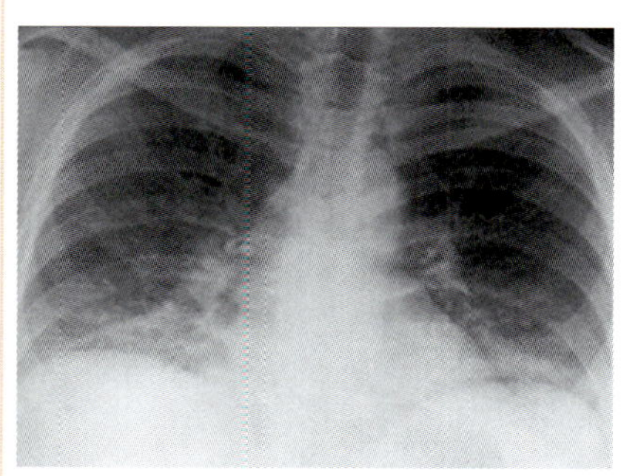 **Figure 12.14:** *Pneumocystis jiroveci* pneumonia *Photo Courtesy:* Ira Shah, Mumbai	*Pneumocystis jiroveci* pneumonia (PCP) (Fig. 12.14) is described below: • *Underlying immunodeficiency*: HIV infection.	*Treatment*: Cotrimoxazole-trimethoprim for 21 days.

Picture	Note	Management

Scrofuloderma

Picture	Note	Management
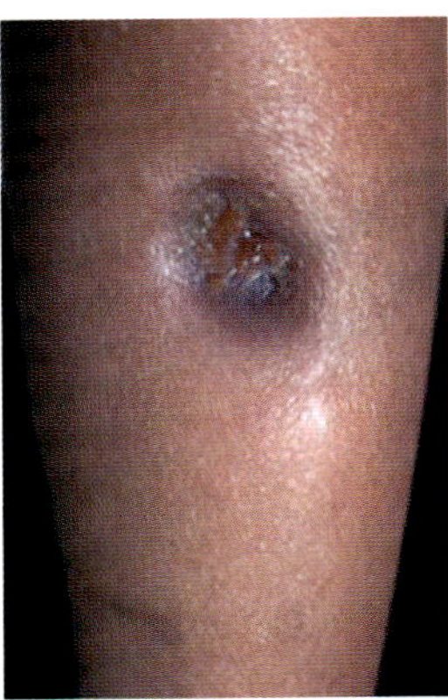 **Figure 12.15:** Scrofuloderma *Photo Courtesy:* Ira Shah, Mumbai	Scrofuloderma (Fig. 12.15) is described below: • Occurs as a result of tuberculous lymphadenitis with cutaneous extension. • *Etiology*: *Mycobacterium tuberculosis.* • *Underlying immunodeficiency*: HIV infection.	• Antimycobacterial therapy (HRZE) for 6 months. • Treatment of underlying immuno-deficiency.

Herpes Zoster

Picture	Note	Management
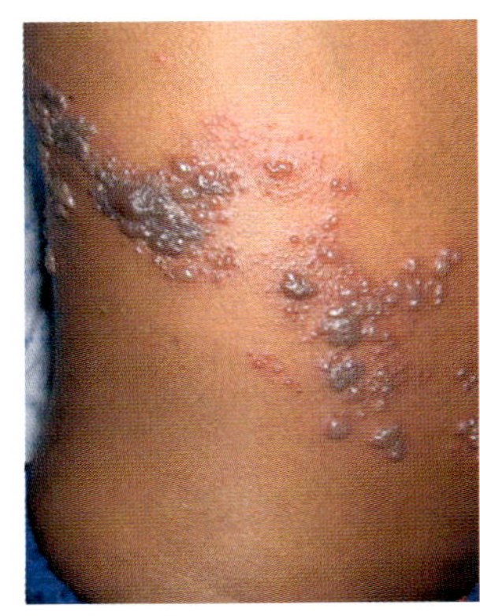 **Figure 12.16:** Herpes zoster *Photo Courtesy:* Preethy Harrison, Bengaluru	Herpes zoster (Fig. 12.16) is described below: • Occurs in children previously exposed to varicella zoster virus. There is a clear dermatomal distribution. • *Underlying immunodeficiency*: HIV	Intravenous acyclovir for 7–14 days. For mild disease, oral acyclovir for 7 days.

Axillary Lymphadenopathy

Picture	Note	Management
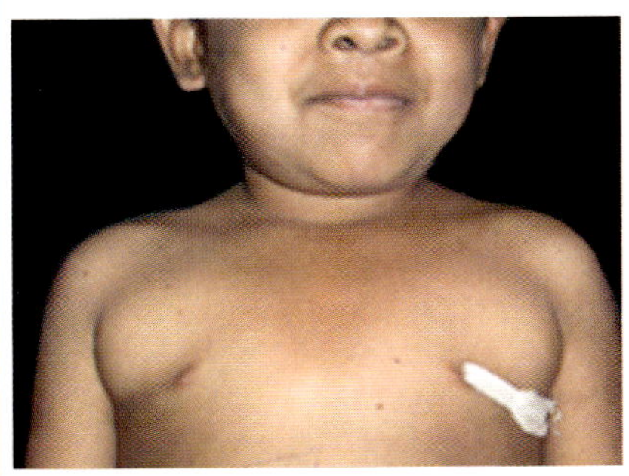 **Figure 12.17:** Axillary lymphadenopathy *Photo Courtesy:* Ira Shah, Mumbai	Axillary lymphadenopathy (Fig. 12.17) is described below: Generalized lymphadenopathy (enlargement of cervical, axillary and inguinal lymph nodes) is one of the earliest features of HIV infection.	• Treatment of underlying infection, i.e. antiretroviral therapy. • In case of tender lymphadenitis antibiotics may be helpful.

Picture	Note	Management

Oral Candidiasis

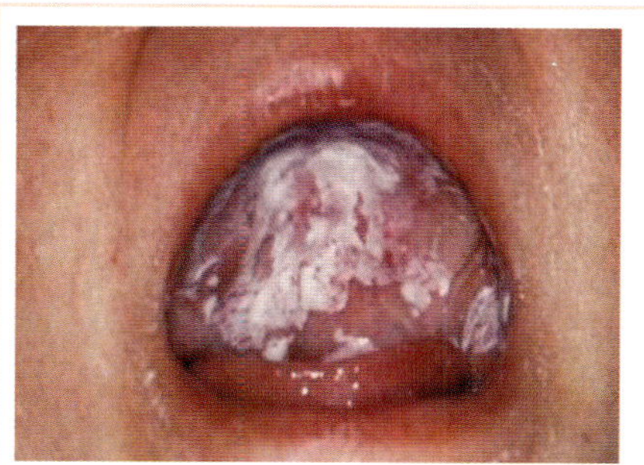 **Figure 12.18:** Oral candidiasis *Photo Courtesy:* Preethy Harrison, Bengaluru	Oral candidiasis (Fig. 12.18) is described below: Caused by the fungus, *Candida albicans*. Esophageal candidiasis can be seen in severe cases. *Underlying immunodeficiency*: HIV	Clotrimazole lotion for local application in mild cases. For severe and extensive candidiasis, oral or intravenous fluconazole can be given for 7–14 days.

Index

Page numbers followed by *f* refer figure